The Social Organization
of Sports Medicine

T0271940

Routledge Research in Sport, Culture and Society

The Social Organization of Sports Medicine
Critical Socio-Cultural Perspectives

**Edited by Dominic Malcolm
and Parissa Safai**

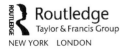
Routledge
Taylor & Francis Group
NEW YORK   LONDON

First published 2012
by Routledge
711 Third Avenue, New York, NY 10017

Simultaneously published in the UK
by Routledge
2 Park Square, Milton Park, Abingdon, Oxfordshire OX14 4RN

First issued in paperback 2014

*Routledge is an imprint of the Taylor & Francis Group,
an informa business*

© 2012 Taylor & Francis

The right of Dominic Malcolm and Parissa Safai to be identified as the
authors of the editorial material, and of the authors for their individual
chapters, has been asserted in accordance with sections 77 and 78 of the
Copyright, Designs and Patents Act 1988.

All rights reserved. No part of this book may be reprinted or reproduced or
utilised in any form or by any electronic, mechanical, or other means, now
known or hereafter invented, including photocopying and recording, or in
any information storage or retrieval system, without permission in writing
from the publishers.

Trademark Notice: Product or corporate names may be trademarks or
registered trademarks, and are used only for identification and explanation
without intent to infringe.

Library of Congress Cataloging-in-Publication Data
   The social organization of sports medicine : critical socio-cultural
perspectives / edited by Dominic Malcolm and Parissa Safai.
      p. cm. — (Routledge research in sport, culture and society 14)
      Includes bibliographical references and index.
   1.   Sports medicine. 2.   Sports—Sociological aspects. 3.   Sports—
Anthropological aspects.   I. Malcolm, Dominic, 1969–   II. Safai,
Parissa.
   RC1210.S624 2012
   617.1'027—dc23
   2011051528

ISBN 978-0-415-88444-0 (hbk)
ISBN 978-1-138-80947-5 (pbk)
ISBN 978-0-203-11340-0 (ebk)

Typeset in Sabon
by IBT Global.

For Liz, Lucy and Lottie — DM

For John and Kiana — PS

Contents

1 Introduction

The Social Science of Sports Medicine

Dominic Malcolm and Parissa Safai

This book examines sports medicine from a variety of social scientific perspectives. Although the dominant approach in this volume is sociology, being the home discipline of both editors and the majority of contributors, reflective of the growth of inter- and multidisciplinary research the collection also includes contributions from historians, policy analysts, philosophers and ethicists, social psychologists and those whose disciplinary influences are more eclectic. Our aim in producing this collection is to consolidate recent advances in this area of study in order to establish a basis for future development. This book is partly an attempt to undergo a "stocktaking" process, but in itself (we hope) has acted, and will in future act, as a stimulus to the field. We see this as a long overdue development and one that has the potential to have a significant impact on the various sport-related subdisciplines. Moreover, by delineating the specificities of sport as a context and focus for medicine, we believe this area has the potential to inform ongoing debates within broader social scientific studies of medicine. A central aim of this introduction, therefore, is to look at the roots of the social scientific investigation of sports medicine and discuss the field's future prospects. Prior to doing this, however, we wish to provide some conceptual clarity by interrogating "sports medicine" as a concept.

WHAT IS SPORTS MEDICINE?

Defining sports medicine may seem a somewhat redundant task given that there are perhaps few words in the English language more widely understood than *sport* and *medicine*. However, as Ingham and Donnelly note, a "taxonomizing propensity" is "characteristic of fields in formation,"[1] and the social scientific study of sports medicine is no exception. It is not our aim here to arrive at a definitive conceptual framework. Rather, in examining the parameters of the field, we hope to reveal something of the dynamic and multifaceted relationship between sport and medicine and their social scientific study.

Sport, Andrews argues, is "a vague and imprecise noun that fails to capture the empirical breadth of the work carried out in the sociology of sport."[2] We think, however, that Andrews is only partially correct in this. Initially sharing Andrews's concerns, early sociologists of sport put considerable effort into defining a concept they recognized was "self-evident until one is asked to define it."[3] The key, Gruneau suggested, was to understand sport's multidimensional character.[4] Recognizing these complexities, we might define sport as historian Allen Guttmann has—organized contests of a playful, nonutilitarian character in which the physical demands outweigh the intellectual components[5]—or follow sociologists like McPherson, Curtis and Loy who define sport as structured, goal-oriented, competitive forms of play.[6] Alternatively, we might eschew a search for "essential" characteristics and, *pace* Elias and Dunning, seek to define sport developmentally, as a group of activities that emerged at a particular time and place (most notably eighteenth-century England) characterized by a particular structure (rule bound, formalized) and function (the generation of pleasurable excitement).[7] Regardless of which approach one adopts, there are criteria available that enable us to distinguish sport from closely related concepts such as exercise, physical activity, leisure and recreation.

Andrews is, however, right to note that sociologists of sport have become increasingly interested in physical activities that are not formally organized (e.g., skateboarding) and are driven by internal rather than shared or formally proscribed competitive goals (e.g., aerobics). They have also exposed some of the highly utilitarian characteristics of modern sport.[8] Thus the sociology of sport is, as Andrews notes, a misnomer. This shift is attributable to the impact of the emergence of the sociology of the body from the 1980s onward,[9] and it is both logically questionable and empirically unrealistic to insist upon a narrow definition of "sport" to the exclusion of a wide variety of physical cultures such as fitness training, dance and bodybuilding. We revisit this empirical shift later but for now it is important to note that sport, and in particular its social scientific study, has become defined in increasingly broad terms in recent years.

The term *sport* is similarly problematic in relation to medicine. Some national bodies refer simply to sports medicine (for instance, the American College of Sports Medicine [ACSM], Sports Medicine Australia, Federación Española de Medicina del Deporte), whereas the titles of other organizations signal a wider remit (e.g., the Japanese Federation of Physical Fitness and Sports Medicine). Debates about the appropriateness of either a narrower (i.e., sport) or wider (exercise, fitness, etc.) focus influenced the establishment of a number of these national bodies. Safai shows how attempts to establish a Canadian branch of the Fédération Internationale de Médecine du Sport (FIMS) was predicated on debates about public health issues rather than sports performance. Doris Plewes, a key advocate in this process, sought to generate support by claiming that sports medicine was "misunderstood by many in the medical profession in Canada" as being focused on elite athletic performance rather than the health of "normal people." Plewes's campaign was successful, but the resultant body was named the Canadian Academy of Sport Medicine (CASM).[10] Similar arguments were expressed in the UK but with a different outcome. Writing an editorial in the *British Medical Journal* in 1997, Batt and Macleod noted: "The terms sports medicine is emotive as it has connotations of care to the sporting elite. This is wrong. More accurately described as sport and exercise medicine, the speciality covers the entire spectrum of human performance and reflects the total medical care of people who exercise."[11] A year later the British Association of Sport and Medicine (BASM) changed its name to the British Association of Sport and Exercise Medicine (BASEM) and, in 2005, Sport and Exercise Medicine was granted medical specialism status by the UK government. By 2010, some were seeking to recognize what they called High-Performance Sports Medicine in an attempt to reassert the distinctiveness of their own work relative to that of clinicians who serve the broader public.[12]

If it is questionable whether sports medicine is simply about sport, it could also be argued that it does not conform to conventional definitions of medicine either. Etymologically and historically, medicine has been defined by attempts to relieve human suffering. Consequently Edwards and McNamee assert that "any practice which does not necessarily aim at relief of suffering cannot count as medicine."[13] Yet both medical bodies like the British Medical Association (BMA) and subdisciplinary specialists define sports medicine as inherently focused on performance enhancement. According to sports medicine's international federation: "The aim of FIMS is to assist athletes in achieving optimal performance by maximising their genetic potential, health, nutrition, and high-quality medical care and training."[14] Clearly these aims exceed the relief of suffering, and, thus, Edwards and McNamee argue, sports medicine encompasses many aspects that are "not medicine."[15] Interviews with those involved in the delivery of sports medicine indicate that such theoretical aims translate directly into practice. Typical of this position is the physician cited by Theberge who suggests that Olympic athletes "measure health . . . by how well they do in performance" (see Scott in this collection).[16] The IOC Medical Commission similarly exceeds the normal boundaries of medicine, being guided by principles that not only include the health of athletes, but also concern equality of opportunity and the ethic of fair play.[17]

A further characteristic that distinguishes sports medicine from conventional understandings of "medicine" is its multidisciplinarity. Medical associations are notoriously exclusionary. For example, at its inaugural meeting in 1847 the American Medical Association (AMA) founded a nationwide standard for preliminary medical education as a way of establishing strict membership criteria. Contemporary organizations continue in a similar vein. The BMA, for instance, describes itself as "the independent trade union and professional association for doctors and medical students,"[18] whereas the AMA argues that its mission is to help "doctors help patients by uniting physicians nationwide to work on the most important professional and public health issues."[19] In contrast, debates about the inclusion/exclusion of multiple health care providers have dogged the development of organizations essentially devoted to "sports medicine." This was evident in relation to BASM/BASEM, which was briefly challenged by the establishment of a body called the UK Association of Doctors in Sports (UKADIS)[20] and the Sports Medicine and Science Council of Canada (SMSCC). In the case of SMSCC, resistance to the inclusion of chiropractors and registered massage therapists from sports medicine physicians, athletics therapists and sport physiotherapists contributed to the dissolution of the council, an organization that, during its tenure, provided the gold standard of care to athletes and was pushing the envelope of innovation in the field of sports medicine nationally and internationally (see also Theberge's contribution to this collection for a discussion of the impact of the SMSCC). Some organizations are explicit in recognizing that their membership incorporates not merely medical practitioners, but also those from allied health professions and beyond. In 1990, for instance, the AMA granted athletic trainers allied health care professional status.[21] Sports Medicine Australia describes itself as "a national multidisciplinary organisation committed to enhancing the health of all Australian's through safe participation in sport, recreation and physical activity."[22] Allan Ryan, former editor of *The Physician and Sportsmedicine*, has even argued that that sports medicine practitioners may include "physicians, coaches, trainers, exercise physiologists, psychologists, sociologists, physical educators and others whose special interests are less well-defined."[23] The distinctions between the practice of sports medicine and the research of sports scientists have also been indistinctly drawn. Williams and Sperryn, two of the founders of sports medicine in Britain, have defined the area as "an integrated multi-disciplinary field embracing the relevant areas of clinical medicine (sports traumatology, the medicine of sport and sports psychiatry) and the appropriate allied scientific disciplines (including physiology, psychology and biomechanics)."[24] *Sports medicine*, therefore, can refer to both an empirically narrow yet holistic medical specialty as has existed in the UK since 2005 or as "a set of fractured subdisciplines" as is the case in the US.[25]

A comparison with other branches or specialties within medicine further illustrates the unusual structure of sports medicine. Medical subdisciplines tend to focus on particular technical interventions (e.g., surgery, anesthesiology); organs or organ systems (cardiology, nephrology); or physical states (oncology, obstetrics). Others focus on health issues related to particular demographic groups (pediatrics, geriatrics) or particular social contexts (occupational and environmental medicine). Sports medicine does not fit neatly into any of these categories. Orthopedics is often seen as foundational to sports medicine, but a sports medicine specialist would also be likely to incorporate aspects of nutrition, epidemiology, traumatology and, in the case of high-impact sports, neurology. Some definitions of sports medicine, like that of Williams and Sperryn cited above, illustrate the potential breadth of treatment interventions in the subdiscipline by incorporating aspects of psychology. Some claim that sports medicine is inherently related to particular skills but, tellingly, these skills stem from an understanding of the practice of sport rather than the practice of medicine.[26] Perhaps, as Kotarba has argued, the area has the greatest similarity to occupational medicine,[27] but the particular demographic group serviced by sports medicine is diverse and often not subject to similar workplace or environmental conditions. Such a comparison is therefore problematic.

Consequently, sports medicine is confined neither to sport nor the aims/knowledge/techniques that have traditionally defined medicine. Its definitional parameters are, both logically and in practice, drawn according to different and distinct criteria. This is not to say that sports medicine defies any common-sense understanding of that term—that is, relieving the suffering and contributing to the health of those who participate in sport—simply to acknowledge that the breadth of the subdiscipline, and thus our interest in this volume, is both somewhat broader and has its own context-specific dynamics.

To capture this breadth, sports medicine needs to be viewed as socially constructed and comprehensible only through interpreting the thoughts and actions of humans. Both Vertinsky and Theberge have argued that the consumption of sports medicine is significant in this regard.[28] Both note that sports medicine is shaped by the consumptive demands of athletes who seek assistance for reasons ranging from enabling participation to enhancing athletic performance. But sports medicine is also shaped by the sports clubs/teams that consume sports medicine in order to advance their own competitive and/or commercial success, the governments and international bodies for which sports (and exercise) medicine is an adjunct to the encouragement of populations to "consume" physical activity in the pursuit of "health" and sports federations that look to medical science to help them establish the "fair" conditions of competition. There can be few other fields of social life in which competing forms of consumption pull medicine in so many different directions.

Equally, sports medicine can only be comprehended as a manifestation of an identity. While this may be true of all professions, it is perhaps particularly marked in the case of sports medicine. People have always taken part in sport (or sport-like activities), and there have always been injury-related consequences of sports participation. In this sense sports medicine is as old as medicine itself. For instance, Herodicus, the teacher of Hippocrates (460–370 BC), spoke of the therapeutic and health-related benefits of exercise and has been described as a "gymnastics master." Galen (AD 129–210) worked for three years as a physician in a gladiator school.[29] Yet because practitioners of medicine in the sports context neither operate a monopoly of knowledge nor possess esoteric skills, the ideas (bodies of knowledge) and actions (practice) that could in theory form sports medicine have normally been enveloped within other branches of health care. At the point at which physical ailments become defined as sport related—indicative examples include the use of the terms *punch-drunk* to describe a dazed or confused manner, *athlete's foot* to describe a fungal foot infection and *tennis elbow* to describe tendon inflammation—sports medicine becomes more of a possibility as the provision of treatment is seen to depend upon or be enhanced by knowledge of an identifiable sports "specialism." Crucially, however, it is not until clinicians detect the potential for individual and collective gain that a sense of identity emerges from which member organizations, proscribed qualifications and a formalized body of knowledge collated in specialist publications are formed. At this point, sports medicine becomes *feasible*.

The preconditions of consumption and identity mean that a sports-related specialism is a relatively recent development within medicine. The British, American and Canadian medical associations were founded in 1832, 1847 and 1876, respectively; however, their sport-specific counterparts were all established approximately one hundred years later (1952, 1954 and 1970; for more detailed discussions of the American and British cases, see Berryman and Carter's respective contributions in this collection). The first university lecture course on sports medicine and the first sports medicine journal were founded in 1919 and 1924, respectively.[30] An international body for sports medicine, the Association Internationale Medico Sportive (AIMS), was founded following a meeting of physicians attending the 1928 St. Moritz Winter Olympics, many of whom were present as competitors or spectators rather than in any medical capacity. AIMS changed its name to FIMS in 1934, and now has 137 member states, eight multinational organizations and four continental associations.[31] As a number of studies show, the issues of doping, sex-testing and exercising at altitude that converged around the 1968 Mexico Olympics acted as a significant stimulus to the development of sports medicine.[32]

Although increasing in organizational coherence in recent years, sports medicine remains diffuse. In attempting to understand the breadth of our focus we suggest that a number of dimensions of sports medicine need to be considered. Implied by the intentionally loose term *social organization*, a comprehensive understanding of sports medicine would encompass (but not be limited to): a field of innovative and, particularly in the case of the development of performance-enhancing drug use, exploratory scientific *research*; a system of *professions* with their own organizations and dynamic power relations; a form of *practice*, structured in specific ways by particular clients and particular contextual demands; and, as evidenced by the classificatory systems in sport that determine the rights of individuals to take part in particular competitive events (i.e., males and females, the able-bodied and those with disabilities), a form of *regulation*. It is a field that has its own ethical and legal considerations,[33] has a distinct organizational and social history,[34] is implicated in its own nexus of policy-making considerations[35] and faces its own unique set of challenges for the future. The cross-cultural variation in its manifestations call for an international perspective. Underpinning the complexity of the area is the fact that, concurrently, medical personnel actively promote sport for its health-enhancing qualities; are seen as a necessary adjunct to its relatively safe practice; are called upon to establish the criteria of equitable competition; and, as in the case of boxing, actively campaign against its legal status. Having identified the parameters of the field, we can begin to look at the existing social science literature that examines sports medicine.

THE SOCIAL SCIENTIFIC ANALYSIS OF SPORTS MEDICINE

It seems to us that social scientists of medicine have largely overlooked the study of sport, and that sports studies researchers have, perhaps more surprisingly, neglected aspects of medicine. Examination of any number of textbooks or readers on the history or sociology of medicine and health reveals a dearth of studies relating to sport. Indeed, of those authors known primarily for their focus on health and medical issues, Kotarba's study of the sports medicine provision in professional rodeo and wrestling stands out as unique. Graham Scambler has written extensively on the sociology of medicine,[36] and has also written about sport,[37] but his work on sport does not focus on medicine, and his work on medicine does not embrace sport.

Table 1.1 Sport-Related Research within Social Scientific Medical Journals

	Volumes	Physical Activity	Exercise	Sport
Social Science & Medicine	71	4,810	2,927	801
Journal of Health & Social Behavior	51	220	77	21
Medical Humanities	36	220	77	21
Sociology of Health & Illness	32	593	282	139
Journal of Medical Humanities	31	97	101	29
Social History of Medicine	23	1,076	357	82
Qualitative Health Research	20	648	424	117

Table 1.2 Chronological Trends in Sport-Related Research

	Physical Activity	Exercise	Sport
2001–2010	44	44.5	54
1991–2000	31	31.5	27
Pre-1990	25	24	19
Total	100	100	100

Table 1.3   Selected Sport-Related Readings in Social Scientific Medical Journals

Author	Title	Journal	Year
Malcolm and Scott	"Professional Relations in Sport Healthcare: Workplace Responses to Organizational Change"	*Social Science & Medicine*	2010
Lunn	"The Sports and Exercise Life-Course: A Survival Analysis of Recall Data from Ireland"	*Social Science & Medicine*	2010
Heggie	"A Century of Cardiomythology: Exercise and the Heart c.1880–1980"	*Social History of Medicine*	2010
Carter	"The Rise and Fall of the Magic Sponge: Medicine and the Transformation of the Football Trainer"	*Social History of Medicine*	2010
Smith and Sparkes	"Changing Bodies, Changing Narratives and the Consequences of Tellability: A Case Study of Becoming Disabled through Sport"	*Sociology of Health & Illness*	2008
Theberge	"The Integration of Chiropractors into Healthcare Teams: A Case Study from Sport Medicine"	*Sociology of Health & Illness*	2008
Roderick	"Adding Insult to Injury: Workplace Injury in English Professional Football"	*Sociology of Health & Illness*	2006
Sparkes and Smith	"When Narratives Matter: Men, Sport, and Spinal Cord Injury"	*Medical Humanities*	2005
Smith and Sparkes	"Men, Sport, Spinal Cord Injury, and Narratives of Hope"	*Social Science & Medicine*	2005
Andrews and Andrews	"Life in a Secure Unit: The Rehabilitation of Young People through the Use of Sport"	*Social Science & Medicine*	2003
Kotarba	"Conceptualizing Sports Medicine as Occupational Health Care: Illustrations from Professional Rodeo and Wrestling"	*Qualitative Health Research*	2001
Lamb, Roberts and Brodie	"Self-Perceived Health among Sports Participants and Non-Sports Participants"	*Social Science & Medicine*	1990
Lamb, Dench, Brodie and Roberts	"Sports Participation and Health Status: A Preliminary Analysis"	*Social Science & Medicine*	1988
Riordan	"Sports Medicine in the Soviet Union and German Democratic Republic"	*Social Science & Medicine*	1987

A keyword search of social science journals devoted to research on medicine, health and illness underscores this lacuna. From the quantitative data in Table 1.1, it is clear that there has been considerably more interest in the health-related aspects of *physical activity* and *exercise* than there has been in sport per se. From this we can conclude that the organizational, performance-based or regulative aspects of sports medicine have been little researched. It is also apparent that what little interest there is in sport is a relatively recent phenomenon. Table 1.2 illustrates trends in sport-related research over time and suggests that the majority of work related to sport (narrowly defined) has been produced in the last decade. Finally, Table 1.3 presents the findings of a qualitative survey of the contents of these journals and provides a stark illustration of the limited engagement with sports medicine as a field of empirical enquiry among social scientists of medicine. Only a handful of the authors featured in this table do not come from a 'sports studies' background.

The neglect of sport among medical social scientists is not wholly surprising. As noted earlier, in terms of consumption, identification and institutionalization, sports medicine is a relatively recent development. Furthermore, as Waddington, Loland and Skirstad note, a central feature of early work in medical sociology was a strong focus on "illness behaviour."[38] The merits of this approach were that it enabled an emerging subdiscipline to establish legitimacy, acquire recognition and exert influence. However, an unintended consequence of this trend was that research agendas were dominated by the interests of medicine rather than of sociology. We suggest that this partly accounts for the neglect of sport. If, as appears to have been the case, mainstream medicine was ambivalent—hostile even—to sports medicine,[39] it was unlikely that social scientists of medicine would see much value in swimming so evidently against the tide. However, expanding beyond this initial narrow focus medical sociology, as Nettleton has recently argued, retains this "problem-solving" orientation, to the point that the intellectual rigor of the subdiscipline is seen to be threatened.[40] Research driven by an interest in sport-related aspects of medicine has not been viewed as a priority because sports medicine was not viewed as a problem.

The degree of neglect of medicine in the social scientific analysis of sport is more difficult to explain partly because it varies across subdisciplines. There are, for instance, a number of very good historically oriented studies of the relationship between sport and medicine. Notable in this regard are Vertinsky's work on the medical establishment's contribution to social attitudes toward female participation in sport and exercise,[41] Berryman's history of the American College of Sports Medicine[42] and Berryman and Park's edited collection, which includes a number of sports science/sports medicine articles previously published in the *Journal of Sport History*.[43] The historical study of sports medicine in Britain is growing rapidly with monographs by Heggie and Carter published in 2011 and 2012, respectively.[44] The history of medical involvement in the supply and use of

performance-enhancing drugs and techniques has also attracted considerable attention, exemplified in Hoberman's seminal *Mortal Engines*.[45]

Where sociologists of sport have addressed sports medicine, they have
tended to do so less directly. Waddington addresses various aspects of medicine—epidemiological studies informing the promotion of sport for health,
the historical role of doctors in performance enhancement and the "dilemmas" doctors face when practicing in sport—within a broader discussion of
Sport, Health and Drugs.[46] Beamish and Ritchie examine the role of medicine within the contribution of sports science to, and revolution in, high-performance sport,[47] and Howe's *Sport, Professionalism and Pain* and Young's
edited collection *Sporting Selves, Damaged Bodies* focus on the illness experiences of athletes.[48] Loland, Skirstad and Waddington's *Pain and Injury in
Sport* again priorities athletes' experiences but from both social and ethical
perspectives.[49] Most of the philosophical works addressing medical issues in
sport focus on drug-related issues (e.g., Miah's *Genetically Modified Athletes*; Moller's *The Ethics of Doping and Anti-Doping)*.[50]

A number of journal articles that focus more directly on the actions and
experiences of those who practice in sports settings have, however, begun
to appear. Among sociologists of sport, Walk's examination of the role of
student athletic trainers in US colleges led the way.[51] Subsequent works of
note include research by Waddington and colleagues examining the role of
doctors and physiotherapists practicing in English professional football;[52] a
parallel study by Malcolm and Sheard focusing on English rugby union;[53]
Safai's examination of sports medicine provision in Canadian sport;[54] Theberge's investigation of the multidisciplinary medical teams devoted to
Canada's elite athletes;[55] and Scott's research on the occupational practices of sports clinicians working with British Olympic athletes.[56] Equiva-
lent works by sports historians include Carter's work on the history of the
role of football trainers and football club doctors,[57] and Heggie's work on
medical interest in the effects of exercise on the heart and of competing
at altitude.[58] In 2007 the *Journal of Sport History* dedicated a forum to
sports medicine that, in addition to Carter's work, contained analyses of
the development of sports medicine in Britain, the historical connections
between athletic trainers and physical educators in the US and an examination of the changing composition of sports medicine support to Canadian
Olympic teams during the twentieth century.[59]

The late development of sports medicine again partly explains the relative
neglect of medicine within the sport subdisciplines. It is interesting to note
that perhaps *the* first article to directly address sports medicine was written
by Jim Riordan, a specialist on sport in the Soviet Union and allied communist states (see Table 1.3). For a period of time, sports medicine was perceived
as something inherently linked to "deviant" communist sports systems and
thus unworthy of investigation by sociologists of Western sport.

But the relatively small number of works listed here belies the historical
links between medicine and physical education.[60] A close alliance between

the subjects began to weaken as physical education fragmented in the mid-1960s following Franklin Henry's seminal publication, "Physical Education: An Academic Discipline."[61] From this point various sport-related subdisciplines, such as sports history, the sociology of sport, sports biomechanics and so on, began to emerge. It was in this context that social scientists abandoned the essentially "corporeal" basis of their subdisciplines for, in contrast to the founders of the sociology of medicine who sought to legitimize their emerging area through allegiances with the medical profession, the dominant voices among the founders of the sociology of sport sought to establish legitimacy through emphasizing their *sociological* credentials. The somewhat ambivalent reception this emerging community of scholars gave to Ernst Jokl's *Medical Sociology and Cultural Anthropology of Sports and Physical Education* illustrates this point.[62] Remarkably, this text, published in 1964, was the first English-language text to combine the words *sociology* and *sport* in its title. It predated the establishment of the International Committee for the Sociology of Sport (formed around 1965) yet it was never mentioned in any of the early programmatic statements that sought to establish the sociology of sport field.[63] Push and pull factors influenced this response. First, in seeking to distance themselves from the other subdisciplines emerging from physical education, sociologists of sport were keen to focus primarily on social rather than physical aspects of sport. Second, in seeking to align the sociology of sport with the sociological "mainstream," this community sought to replicate the theoretical, methodological and empirical principles that dominated sociology at this time, and thus contributed to a discipline that later researchers were to criticize for its "disembodied" character.[64] Similar remarks have been made about the development of sports history where the subdiscipline has been described as like "watching 'Hamlet without the Prince' . . . [where] context becomes all and sport is seen only in terms of something outside of itself."[65]

Sociologists of sport did not to return to medical aspects of sport until the early 1990s. The works of Nixon and Young et al. were particularly influential.[66] Waddington, Loland and Skirstad have suggested that this development was considerably influenced by the commercialization of sport and the increasing economic impact of injuries to athletes.[67] This might explain why the initial work was conducted in North America (where many commercial sporting practices are pioneered), though perhaps not why research tended to focus on college and nonelite or retired sportspeople. Young alternatively suggests that the development of the sociology of the body was particularly influential and this is corroborated by the enthusiasm with which sociologists of sport greeted the emergence of this research area. The sociology of sport, Maguire argued, was in a "unique position to emphasize to the parent discipline the importance of the body." Potentially, "not only would the subject of the body become more central to the concerns of sociology, but the marginal status of the sociology of sport could be shed."[68] Ironically, while the sociology of medicine, health and illness

was seen as a significant catalyst to the sociology of the body,[69] the sociology of the body has been a significant catalyst to the development of the
sociological analysis of sports medicine.

The development of an increasing critical sociology of sport has also
contributed to the growing focus on sports medicine. Dunning refers to this
as a "left-radicalization" that occurred in the 1970s and 1980s.[70] Inspired
by the growing use of Marxism and cultural studies in the subdiscipline,
research increasingly focused on critiquing sport as a social institution. As
part of this development, feminist critiques demonstrated sport's gendered
and gendering properties. Females were excluded from sport, and gender
roles were recreated through female (non)participation. These works were
followed by pro-feminist studies that examined the affects of sports participation on the men who were *not* excluded. Questions were asked about
the socialization processes that led men to be tolerant of, or at least seek to
conceal, pain and injury from each other (and by inference, medical personnel).[71] In this respect, the sociology of sport has developed in the way
leading proponents of the sociology of medicine have wished for their own
subdiscipline. While Nettleton, for instance, has argued that if medical
sociology is to have an enduring influence, a greater theoretical orientation and more nonapplied research is required,[72] an increasing amount of
sport-related research has become theoretically oriented. Researchers have
become sociologists *of* sport rather than sociologists *in* sport. This increasingly critical trend has developed in parallel with the empirical shift in the
sociology of sport away from sport as narrowly defined. The view of sport
as a social construction that is neither politically neutral nor ideologically
uncontested has led sociologists of sport to embrace related physical cultures in an attempt to be more inclusive. The more widely defined remit of
sports and exercise medicine is therefore of as much interest to sociologists
of sport as the area more narrowly defined.

The preceding wide-ranging discussion clearly demonstrates the intri-
cate and fluid nature of both the social phenomena we recognize today as
sports medicine as well as the emergent field of academic study we refer to
as the social organization of sports medicine. As noted already, the aim of
this collection is to pull together work from an international cadre of scholars who examine and provide (interdisciplinary) analysis of the dynamic
and multifaceted relationships between sports and medicine and within
sports medicine. The chapters in this collection chart changing perceptions
of sport within medical discourse, attempts by sports medicine providers to
forge professional identities in response to these processes, the day-to-day
experiences of deliverers of sports medicine and the reactions of recipients
of that health care.

Organized into four sections, the contributions in this collection speak
to the multidimensionality and complexity of the sport and medicine relationship. The chapters in the first part, entitled "Sports Medicine Conceived," explore the social and historical development of sports medicine

in Canada (Mason), the US (Berryman) and United Kingdom (Carter). In doing so, each author adds to our discussion of the way in which sports medicine has been envisaged over time through competing ideas about the nature and purposes of sports medicine and the medical use of sport. In his examination of the ACSM, Jack Berryman demonstrates that the roots of the association—and, in turn, the field of sports medicine in the US— rested not in sports or in the treatment of sports injury per se but rather in cardiology and physiology. Furthermore, as Berryman describes in detail, the impetus for the founding and development of ACSM among these cardiologists and physiologists arose from a concern for the nation's health and fitness, particularly among youth. This dovetails with Neil Carter's account of the development of BASEM. Carter centers his focus on the struggle among physicians to carve out a professional identity for themselves as sports medicine practitioners. Similar to Berryman's analysis of ACSM, of note for Carter is that the demand for specialist sports medicine services grew both within elite sport and from the government that came to see sport and exercise as a form of medicine to improve the population's fitness. This led to the recognition of sports medicine as a fully fledged medical specialty within the British National Health Service. In the final chapter of this section, Fred Mason explores the sociohistorical development of sports medicine for people with disabilities, with particular attention to developments in Canada. In offering a periodization of sports medicine for athletes with disabilities, Mason demonstrates that the development of a performance-oriented sports medicine for athletes with disabilities was hampered by the traditional therapeutic orientation of medicine and stereotypical conceptions of people with disabilities. As a result, tangible developments in this area did not occur until the 1980s, spurred more by sports medicine physicians than by those specialties traditionally involved with disability sport (e.g., neurology and physical medicine).

The second part, "Sports Medicine Organized," offers four readings on the ways in which sports medicine is structured. Contributions examine gender inequalities in elite sports medicine (Kotarba), the implications of attempting to balance participant and broader public health concerns (Paraschak), the coalescence of traditional medical models and complementary and alternative medicine (Pike) and the social and political factors shaping the integration of sports science and sports medicine (Theberge). In the first chapter of this section, Joseph Kotarba offers a case study of the Houston Pinks, a professional women's football team, and examines the (lack of) sports medicine provision for women athletes, as well as the athletes' negotiation of access to supplementary forms of health care support. Kotarba does this through the analytical lens of community (e.g., the informal community of teammates, the formal team organization) and contends that, although female athletes do not receive the quality of care men receive, they do assemble support among one another to take care of themselves in the absence of, or in complement to, formal sports medicine. In the second chapter, Vicky Paraschak also explores notions of community—in this case, the community of Olympic Games' participants in contrast to the community of nonparticipants (i.e., the public at large)—in her case study of the 2007 Canada Winter Games (CWG) held in Whitehorse, Yukon. Paraschak demonstrates that despite the promotion of the Games as healthful for all, including for the community hosting the event, health care practices were well developed only with regard to the acute health care of "participants," were less-well-developed for "nonparticipants" and were underdeveloped and at times oppositional when linked to public health concerns such as increasing cases of respiratory infections and norovirus-like symptoms.

The third and fourth chapters in this part shift our focus to the rationalization of sports medicine (including its professionalization and bureaucratization) in the sport community and beyond, and the impact of these processes on health care disciplines often located at (or, rather, relegated to) the periphery of orthodox (sports) medicine. In her examination of complementary and alternative medicines (CAM), Elizabeth Pike argues that despite CAM's positive reception among athletes, the privileging of evidence-based medicine (EBM) as underpinned by a positivist scientific paradigm reinforces orthodox medicine's hegemonic position and constrains athletes' abilities to utilize CAM as part of their health care practices. Pike furthers argues that this hinders an inclusive health care system that must respond to and be informed by the voices of both service providers and users. Nancy Theberge similarly explores the rationalization of sports medicine yet her focus is on massage therapy in the Canadian sports medicine context. Her discussion addresses the challenges of identifying and implementing an effective sports medicine delivery model, as understood by administrators, coaches, health care providers and athletes. Massage therapy is offered as a case study of these challenges as it has become established within the system of sports medicine professions despite ongoing debate about its benefits fueled by the evidence-based sports medicine orthodoxy. Theberge acknowledges that athletes' support/demand for massage therapy—a marker of the client-centered nature of sports medicine—has challenged sport administrators in their negotiation over which professions and which professional services be supported in the high-performance sports medicine system.

The third part looks at the way in which sports medicine is *practiced*. It examines the response of athletes to their exposure to sports medicine (Thing), the constraints on practitioners in responding to their client athletes (Waddington, Scott) and, consequently, practitioners' involvement in illegal performance enhancement (Hoberman). With a focus on the patient, Lone Thing explores injured athletes' experiences with sports medicine clinicians and with sports medicine technology in the first chapter in this part. In questioning the docility or reflexivity of patient-athletes, Thing examines patient-athletes' narratives of illness and choice making over competing forms of treatment such as surgery. She concludes by arguing that health care institutions should more seriously consider questions of user democracy and dialogue. In his exploration of the client-centered nature of sports medicine in professional sport, Ivan Waddington suggests that the values associated with sport performance and success in professional sport inform the context within which sports medicine physicians practice and frame the ways in which sports medicine physicians are able to negotiate with their patient-athletes. Waddington argues that we must be cognizant of the ways in which sports medicine physicians, as a function of their "everyday work settings," are constrained to respond to the demands of their clients, even when this runs counter to their ethic of care. In the third chapter of this part, Andrea Scott continues to examine the health–performance tension that distinguishes the working environment of sports medicine physicians and sport physiotherapists in British Olympic sports. Drawing upon interview data, Scott echoes a number of the same themes raised by Waddington, including the constraints on sports medicine clinicians. In contrast to Waddington, who stresses that ethically dubious practice is primarily a consequence of clinicians' capitulation to pressure exerted by owners and management, Scott emphasizes the prevalence of the ethically less problematic situation, in which clinicians' counsel against yet ultimately sanction practices they consider are not in the athletes' "best interests" due to pressure from the athletes themselves. In the final chapter of this part, John Hoberman continues to examine the client-centered nature of sports medicine but, in this case, through an exploration of physicians' involvement with doping. As Hoberman demonstrates, the involvement of doctors with the doping practices of elite athletes is, although not a recent phenomenon, one that has become increasingly more complex and widespread. A critical analysis of doping doctors—whether positioned as medical mercenaries or as entrepreneurial physicians—encourages us to further question the health–performance tension in sport as collaborations between doctors and patients have long raised fundamental questions about the relationship between doctors and "patients" whose "medical" priority is their level of performance rather than their health.

The fourth part, "Sports and Medicine Contested," looks at the way in which sports medicine is challenged, examining the resistance to the dominance of traditional medical models posed by lay medical practice (Atkinson), the legal and ethical considerations that underpin the introduction (or nonintroduction) of particular health care policies (Müller) and the blurring distinctions between therapy and enhancement (Kondo and McNamee). Drawing on personal experiences as well as interview data with (other) triathletes, Michael Atkinson examines ethno-pharmacological practices around food, drugs and nutrition regimes. He demonstrates the contestation of "scientifically validated" knowledge and authority by athletes' uptake of, and preference for, local or lay knowledge. In doing so, Atkinson illustrates a subversion of "evidence-based" health care—in this case, the triathletes' lay knowledge becomes the evidence on which health claims and practices are made. Arno Müller explores the tensions associated with the practice of mass heart screening of high-performance athletes. Although initially discussing the contexts within which mass screening of athletes is supported (e.g., Italy) and not supported (e.g., the US), Müller's analysis develops the broader debates and implications of screening, asking such questions as: Should genetic testing also be considered and would it improve or provide a differential diagnosis? Could cascade screening (i.e., the testing of family members of a person at risk) help to reduce the numbers of sudden death in athletes and at the same time reduce the costs? What other legal and ethical aspects are relevant? Is it purely a factual disagreement or is there a moral divergence behind the opposing views in Italy and the US? Is the opposition to a mass screening the result of the litigious nature of the US health care system? Do the athletes have a voice in this process? Do athletes have a *right to know* and/or a *right not to know* about their medical condition? Yoshitaka Kondo and Michael McNamee further explore the ethical frontiers of sports medicine in the third chapter in this part, but do so through a literary turn in their analysis of genetic doping and enhancement. In discussing Danish athlete-turned-writer Knud Lundberg's *The Olympic Hope*, they assert that a critical analysis of sports medicine—including a recent US government position paper on genetic therapy—must be multidisciplinary in nature, extending (at least) to historical, literary and philosophical scholarship. Such wide-ranging sources, they argue, fuel our imagination and provoke discussion of what sports medicine currently means and what it can become.

Through each contribution in this book, we see the dynamic, ever-changing nature of contemporary sports medicine—whether through the voices of athletes negotiating sports medicine in their lives; the observations of clinicians and other sport professionals/administrators charged with managing sports medicine support for athletes; or through broader political, ethical and philosophical debates and discussions of the health–performance paradox. In all, these chapters offer us rich food for thought and, in this vein, the words of Donnelly remain prophetic. Stimulated by his experience of attending the 1999 ACSM annual meeting, Donnelly noted, "rarely have we 'studied up' on sport science [or] sport medicine."[73] He concluded: "It is clear that we, as sport sociologists, need to develop our sociology of sport science and our sociology of sports medicine."[74] Over a decade later this statement remains true. Our aim in producing this collection is to go some way to answering this call, and to go beyond it by developing a more broadly social scientific analysis of a rapidly developing and increasingly significant social institution in the contemporary world.

NOTES

1. Ingham and Donnelly, "Sociology of North American Sociology," 367.
2. Andrews, "Kinesiology's Inconvenient Truth," 50.
3. Snyder and Spreitzer, "Sociology of Sport," 17.

4. Gruneau, "Sport as an Area," 12.
5. Guttmann, *From Ritual to Record.*
6. McPherson, Curtis and Loy, "Defining Sport."
7. Elias and Dunning, *Quest for Excitement.*
8. See, e.g., Roderick, *Work of Professional Football*; Beamish and Ritchie, *Fastest, Highest, Strongest.*
9. Andrews, "Kinesiology's Inconvenient Truth," 52.
10. Safai, "Critical Analysis."
11. Batt and Macleod, "Coming of Age," 621.
12. See, e.g., Speed and Jacques, "High-Performance Sports Medicine."
13. Edwards and McNamee, "Why Sports Medicine Is Not Medicine," 105.
14. See http://www.fims.org/en/general/history-and-purpose/ (accessed 18 January 2011).
15. Edwards and McNamee, "Why Sports Medicine Is Not Medicine," 106.
16. Theberge, "'It's Not about Health," 180–181.
17. Wrynn, "Human Factor."
18. See http://www.bma.org.uk/ (accessed 18 January 2011).
19. See http://www.ama-assn.org/ama/pub/about-ama/our-mission.shtml (accessed 18 January 2011).
20. Reynolds and Tansey, *Development of Sports Medicine*; Heggie, "Specialization without the Hospital."
21. Vertinsky, "Commentary," 94.
22. See http://sma.org.au/ (accessed 18 January 2011).
23. Ryan, "Sports Medicine," 13.
24. Williams and Sperryn, *Sports Medicine*, ix; cited in Waddington, *Sport, Health and Drugs*, 121.
25. Heggie, "Specialization without the Hospital," 474.
26. Kennedy, "Team Doctor."
27. Kotarba, "Conceptualizing Sports Medicine."
28. Vertinsky, "Commentary"; Theberge, "Integration of Chiropractors."
29. We are grateful to Alan Bairner for providing these biographical insights into the lives of some of medicine's founding fathers.
30. Hoberman, "Early Development," 240.
31. See http://www.fims.org/en/associations/info/ (accessed 18 November 2011). Since the beginning of 2011, twenty-four new member states have joined FIMS.
32. Wrynn, "Human Factor"; Safai, "Critical Analysis"; Heggie, "Only the British."
33. Anderson, "Writing a New Code"; Waddington and Roderick, "Management of Medical Confidentiality."
34. Heggie, "Specialization without the Hospital;" Safai, "Critical Analysis."
35. Malcolm, "Medical Uncertainty"; Cavanaugh and Sykes, "Transsexual Bodies"; Houlihan, "Civil Rights."
36. Scambler, *Sociology.*
37. Scambler, *Sport in Society.* See also Scambler and Jennings, "On the Periphery."
38. Waddington, Loland and Skirstad, "Introduction."
39. Reynolds and Tansey, *Development of Sports Medicine*, xxviii.
40. Nettleton, "Retaining the Sociology," 2409.
41. Vertinsky, *Eternally Wounded Woman.* It would be remiss not to mention the significant work Vertinsky has also published on gender and exercise in a range of health and medical social science journals not covered in the quantitative analysis in this chapter.
42. Berryman, *Out of Many, One.*

43. Berryman and Park, *Sport and Exercise Science.*
44. Carter, *Medicine, Sport and the Body*; Heggie, *History of British Sports Medicine.*
45. Hoberman, *Mortal Engines.*
46. Waddington, *Sport, Health and Drugs.*
47. Beamish and Ritchie, *Fastest, Highest, Strongest.*
48. Howe, *Sport, Professionalism and Pain*; Young, *Sporting Selves, Damaged Bodies.*
49. Loland, Skirstad and Waddington, *Pain and Injury in Sport.*
50. Miah, *Genetically Modified Athletes*; Moller, *Ethics of Doping.*
51. Walk, "Peers in Pain."
52. Waddington, *Sport, Health and Drugs* and "Jobs for the Boys?"; Waddington and Roderick, "Management of Medical Confidentiality"; Waddington, Roderick and Naik, "Methods of Appointment."
53. Malcolm and Sheard, "Pain in the Assets"; Malcolm, "Unprofessional Practice?"; "Sports Medicine"; "Medical Uncertainty."
54. Safai, "Healing the Body" and "Critical Analysis."
55. See Theberge's "'It's Not about Health"; "We Have All the Bases Covered"; "Professional Identities."
56. Scott, "More Professional?"; Malcolm and Scott, "Professional Relations."
57. Carter, "Metatarsals and Magic Sponges"; "Mixing Business with Leisure?"; "Rise and Fall."
58. Heggie, "Century of Cardiomythology"; "Only the British."
59. Cronin, "Not Taking the Medicine"; Wrynn, "Under the Showers"; Teetzel, "Sports, Medicine."
60. Vertinsky, "Commentary," 94.
61. Henry, "Physical Education."
62. Jokl, *Medical Sociology.*
63. These points are developed in more detail in Malcolm, *Sport and Sociology.*
64. Frank, "Bringing Bodies Back In"; Turner, *Body and Society.*
65. Holt, "Sport and History," 17.
66. Nixon, "Social Network Analysis"; "Accepting the Risks"; "Coaches' Views of Risk"; Young, "Violence, Risk and Liability"; Young and White, "Sport, Physical Danger and Injury"; Young, White and McTeer, "Body Talk."
67. Waddington, Loland and Skirstad, "Introduction."
68. Maguire, "Bodies, Sportscultures and Societies," 33.
69. Scott and Morgan, *Body Matters.*
70. Dunning, "Sociology of Sport."
71. Messner, *Power at Play.*
72. Nettleton, "Retaining the Sociology."
73. Donnelly, "Gulliver's Travels," 455.
74. Ibid., 457.

BIBLIOGRAPHY

Anderson, Lynley. "Writing a New Code of Ethics for Sports Physicians: Principles and Challenges." *British Journal of Sports Medicine* 43 (2009): 1079–1082.
Andrews, David. "Kinesiology's Inconvenient Truth and the Physical Cultural Studies Imperative." *Quest* 60 (2008): 45–62.
Andrews, Justin and Andrews, Gavin. "Life in a Secure Unit: The Rehabilitation of Young People through the Use of Sport." *Social Science & Medicine* 56, no. 3 (2003): 531–550.

Batt, Mike, and Donald A. Macleod. "The Coming of Age of Sports Medicine." *British Medical and Journal* 314 (1997): 621.

Beamish, Rob, and Ian Ritchie. *Fastest, Highest, Strongest: A Critique of High Performance Sport*. London: Routledge, 2006.

Berryman, Jack. *Out of Many, One: A History of the American College of Sports Medicine*. Champaign, IL: Human Kinetics, 1995.

Berryman, Jack, and Roberta Park, eds. *Sport and Exercise Science: Essays in the History of Sports Medicine*. Chicago: University of Illinois Press, 1992.

Carter, Neil. *Medicine Sport and the Body: A Historical Perspective*. London: Bloomsbury, 2012.

———. "Metatarsals and Magic Sponges: English Football and the Development of Sports Medicine." *Journal of Sport History* 34, no. 1 (2007): 53–74.

———. "Mixing Business with Leisure? The Football Club Doctor, Sports Medicine and the Voluntary Tradition." *Sport in History* 29, no. 1 (2009): 69–91.

———. "The Rise and Fall of the Magic Sponge: Medicine and the Transformation of the Football Trainer." *Social History of Medicine* 23, no. 2 (2009): 261–279.

Cavanaugh, Sheila, and Heather Sykes. "Transsexual Bodies at the Olympics: The International Olympic Committee's Policy on Transsexual Athletes at the 2004 Athens Summer Games." *Body and Society* 12, no. 3 (2006): 75–102.

Cronin, Mike. "Not Taking the Medicine: Sportsmen and Doctors in Late Nineteenth Century Britain." *Journal of Sport History* 34, no. 1 (2007): 23–36.

Donnelly, Peter. "Gulliver's Travels: A Sport Sociologist among the Labcoats." *Journal of Sport & Social Issues* 24, no. 3 (1999): 455–458.

Dunning, Eric. "Sociology of Sport in the Balance: Critical Reflections on Some Recent and More Enduring Trends." *Sport in Society* 7, no. 1 (2004): 1–24.

Edwards, Steven, and Mike McNamee. "Why Sports Medicine Is Not Medicine." *Health Care Analysis* 14 (2006): 103–109.

Elias, Norbert, and Eric Dunning. *Quest for Excitement*. Oxford: Basil Blackwell, 1986.

Frank, Arthur. "Bringing Bodies Back In: A Decade Review." *Theory, Culture and Society* 7 (1990): 131–162.

Gruneau, Richard. "Sport as an Area of Sociological Study: An Introduction to Major Themes and Perspectives." In *Canadian Sport: Sociological Perspectives*, edited by R. Grunean and J.G. Albinson, 8–30. Reading, MA: Addison Wesley, 1976.

Guttmann, Allen. *From Ritual to Record: The Nature of Modern Sport*. New York: Columbia University Press, 1978.

Heggie, Vanessa. "A Century of Cardiomythology: Exercise and the Heart c. 1880–1980." *Social History of Medicine* 23, no. 2 (2009): 280–298.

———. *A History of British Sports Medicine*. Manchester: Manchester University Press, 2011.

———. "'Only the British Appear to be Making a Fuss': The Science of Success and the Myth of Amateurism at the Mexico Olympiad, 1968." *Sport in History* 28 (2008): 213–235.

———. "Specialization without the Hospital: The Case of British Sports Medicine." *Medical History* 54 (2010): 457–474.

Henry, Franklin M. "Physical Education: An Academic Discipline." *Journal of Health, Physical Education, and Recreation* 35 (1964): 32–33.

Hoberman, John. "The Early Development of Sports Medicine in Germany." In *Sport and Exercise Science: Essays in the History of Sports Medicine*, edited by Jack Berryman and Roberta Park, 233–282. Chicago: University of Illinois Press, 1992.

———. *Mortal Engines: The Science of Performance and the Dehumanization of Sport*. New York: Free Press, 1992.

20   *Dominic Malcolm and Parissa Safai*

Holt, Richard. "Sport and History: British and European Traditions." In *Taking Sport Seriously*, edited by Lincoln Allison, 7–30. Aachen: Meyer and Meyer, 1998.

Houlihan, Barrie. "Civil Rights, Doping Control and the World Anti-Doping Code." *Sport in Society* 7, no. 3 (2004): 420–437.

Howe, P. David. *Sport, Professionalism and Pain: Ethnographies of Injury and Risk*. London: Routledge, 2004.

Ingham, Alan, and Peter Donnelly. "A Sociology of North American Sociology of Sport: Disunity in Unity, 1965 to 1996." *Sociology of Sport Journal* 14, no. 4 (1997): 362–418.

Jokl, Ernst. *Medical Sociology and Cultural Anthropology of Sports and Physical Education*. Springfield, IL: Thomas, 1964.

Kennedy, Ken W. "The Team Doctor in Rugby Union Football." In *Medicine, Sport and the Law*, edited by S.D.W. Payne, 315–323. Oxford: Blackwell, 1990.

Kotarba, Joseph. "Conceptualizing Sports Medicine as Occupational Health Care: Illustrations from Professional Rodeo and Wrestling." *Qualitative Health Research* 11 (2001): 766–779.

Lamb, Kevin, Dench, S., Brodie, D. and Roberts, K. "Sports Participation and Health Status: A Preliminary Analysis." *Social Science & Medicine 25, no. 1 (1987): 19–26*.

Lamb, Kevin, Roberts, K. and Brodie, D. "Self-Perceived Health among Sports Participants and Non-Sports Participants." *Social Science & Medicine 31, no. 9 (1990): 963–969*.

Loland, Sigmund, Berit Skirstad and Ivan Waddington, eds. *Pain and Injury in Sport: Social and Ethical Analysis*. London: Routledge, 2006.

Lunn, Peter. "The Sports and Exercise Life-Course: A Survival Analysis of Recall Data from Ireland." *Social Science & Medicine 70, no. 5 (2010): 711–719*.

Maguire, Joseph. "Bodies, Sportscultures and Societies: A Critical Review of Some Theories in the Sociology of the Body." *International Review for the Sociology of Sport* 28, no. 1 (1993): 33–51.

Malcolm, Dominic. "Medical Uncertainty and Clinician–Athlete Relations: The Management of Concussion Injuries in Rugby Union." *Sociology of Sport Journal* 26, no. 2 (2009): 191–210.

———. *Sport and Society*. London: Routledge, 2012.

———. "Sports Medicine: A Very Peculiar Practice? Doctors and Physiotherapists in Elite English Rugby Union." In *Pain and Injury in Sport: Social and Ethical Analysis*, edited by S. Loland, B. Skirstad and I. Waddington, 165–181. London: Routledge, 2006.

———. "Unprofessional Practice? The Status and Power of Sports Physicians." *Sociology of Sport Journal* 23 (2006): 376–395.

Malcolm, Dominic, and Andrea Scott. "Professional Relations in Elite Sport Healthcare: Workplace Responses to Organizational Change." *Social Science & Medicine* 72 (2011): 513–520.

Malcolm, Dominic, and Ken Sheard. "'Pain in the Assets': The Effects of Commercialization and Professionalization on the Management of Injury in English Rugby Union." *Sociology of Sport Journal* 19 (2002): 149–169.

McPherson, B.D., J.E. Curtis and J.W. Loy. "Defining Sport." In *The Social Significance of Sport*, edited by B.D. McPherson, J.E. Curtis and J.W. Loy, 15–17. Champaign, IL: Human Kinetics, 1989.

Messner, Michael. *Power at Play: Sport and the Problem of Masculinity*. Boston: Beacon Press, 1995.

Miah, Andy. *Genetically Modified Athletes; Biomedical Ethics, Gene Doping and Sport*. London: Routledge, 2004.

Moller, Verner. *The Ethics of Doping and Anti-Doping*. London: Routledge, 2009.

Nettleton, Sarah. 'Retaining the Sociology in Medical Sociology', *Social Science & Medicine*, 65 (2007): 2409–2412

Nixon, Howard L., II. "Accepting the Risks of Pain and Injury in Sport: Mediated Cultural Influences on Playing Hurt." *Sociology of Sport Journal* 10 (1993): 183–196.

———. "Coaches' Views of Risk, Pain, and Injury in Sport, with Special Reference to Gender Differences." *Sociology of Sport Journal* 11 (1994): 79–87.

———. "A Social Network Analysis of Influences of Athletes to Play with Pain and Injury." *Journal of Sport & Social Issues* 16 (1992): 127–135.

Reynolds, Lois, and Tilli Tansey, eds. *The Development of Sports Medicine in Twentieth Century Britain*. London: Wellcome Trust Centre, 2009.

Roderick, Martin. *The Work of Professional Football*. London: Routledge, 2006.

———. "Adding Insult to Injury: Workplace Injury in English Professional Football." *Sociology of Health & Illness* 28, no. 1 (2006): 76–97.

Riordan, James. "Sports Medicine in the Soviet Union and German Democratic Republic."
Social Science & Medicine 25, no. 1 (1987): 19–26.

Ryan, Allan J. "Sports Medicine in the World Today." In *Sports Medicine*, edited by A.J. Ryan and F.L. Allman, 3–21. San Diego, CA: Academic Press, 1989.

Safai, Parissa. "A Critical Analysis of the Development of Sport Medicine in Canada, 1955–1980." *International Review for the Sociology of Sport* 42, no. 3 (2007): 321–341.

———. "Healing the Body in the 'Culture of Risk': Examining the Negotiation of Treatment between Sports Medicine Clinicians and Injured Athletes in Canadian Intercollegiate Sport." *Sociology of Sport Journal* 20 (2003): 127–146.

Scambler, Graham. *Sociology as Applied to Medicine*. 6th ed. London: Saunders Elsevier, 2008.

———. *Sport and Society: History, Power and Culture*. Maidenhead: Open University Press, 2005.

Scambler, Graham, and M. Jennings. "On the Periphery of the Sex Industry: Female Combat, Male Punters and Feminist Discourse." *Journal of Sport & Social Issues* 22 (1998): 414–427.

Scott, Andrea. "'More Professional?' The Occupational Practices of Sports Medicine Clinicians Working with British Olympic Athletes." Unpublished PhD thesis, Loughborough University, 2010.

Scott, Sue, and David Morgan. *Body Matters: Essays on the Sociology of the Body*. London: Falmer Press, 1993.

Smith, Brett and Sparkes, Andrew. "Men, Sport, Spinal Cord Injury, and Narratives of Hope." *Social Science & Medicine* 61, no. 5 (2005): 1095–1105.

———. "Changing Bodies, Changing Narratives and the Consequences of Tellability: A Case Study of Becoming Disabled through Sport." *Sociology of Health & Illness* 30, no. 2 (2008): 217–236

Snyder, E., and E. Spreitzer. "Sociology of Sport: An Overview." *Sociological Quarterly* 15 (1974): 467–487.

Sparkes, Andrew and Smith, Brett. "When Narratives Matter: Men, Sport, and Spinal Cord Injury." *Medical Humanities* 31 (2005): 81–88

Speed, Cathy, and Rod Jacques. "High Performance Sports Medicine: An Ancient but Evolving Field." *British Journal of Sports Medicine* 45 (2010): 81–83.

Teetzel, Sarah. "Sports, Medicine, and the Emergence of Sports Medicine in the Olympic Games: The Canadian Example." *Journal of Sport History* 34, no. 1 (2007): 75–86.

Theberge, Nancy. "The Integration of Chiropractors into Healthcare Teams: A Case Study from Sports Medicine." *Sociology of Health & Illness* 30 (2008): 19–34.

———. "'It's Not about Health, It's about Performance.' Sport Medicine, Health and the Culture of Risk in Canadian Sport." In *Physical Culture, Power and the Body*, edited by J. Hargreaves and P. Vertinsky, 176–194. London: Routledge, 2007.

———. "Professional Identities and the Practice of Sport Medicine in Canada: A Comparative Analysis of Two Sporting Contexts." In *Sport and Social Identities*, edited by Jon Harris and Andrew Parker, 49–69. Basingstoke, UK: Palgrave, 2009.

———. "'We Have All the Bases Covered.' Constructions of Professional Boundaries in Sport Medicine." *International Review for the Sociology of Sport* 44 (2009): 265–282.

Turner, Bryan S. *The Body and Society: Explorations in Social Theory*. Oxford: Basil Blackwell, 1984.

Vertinsky, Patricia. *The Eternally Wounded Woman: Women, Doctors and Exercise in the Late Nineteenth Century*. Manchester: Manchester University Press, 1990.

———. "Commentary: What Is Sports Medicine?" *Journal of Sport History* 34, no. 1 (2007): 87–95.

Waddington, Ivan. "Jobs for the Boys? A Study of the Employment of Club Doctors and Physiotherapists in English Professional Football." *Soccer & Society* 3 (2002): 51–64.

———. *Sport, Health and Drugs: A Critical Sociological Investigation*. London: E & FN Spon, 2000.

Waddington, Ivan, Sigmund Loland and Berit Skirstad. "Introduction." In *Pain and Injury in Sport: Social and Ethical Analysis*, edited by Sigmund Loland, Berit Skirstad and Ivan Waddington, 1–13. London: Routledge, 2006.

Waddington, Ivan, and Martin Roderick. "The Management of Medical Confidentiality in English Professional Football Clubs: Some Ethical Problems and Issues." *British Journal of Sports Medicine* 36 (2002): 118–123.

Waddington, Ivan, Martin Roderick, and Rav Naik. "Methods of Appointment and Qualifications of Club Doctors and Physiotherapists in English Professional Football: Some Problems and Issues." *British Journal of Sports Medicine* 35 (2001): 48–53.

Walk, Stephan R. "Peers in Pain: The Experiences of Student Athletic Trainers." *Sociology of Sport Journal* 14 (1997): 22–56.

Williams, John, and Peter Sperryn, eds. *Sports Medicine*. 2nd ed. London: Edward Arnold, 1976.

Wrynn, Alison. "The Human Factor: Science, Medicine and the International Olympic Committee, 1900–1970." *Sport in Society* 7, no. 2 (2004): 211–231.

———. "'Under the Showers': An Analysis of the Historical Connections between American Athletic Training and Physical Education." *Journal of Sport History* 34, no. 1 (2007): 37–52.

Young, Kevin, ed. *Sporting Bodies Damaged Selves: Sociological Studies of Sports Related Injuries*. Oxford: Elsevier Press, 2004.

———. "Violence, Risk and Liability in Male Sports Culture." *Sociology of Sport Journal* 10 (1993): 373–396.

Young, Kevin, and Philip White. "Sport, Physical Danger and Injury: The Experiences of Elite Women Athletes." *Journal of Sport & Social Issues* 19 (1993): 45–61.

Young, Kevin, Philip White and William McTeer. "Body Talk: Male Athletes Reflect on Sport, Injury and Pain." *Sociology of Sport Journal* 11 (1994): 175–194.

Part I
Sports Medicine Conceived

2 The Role of Physiology and Cardiology in the Founding and Early Years of the American College of Sports Medicine

Jack W. Berryman

The American College of Sports Medicine (ACSM) is the largest and most active sports medicine organization in the world with a membership over twenty thousand. Approximately twenty-four hundred are international members from nearly seventy-five different countries. Throughout its history, ACSM has been the recognized authority on issues in sports medicine and exercise science through its position stands, opinion statements, certifications, journals, books, newsletter, lecture tours, media education, regional chapters, clinical programs and annual meetings. The College has also been a respected partner with other national organizations like the American Heart Association and the Centers for Disease Control and Prevention, among numerous others, to implement policy change and legislation. More than any other professional association, ACSM has been a pioneer in advocating the importance and necessity of studying exercise and its many ramifications.[1]

For ACSM, sports medicine itself, defies definition as a specific discipline. Instead, it represents a convergence of different fields in a common focus. Accordingly, ACSM divides its membership into three core groups—basic and applied science; medicine; and, allied health and education—each contributing to sports medicine as a totality. Typical professionals in the basic and applied science area are physiologists, biomechanists and biochemists. The medical group is composed of licensed professionals engaged in patient care, including orthopedists, podiatrists, pediatricians and internists, among others. Common professionals in the allied health and education area are physical educators, athletic trainers, nurses, nutritionists, physical therapists, exercise program directors and recreation leaders. This diversity has always been ACSM's strength and has been used as the rationale for the College's existence as well as its success. ACSM's unique interdisciplinary nature and broad spectrum of fields united for shared goals, is also the College's unique heritage that slowly developed during the first half of the twentieth century.

ACSM'S FOUNDING AND EARLY YEARS

The founding meeting of the "Federation of Sports Medicine" took place in New York City at the Hotel Statler on 22 April 1954 as part of the afternoon program of the American Association for Health, Physical Education, and Recreation (AAHPER).[2] The following year, the ACSM was officially incorporated and eleven individuals were designated as founders.[3] This group was composed of seven men and one woman with careers in physical education, and three physicians. The title chosen by the founders for this new organization, the ACSM, represented a definition of sports medicine unlike that in other countries. ACSM included as founders and charter members and eventual members those without medical degrees, whereas all of the members of the Federation Internationale de Medecine Sportive (FIMS) were physicians. Sports medicine, as defined by ACSM, was a unique blend of physical education, medicine and physiology, much as it was in ancient Greece. Whereas countries like Germany developed formal divisions of medicine devoted to sports by the early 1900s, sports medicine in the US did not become recognized in the same way until the 1950s.[4]

It was evident that the organizational meeting in 1954 was a result of several interrelated events that occurred throughout the first half of the twentieth century. The ACSM evolved from this milieu, which saw an increased interest in exercise and health within the professions of physical education, physiology and medicine, especially cardiology. Two interrelated activities—the development and measurement of physical fitness and the physical training and rehabilitation of soldiers—along with other types of military research, served as common areas of interest for all three professional groups from World War I onward. Important, too, was the developing field of physical activity epidemiology, initiated by those studying coronary heart disease. ACSM also came about because of the special vision and work of key individuals: Joseph Wolffe (founder and first president of ACSM), Grover Mueller, Ernst Jokl, Arthur Steinhaus and Albert Hyman, in particular.

EXERCISE, SPORT AND MEDICINE PRE-ACSM

The connection between sports and medicine, or at least exercise and medicine, originated out of the tradition of the "six things nonnatural," dating to the time of Hippocrates and Galen. While the tradition linking medicine and exercise continued into nineteenth-century American medicine, guidelines for exercise and formal exercise instruction became more and more associated with physical education. By the 1880s, several different exercise systems were used in both private and public education, and more professionals were trained in nonmedical degree programs to teach exercises. Also by this time, organized college sports were becoming popular in the

US. The success and widespread interest in athletics at universities began to direct the physical educator's attention away from various exercise systems and calisthenics to games and sports at the expense of health and fitness. Similarly, mainstream medicine abandoned its long-standing central component of prevention in favor of new techniques of therapy that were dependent on drugs and surgery. Accordingly, by the middle of the twentieth century, a few visionaries saw the need for an organization like ACSM to combine the expertise of physical education, physiology and medicine and direct it toward the goal of national health and fitness. This redirection coincided with the era when health was beginning to be defined as a state of wellness or wholeness instead of the mere absence of disease.[5]

Exercise and sports and the medical profession in American society also had a cautious and sometimes strained relationship during the late nineteenth and early twentieth centuries. Those with medical training who had once led the movement for systematic exercise moved into mainstream therapy as a career rather than dwelling on the preventive tactics that were so popular before new drugs and surgeries were developed. Also, with the coming of high-level sporting competition and the intense training accompanying it, physicians in general tended to look with suspicion at any activity that put the body in a stressful situation or taxed one's physiological systems beyond normal limits. Those physicians who did get involved with exercise and sport, however, usually did so as health officers at universities or colleges that were involved in intercollegiate sports.[6]

At about the same time, physiologists realized that the study of physiological responses to exercise provided a unique opportunity to understand how the body's control mechanisms reacted to diverse circumstances. They also found it to be a good way to discover more about the overall process of physiological adaptation. Others with interests in physiology began to study athletes to better understand and extend the limits of human performance. These were the beginnings, at least in early twentieth-century America, of the fields of physiology of exercise and exercise physiology.[7]

The founders and charter members of ACSM were keenly aware that the distinguishing feature of health problems was their association with habits and lifestyle, particularly stress, smoking, poor nutrition and lack of exercise. They also believed prevention rather than treatment showed more potential for success, and that if prevention were to be effective, it had to begin at a young age. Consequently, ACSM and its membership were at the forefront of a surge in health-related exercise research. Not surprising, given Joseph Wolffe's background in cardiology and the preponderance of heart disease in America, this early research first focused on cardiovascular disease and youth fitness.

Their emphasis within sports medicine was unique, and much different from that of traditional therapeutic medicine or mainstream physiology. The founders reveled in the idea of studying the healthy as opposed to working with the ill. They also valued research on ultrahealthy individuals, usually high-level athletes, to better understand lower versus higher levels of performance capability. By researching the physiology of exercise, they had a better understanding of what could be accomplished by physical training. In particular, they hoped to discover physical training regimens that would help humans cope with the serious onslaught of diseases of the lungs and heart. Also of particular interest to the founders was the challenge of keeping healthy people healthy and possibly even improving their physical status or returning the sick, weak or injured to a state of normalcy.

It was a combination of these interests and motives that led several of the founders to attempt the formation of centers, federations or associations to focus on fitness, cardiac rehabilitation or physical therapy, among others. Rather than continue to emphasize studies of physiological mechanisms and their application to work and the environment, the founders chose to dwell more on the relationship of physical activity to health. Not surprisingly, then, the first area of health-related exercise research focused on cardiovascular disease. Some plans did not materialize, but others did. After attempts to begin an "American Association of Sportmedicine" in 1952, the founding meeting of the "Federation of Sports Medicine" was eventually held in 1954. The following year, the Federation became the ACSM or, as it was sometimes called in the early years, the American Chapter of FIMS.[8]

What follows then, in this chapter, is an in-depth description of the key individuals and events in cardiology and physiology that eventually led to the creation of ACSM. All of the presidents of ACSM from its founding through 1966, were either cardiologists or physiologists. Each had a specific interest in exercise, cardiovascular health and physical fitness. Accordingly, it was this unique blend of contributions from a handful of ACSM founders and charter members that established sports medicine in the US.

THE ROLE OF PHYSIOLOGY
AND ITS INFLUENCE ON ACSM

Four of the founders of ACSM, although employed in departments of physical education or working in that field, were primarily engaged in physiological research. Arthur Steinhaus was at George Williams College near Chicago; Leonard Larson began his research at Springfield College in Massachusetts and moved to New York University; Peter Karpovich was at Springfield College; and Ernst Jokl was at Witwatersrand Technical College in Johannesburg, South Africa. Several charter members were also engaged in physiological research in departments of physical education, departments of physiology or private laboratories before 1953. Most notable in this group were David Brace, Lucien Brouha, Thomas Cureton, Jr., D. Bruce Dill, Anna Espenschade, Creighton Hale, Ancel Keys, Leon Kranz, Ulrich Luft, Charles McCloy, Henry Montoye and Raymond Weiss.

William H. Byford had published "On the Physiology of Exercise" in 1855 in the *American Journal of Medical Sciences*; Austin Flint, a New York physician, had written several articles in the 1870s, including "Influence of Excessive and Prolonged Muscular Exercise" and "On the Source of Muscular Power"; and Edward Mussey Hartwell, a leading physical educator, had written a two-part series, "On the Physiology of Exercise," for the *Boston Medical and Surgical Journal* in 1887. However, the first important book on the subject did not appear until 1888, when Fernand Lagrange's *Physiology of Bodily Exercise* was published.[9] Despite the good intentions of the physician Byford, both the medical and physical education professions were largely unconcerned with the scientific analysis of exercise. Byford tried to account for this lack of interest and encourage his colleagues to do more research in the area:

> Although the importance of voluntary exercise has been recognized for centuries and prescribed to its most useful extent by many of the profession, its great practical advantages in a large number of diseases have not been appreciated to their full extent by all. The only reason I can ascribe for this is that its effects upon the animal economy have not been thoroughly investigated and understood. It is with a view to draw the attention of the profession to the importance of more research in this direction, that I wish to record my views upon the subject.[10]

Despite the fact that Byford's plea was published in 1855, it would take at least another half century for any real interest to be shown in the physiology of exercise.

A few physical educators, physiologists and physicians published articles on related topics in the *American Physical Education Review*, the *Boston Medical and Surgical Journal* and the *American Journal of Physiology* during the early 1900s, and George W. Fitz of Harvard published his *Principles of Physiology and Hygiene* in 1908. Fitz also established a physiology of exercise laboratory within Harvard's Department of Anatomy, Physiology and Physical Training in the early 1890s. R. Tait McKenzie's *Exercise in Education and Medicine* appeared in 1909 and was followed by Francis G. Benedict and Edward P. Cathcart's *Muscular Work, A Metabolic Study with Special Reference to the Efficiency of the Human Body as a Machine* in 1913, and by H.M. Smith's *Gaseous Exchange and Physiological Requirements for Level and Grade Walking* in 1922. During the following year, F.A. Bainbridge of the University of London published the classic *Physiology of Muscular Exercise* and in 1924, James H. McCurdy of Springfield College published *The Physiology of Exercise*.[11]

In 1923, the year Archibald V. Hill was appointed Joddrell Professor of Physiology at University College, London, the physiology of exercise acquired one of its most respected researchers and staunchest supporters.

In his inaugural address in October, Hill explained why his type of research was important:

> Quite apart from direct physiological research on man, the study of instruments and methods applicable to man, their standardization, their description, their reduction to a routine, together with the setting up of standards of normality in man, are bound to prove of great advantage to medicine; and not only to medicine but to all those activities and arts where normal man is the object of study. Athletics, physical training, flying, working, submarines or coal-mines, all require a knowledge of the physiology of man, as does also the study of conditions in factories. The observation of sick men in hospitals is not the best training for the study of normal man at work. It is necessary to build up a sound body of trained scientific opinion versed in the study of normal man, for such trained opinion is likely to prove of the greatest service, not merely to medicine, but in our ordinary social and industrial life.[12]

Hill published his landmark book, *Muscular Activity*, in 1926, and during the previous year, his presidential address at the Annual Meeting of the British Association for the Advancement of Science on "The Physiological Basis of Athletic Records," had appeared in *Lancet*.[13] Hill was a visiting lecturer at Cornell University in 1926 and also became acquainted with Arlie Bock's laboratory at Massachusetts General Hospital. The following year, Hill published *Living Machinery* and *Muscular Movement in Man: The Factors Governing Speed and Recovery from Fatigue*, based largely on his lectures before audiences at the Lowell Institute in Boston and the Baker Laboratory of Chemistry in Ithaca, New York.[14] Ernst Jokl, one of the founders of ACSM, identified Hill's 1925 address as "the beginning of exercise physiology as a subject of its own," and ACSM charter member D. Bruce Dill credited Hill's "bold attack . . . on the physiology of sport" for inspiring his work and that of his colleague, Arlie Bock.[15]

Several leading physiologists besides A.V. Hill were interested in the human body's response to unnatural situations, especially activities involving endurance, strength, altitude, heat and cold. Consequently, these scientists studied soldiers, athletes, aviators and mountain climbers as the best models for acquiring data. Research of this nature was centered in the Boston area, first at the Carnegie Nutrition Laboratory in the 1910s and later at the Harvard Fatigue Laboratory, which was established under the leadership of Lawrence J. Henderson in 1927. At the Carnegie Nutrition Laboratory, Francis G. Benedict and Edward P. Cathcart used a motor-driven treadmill and bicycle ergometers to study human physiology at rest and in exercise, and were joined later by H.M. Smith and Thorne M. Carpenter. Their writings on "the efficiency of the human body as a machine," "the bicycle ergometer with an electric brake," "energy transformations during horizontal walking" and "gaseous exchange and physiological requirements for level and grade walking," were published by the Carnegie Institution of Washington DC between 1912 and 1922. When Benedict retired in 1937, Carpenter was appointed director, and the Carnegie Nutrition Laboratory continued until Carpenter retired in 1945. At the Harvard Fatigue Laboratory, Henderson was joined by numerous coworkers over the years, including D. Bruce Dill, J.H. Talbott, Arlie Bock, W.H. Forbes and R.C. Darling. Dill became a charter member of ACSM. He and Bock rewrote Bainbridge's *The Physiology of Muscular Exercise*, and the third edition appeared in 1931. It contained much updated material, including results of the work done at the Fatigue Laboratory.[16] Besides his work with Bock, Dill published a major review, "The Economy of Muscular Exercise," in *Physiological Reviews* in 1936; a book, *Life, Heat and Altitude*, in 1938; and another review, "Applied Physiology," in the inaugural issue of *Annual Reviews of Physiology* in 1939.[17]

Lucien Brouha, also a charter member of ACSM, spent time at the Fatigue Laboratory while visiting from Belgium; Ancel Keys, another charter member, also did research there. Charter member Ashton Graybiel, a cardiologist, also worked with several different researchers at the Fatigue Laboratory. Other scientists associated with the Fatigue Laboratory who went on to be influential members of ACSM were Laurence Morehouse and Dill's doctoral students Sid Robinson and Steven Horvath.[18]

Henderson died in 1942, and the Harvard Fatigue Laboratory closed for good in 1947. Yet, its influence lived on through the work of those who had been associated with it. Ancel Keys and his student Henry L. Taylor established the Laboratory of Physiological Hygiene at the University of Minnesota and Ashton Graybiel became the director of research for the Naval School of Aviation Medicine in Pensacola, Florida. D. Bruce Dill was appointed scientific director of the Medical Laboratories of the Army Chemical Corps, and Lucien Brouha established a fitness research unit at the University of Montreal before taking charge of physiological research at the Haskell Laboratory for Toxicology and Industrial Medicine. Laurence Morehouse was appointed to a faculty position in the Department of Physical Education at the University of Southern California. Sid Robinson organized a laboratory of exercise physiology at Indiana University, and Steven Horvath worked at the Army Medical Research Laboratory at Fort Knox and at the University of Iowa. Robert Darling became a professor of physical medicine at Columbia University's College of Physicians and Surgeons. These individuals, along with a few others, continued researching and publishing on exercise physiology, which helped establish it as a respectable field of study.[19]

Work in the burgeoning field of exercise physiology continued during the time of the Harvard Fatigue Laboratory in other professions and in other parts of the country. J.H. McCurdy issued the second edition of *The Physiology of Exercise* in 1928, and Edward C. Schneider wrote *Physiology of Muscular Activity* in 1931. Adrian G. Gould and Joseph A. Dye published *Exercise and Its Physiology* in 1932; the following year ACSM founder Peter Karpovich published *Physiology of Muscular Activity* and founder Arthur Steinhaus wrote an extensive article, "Chronic Effects of Exercise," in *Physiological Reviews*. Percy Dawson wrote *The Physiology of Physical Education for Physical Educators and Their Pupils* in 1935, E.C. Schneider wrote a new edition of *Physiology of Muscular Activity* in 1939 and McCurdy's third edition appeared that same year with ACSM founder Leonard Larson as coauthor.[20] Although founder Ernst Jokl was publishing in Germany during the 1930s, his physiological research was introduced to the English-speaking world in 1941 via his articles "On Indisposition after Running" in the *Research Quarterly* and "Physical Fitness" in the *Journal of the American Medical Association* and his book, *The Medical Aspects of Boxing*.[21]

Activities surrounding World War II greatly influenced the research in exercise physiology and several laboratories, including the Harvard Fatigue Laboratory, began directing their efforts toward topics of importance to the military. The different branches of the military also established their own research centers and acquired the services of many leading physiologists. The other national concern that created much interest among physiologists was the fear that American children were less "fit" than their European counterparts. Research was directed toward an analysis of the concept of fitness in growth and development, ways to measure fitness and the various components of fitness.

George Brooks, an exercise physiologist at the University of California, Berkeley, noted in 1987: "Exercise physiology attracts a wide range of practitioners and scientists who are unified only in that they have a common interest either in using exercise to understand physiology or using physiology to understand exercise."[22] This was particularly true during the twenty years preceding the founding of ACSM. Research pertaining to the physiology of exercise was being conducted in departments of physiology by D. Bruce Dill at Harvard University, Eugene Howe at Wellesley College, Sid Robinson at Indiana University, Percy Dawson at the University of Wisconsin, W.W. Tuttle at the University of Iowa and E.C. Schneider at Wesleyan University.[23] Charter member Ulrich Luft left Germany in 1947 and joined the staff of the US Air Force School of Aviation Medicine, at Randolph Field, San Antonio, Texas, as a research physiologist and associate professor. In 1954, Luft became chair of the Department of Physiology at the Lovelace Foundation for Medical Education and Research, Albuquerque, New Mexico.[24]

Departments of physical education located at major universities also had separate exercise physiology laboratories. A survey completed in 1950 indicated that of the sixteen colleges reporting laboratories in physical education, fifteen were devoted to physiological research. Those institutions that had physiology laboratories and also offered graduate degrees in physical education were Springfield College, George Williams College, University of

California (Berkeley), University of Illinois, Indiana University, New York University, University of Southern California and University of Texas. Several of the exercise physiologists operating laboratories at these universities played significant roles in the founding of ACSM. Among this group were founders Peter Karpovich, Arthur Steinhaus, and Leonard Larson, as well as charter members Thomas Cureton, Jr., Anna Espenschade and Charles McCloy. Other charter members associated with exercise physiology research at major universities were David Brace, Henry Montoye and Raymond Weiss.[25]

Several ACSM founders and charter members held leadership positions in the American Physiological Society. Charter member D. Bruce Dill served as treasurer from 1946 to 1948, was a member of the council from 1948 to 1950 and was president from July 1950 through April 1951. He held the office of past president from July 1951 through 1952. In 1948, Dill and founder Steinhaus were on the initial editorial board of the *Journal of Applied Physiology*, and they were joined by charter members Graybiel and Keys in 1954. During that same year, Dill, Graybiel and Steinhaus also served on the editorial board of the *American Journal of Physiology*.[26]

THE ROLE OF CARDIOLOGY AND ITS INFLUENCE ON ACSM

Three of ACSM's eleven founders were physicians with specific training and expertise in the field of cardiology. Louis Bishop, Albert Hyman and Joseph Wolffe had national reputations as cardiologists. Two other founders with medical credentials were Peter Karpovich and Ernst Jokl. Although neither practiced medicine in the US and both were better known as physiologists, Karpovich wrote "Heart of an Athlete" as early as 1935 and Jokl was writing about the heart and exercise as early as 1936. Jokl also published research in the *American Heart Journal* in 1942.[27] Arthur Steinhaus, although not a physician, also wrote several articles regarding the size of the heart as early as 1931.[28]

At least nine charter members were cardiologists. Ashton Graybiel, Seymour Fiske and Epaminonda Secondari were involved in cardiology at the national level and became associated with the newly formed American College of Cardiology (ACC) in 1949.[29] Sidney Arbeit, William Bean, Burgess Gordon, Nicholas Michelson, Isadore Schlamowitz and Max Walkow all specialized in cardiovascular disease or were members of the American College of Chest Physicians.[30] D. Bruce Dill, another ACSM charter member and physiologist, also became directly involved with the ACC, as did founders Bishop, Hyman and Wolffe.[31]

Physiologists and cardiologists had a very cooperative and supportive relationship in the field of medicine that carried over even more dramatically into sports medicine. Cardiology was the one clinical field in which the pragmatic value of physiology was the most obvious, and physiologists and physical educators looked to cardiologists for scientific information regarding physical exertion, "heart health," heart disease prevention and recovery from heart attacks.[32] Once physiologists began to focus on health-related exercise research in the 1940s and 1950s, they directed their attention to cardiovascular disease first. In an overview of the emergence of exercise physiology in physical education, E.R. Buskirk explained: "The major research impetus has come from work related to the prevention of atherosclerosis and coronary heart disease as well as rehabilitation following myocardial infarction."[33] Just a cursory survey of leading physiology journals during the 1930s through the 1950s and of the *Research Quarterly*, published by AAHPER beginning in 1930, shows a substantial number of articles relating to various aspects of the heart and exercise.

Two early pioneers in the study of the heart and exercise were Sir James Mackenzie of Scotland and R. Tait McKenzie from Philadelphia, who had a major influence on the founders of the ACSM. Both made significant contributions to the study of the function and health of the heart during strenuous exercise and also had indirect but important connections with the three cardiologists who were ACSM founders, especially Wolffe. Sir James Mackenzie published such classic works as *The Study of the Pulse* (1902), *Diseases of the Heart* (1908) and *Principles of Diagnosis and Treatment in Heart Affections* (1916). In his early work on the pulse, Mackenzie described his "polygraph" which enabled him to make important and original distinctions concerning harmless and dangerous types of pulse irregularities. He also drew attention to the heart's capacity for work and the energetics of the heart muscle.[34] In his well-known "Discussion on the Soldier's Heart" in 1916, Mackenzie addressed his colleagues of the Royal Society of Medicine on the value of exercise for the treatment of heart disease and warned them that "too much rest is not beneficial."[35] He continued by saying, "the same measure for restoring a flabby leg muscle applies to a merely flabby heart muscle."[36] At this same time, Mackenzie served as a consultant in England's Military Heart Hospital, an institution he had helped establish. It was here, during World War I, that he first met R. Tait McKenzie.

R. Tait McKenzie, in his role as physician, professor of physical education and director of the Department of Physical Education at the University of Pennsylvania, was also very interested in the health of athletes as well as the general effects of exercise on the entire student population; he published an article, "Relation of Athletics to Longevity," in 1906.[37] Much of his research dealt with the heart and, in contrast to beliefs of the time that strenuous exercise was detrimental to one's heart, McKenzie claimed there was "no recorded case of rupture of the healthy heart muscle itself, from effort."[38] In 1912, after more research on "athlete's heart," McKenzie announced: "The hour has arrived for a complete reconsideration of the whole question of exercise in relation to the heart."[39] By showing that "cardiac hypertrophy and irregularities of sound and beat were variations within the normal rather than signs of pathology," McKenzie provided evidence that the athletic heart was really a healthy heart.[40] During the same year, he supplied additional support for this claim in his article "Athletes Do Not Die Prematurely from Cardiac Diseases," published in *Medical Times*.[41]

When R. Tait McKenzie went to England during World War I, he was already friends with the notable physician Sir William Osler and met Sir James Mackenzie, one of Osler's colleagues, at the Military Heart Hospital. After Mackenzie retired from practice in 1918, he started the Institute for Clinical Research at St. Andrew's and provided financial support for it up until his death in 1925. Interestingly, at the dedication of the R. Tait McKenzie Gymnasium at his Valley Forge Medical Center and Heart Hospital in 1962, medical director and ACSM founder Joseph Wolffe alluded to his own connections with Sir James Mackenzie and R. Tait McKenzie:

> In 1916, a special hospital was established in England for the study of heart conditions among members of the armed services. Here Tait McKenzie concentrated on one of his favorite projects—an investigation of the effects of exercise on the cardiovascular system. He had the advantage of working closely with such eminent physicians as Sir William Osler, Sir Thomas Lewis, Sir Clifford Albutt and Sir James Mackenzie, whom I, too, was privileged to have had as my teacher and preceptor during a phase of my own medical studies.[42]

Wolffe continued the tradition of Mackenzie and McKenzie in his early research and published "Cardiac Capacity Determined by Standardized Effort" in 1926, in which he explained "cardiac response to exercise" and credited "the earlier works of Sir James Mackenzie."[43] Wolffe, who, also like Mackenzie and McKenzie, wrote about "athlete's heart," was concerned with the effects of exercise on the entire cardiovascular system and opened special hospitals for patients with heart conditions beginning with the Wolffe Clinic in 1933 and, in 1951, the Valley Forge Medical Center and Heart Hospital. He moved his hospital from the city to the country to give his patients the opportunity to exercise in the fresh air on the beautifully landscaped grounds and set up walking trails for patients with differing physical abilities.[44]

A few years after Wolffe had completed his medical degree at Temple University in 1919, he met Grover Mueller, a physical education teacher and well-known basketball coach at South Philadelphia High School for Boys. They cooperated on devising an early type of ergometer to be accompanied by blood pressure and pulse measurements as a test of an individual's cardiovascular capability.[45] Mueller eventually became director of the Division of Physical and Health Education for the Philadelphia Board of Education in 1927, and in 1930, Wolffe accepted a teaching and research position at the Temple University Medical School. He became associate professor and head of the Cardiovascular Division from 1932 to 1947. During this time, Mueller taught afternoon and evening courses in Temple's Physical Education Department, where he had received his master of science degree in 1927. Wolffe opened his group practice, the Wolffe Clinic, in 1933, and he and Mueller continued to discuss their common interests in school health, physical fitness, the hearts of athletes, public recreation, playgrounds and physical examinations for sports throughout these years.[46] It was through the Wolffe Clinic that Wolffe first implemented his philosophy of medical treatment: "No one physician can know all the answers . . . the individual and collective wisdom of the group can be effectively combined to give the whole patient—mind and body—the rounded benefit of total medicine in one place."[47] This philosophy of enlisting the expertise of those with a variety of skills and of treating the "whole man" served to reinforce the friendship of Mueller and Wolffe as well as to convince Wolffe that he and other physicians needed the talents and assistance of health and physical educators.

In 1944, a Committee on the Cardiovascular Study of Athletes was formed by the Philadelphia Association for Health, Physical Education and Recreation and a group of cardiologists. Grover Mueller was appointed chair of the committee, an advisory committee of athletes was appointed and the first roundtable discussion on "Athletics and the Heart" was held at the Wolffe Clinic in December 1945. Over the next few years, they studied men and women who had participated in athletics for several years and compared them to high school cross-country runners, rowers and boys and girls in the Philadelphia public schools in general.[48] Results of their studies were published widely between 1946 and 1949.[49] In one publication, Wolffe emphasized the value of exercise for the cardiac patient and suggested that its "prescription should be given by one experienced in the field of cardiology or medicine at large and carried out by one expert in the field of physical education."[50] In his conclusion, Wolffe recommended that the US adopt a plan similar to the one suggested in the UK's *Report by the Research Board for the Correlation of Medical Science and Physical Education* in 1947, whereby its aims were:

1. To ensure more general recognition of the need for health and physical education in the widest sense.
2. To achieve more general coordination between authoritative groups dealing with various aspects of the subject.
3. To pool the experience of national groups so that it may be of use to all.[51]

These thoughts were very similar to what Mueller and Wolffe and a few others had in mind as they were planning the organization that would eventually become the ACSM.

Both Mueller and Wolffe served in leadership positions in their respective professional groups and helped to introduce each other and their expertise to colleagues in each other's fields. Mueller served as president of the Philadelphia Physical Education Association 1926–1931; president of the Pennsylvania State Association for Health, Physical Education and Recreation 1942–43; and vice president of health education of the Eastern District of AAHPER 1953–1955.[52] Wolffe was a founder and director of the American Association for the Study of Arteriosclerosis in 1947; a founder, trustee and fellow of the ACC in 1949; a fellow of the American College of Angiology; on the board of governors of the Philadelphia Heart Association; and a member of the American Heart Association's Council on Arteriosclerosis, Clinical Cardiology, and Hypertension.[53] In 1948, Wolffe was presented the Layman's Honor Award of the Pennsylvania Association for Health, Physical Education and Recreation by Grover Mueller for his "noteworthy contributions in meeting the health, recreation and physical education needs of individuals in general, and helping to solve problems confronting physical and health educators."[54]

Wolffe continued to seek answers to questions relating to the heart and exercise and tried to bring more cardiologists and physical educators together. He saw some hope in the American Heart Association. In May 1947, Wolffe wrote a long letter to Howard B. Sprague, a leading cardiologist in Boston, Harvard colleague of Paul Dudley White and member of the board of directors of the American Heart Association, urging that the board undertake a national study of "athlete's heart." Wolffe noted that some respected cardiologists still believed that vigorous physical activity would injure the heart. However, he informed Sprague that the Philadelphia heart study of athletes provided no such evidence. Wolffe explained:

> The problem is urgent because of the emphasis put on vigorous physical exercise in our schools. While at one time there was only one team representing each school, we now have as many as four and five teams. Vigorous physical activity is being encouraged throughout this country. Because of it, physical educators, school physicians and particularly anxious parents are pressing for a definite and more authoritative answer. I, therefore, suggest that the problem be submitted to the Board of Directors of the American Heart Association in order to organize a nationwide study of athletes and to enlist as many reasoned medical opinions as possible. Many leaders in allied professions are very much interested and are looking forward to aid such a study.[55]

Since the American Heart Association never took any formal action on Wolffe's request, he tried again in December 1949. He and Mueller invited leading cardiologists, physiologists and physical educators to a meeting at the Philadelphia Board of Education Administration Building to discuss common problems related to the cardiovascular system. Among those present were the president of the American Heart Association and members of the board of directors of the Philadelphia Heart Association.

Another friend of Joseph Wolffe and founder of ACSM was cardiologist Albert Hyman of New York City. Hyman received his medical degree at Harvard and acquired an early interest in studying athletes by doing research on Boston Marathon runners, Harvard athletes and opera singers as early as 1915–1916. Later in his career, Hyman remembered that he had been attracted to athletes because they were examples of perfect health. He said he "wanted a chance to study high level physical performance which is the physiology of well-conditioned and well-trained individuals."[56] Beginning in 1930, Wolffe served as a consultant to the Witkin Foundation for the Study and Prevention of Heart Disease at New York's Beth David Hospital, of which Hyman was the director. They became good friends and Wolffe spent many vacations at Hyman's summer home at Pin Point, near Fairfield, Connecticut, during the 1930s and 1940s. It was also at this time, about 1932, that Hyman made his newly invented pacemaker public by displaying it at the American Congress of Physical Therapy meetings in New York City.[57]

Excerpts from Hyman's book, *Pioneering in Cardiology: My First 50 Years*, provide some interesting information about Hyman, Wolffe and the eventual founding of ACSM. At one of their summer outings at Pin Point in August of 1932, Hyman was joined by his good friend and frequent coauthor Aaron E. Parsonnet, a cardiologist from Newark, New Jersey; John Homer Cudmore, chief of medicine at New York City Hospital; Wolffe; and A. Allen Sussman, a physician from Baltimore. During one of their many discussions, they realized there was little information available about exercises for older men. Wolffe suggested staging a mile run along the beach with data collection before and after the race. This was done and a men's race was run every year from 1932 until 1941, except 1938, when women ran.[58]

Hyman related another incident that took place in August 1939, which had even more far-reaching ramifications. He was joined again at Pin Point by Wolffe, Sussman, Cudmore and Parsonnet. Their discussion turned to exercise for cardiac patients and the recent book by Hyman and Parsonnet, *The Failing Heart of Middle Life*. They also debated about "the diagnosis, prognosis, and treatment in terms of physical exercise." At that point, Sussman remarked:

> It is obvious that no one of us has the information necessary to evaluate these patients. Many types of interest are involved and I would like to suggest a multidiscipline group made up not of cardiologists exclusively but of physiologists, physical educators, [and] physicians who cope with major disabilities in normal healthy people.[59]

Parsonnet followed by suggesting:

What we need then is a group or organization dedicated to the study and understanding of the basic physiology of both normal and abnormal individuals. We do not need more cardiologists, although the heart and blood vessel systems play a great role here, but scientists in other disciplines.[60]

This statement prompted Wolffe to say: "I think that I know just the right people to approach. First, there is Bill Mueller of the Philadelphia School System who is a leading physical educator. Then Peter Karpovich of Springfield College, a really great physiologist."[61] Sussman then asked, "What could we call a society of such mixed-up interests?" Parsonnet suggested "Society of Applied Cardiac Physiology," Hyman liked "Society of Athletic Medicine" and Wolffe thought "the Society of Sports Medicine" would be appropriate.[62]

Hyman was also active in the New York Cardiological Society, which he helped found and incorporate in 1935, and served as its first secretary. He was associate clinical professor of medicine at New York Medical College and was a consulting cardiologist to seven New York City hospitals. He and Wolffe continued as close friends, and Mueller gradually became more active in some of their research. Hyman joined Wolffe as a founder of the ACC in 1949 and they also coauthored at least two studies in 1950 and 1952.[63]

The third founder of ACSM who was a cardiologist was Louis Bishop, also from New York City. A national standard racquets and squash player, Bishop received his medical degree from Yale in 1925 and followed the footsteps of his pioneering father, Louis F. Bishop, Sr.[64] He coauthored "Athletics and the Heart" with his father in 1930 and published articles on "Racquet Games and Circulation," "Preventing Heart Attacks" and "Exercise in the Treatment of Chronic Cardiovascular Disease," in 1932, 1935 and 1938, respectively.[65] Like Hyman, Bishop was a founder of the New York Cardiological Society in 1935 and served as its first vice president. Bishop and his father supported the study of athletes' hearts at Rutgers University in 1937 with the donation of an electrocardiograph machine and X-ray equipment, and, in that same year, he presented a paper, "Exercise in the Treatment of Cardiovascular Disease," at the American Congress of Physical Therapy. In 1940, Bishop was elected president of the American Therapeutic Society; in 1941, at the American Heart Association meetings, he was on the same program with Ashton Graybiel and heard D. Bruce Dill present the Lewis A. Conner Lecture, "The Effect of Physical Strain and High Altitude on the Heart and Circulation."[66]

Bishop was involved in the same type of research as Mackenzie, McKenzie, Wolffe and Hyman, publishing two articles on "Soldier's Heart" in 1941 and 1942. His expertise, as was the case for several other ACSM founders and charter members, was used by the military during World War II. Bishop joined Wolffe and Hyman as a fellow of the ACC and became president of the New York Cardiological Society in 1953. Shortly there-after, Bishop remembered, he and Wolffe devolved specific plans for what would become ACSM "over a six-hour lunch at the Harvard Club." Bishop stressed that "what was innovative about the idea at the time was the bring-ing together of physicians, physiologists, and athletic trainers." He also became president of the ACC in 1960.[67]

Several founders and charter members of ACSM played significant roles in the field of cardiology through leadership positions in the ACC, founded in 1949, and to a lesser extent in the American Heart Association, founded in 1922. In 1951, the year of the ACC's first national meeting, ACSM founders Hyman and Wolffe served on its board of trustees and were accompanied by charter members Seymour Fiske and Epaminonda Secondari. Charter member D. Bruce Dill was a vice president, as was Ash-ton Graybiel. Fiske also held the position of treasurer. During the follow-ing year, although they still held their officers' positions, Dill and Graybiel became members of the board of trustees and board of governors with Fiske, Hyman, Secondari and Wolffe.[68]

Mention was made earlier of the meeting in Philadelphia in 1949 when representatives of the American Heart Association were invited to join physi-ologists and physical educators in an attempt to stimulate cooperative efforts. Apparently, this meeting did not produce the results expected by Wolffe and Mueller, so the newly incorporated ACC appeared to be a viable forum for the collaborative efforts envisioned by these two. Mueller wrote to Wolffe on 8 May 1951, asking: "I have been wondering for some time if there is any category of membership in the American College of Cardiologists to which teachers of health, physical education, and recreation are eligible. Will you please advise."[69] Mueller continued his letter by outlining the scenario of attempted cooperation with the American Heart Association:

> For a long time it was my hope that the American Heart Association would be willing to cooperate with the physical educators, but that hope vanished. You will remember the meeting we held at the Board of Edu-cation Administration Building in December, 1949 . . . We were told that the moneys of the Association were needed for other studies, and I, personally, got the strong impression that not only was relatively little interest shown in the important problems cited at the meeting, but that endless red tape would be involved in any effort to gain cooperation.[70]

In concluding, Mueller stated:

> Knowing very well your personal concern with, and your strong inter-est in, our mutual problems, I am writing this letter to you in the hope that the American College of Cardiologists can be brought to see the desirability of working with the members of my profession. I have been advised that the College is a particularly active and progressive organi-zation, and it is because of this fact that I venture to write to you.[71]

Evidently, no such arrangements ever developed within the ACC either.

Although the ACC never provided a place in their membership for physical and health educators, it is apparent that when the ACSM was eventually incorporated in 1955, the founders drew heavily upon the ACC. Because Wolffe and Hyman were among the original founders of both the ACC and ACSM, their input was particularly important. They were assisted by Bishop, who had played an active role in the New York Cardiological Society, the model used by the ACC when it was incorporated. Just as ACSM borrowed some of its organizational structure from AAHPER, it also relied on the ACC. The name "American College" itself, although used by many other groups in medicine, was patterned after the ACC, as was the plan of incorporation as a nonprofit corporation in Washington DC. The two groups also stated similar objectives and had almost identical constitutions and bylaws. The ACC administrative structure whereby three vice presidents were elected from different areas of expertise, the idea of chapters and the fact that the board of trustees acted as the main decision-making body were also points of commonality. Finally, the ACC held its first national convention at New York's Statler Hotel in 1951, and the founding meeting of ACSM took place at the same hotel three years later.[72]

Ernst Jokl, also a founder of ACSM, was more associated with physical education and physiology, but began publishing his research on the heart and exercise as early as 1936 and became a fellow of the ACC in 1954.[73] At least as early as 1943, and continuing through the 1940s, Jokl communicated with McCloy, Karpovich, Dill and Steinhaus about their common research.[74] In May of 1949, Wolffe wrote Jokl in South Africa with the hope of persuading him to visit the US and be his guest in Philadelphia. After several delays, and through the generous assistance of McCloy and Steinhaus, among others, Jokl finally visited the US in 1952. He made numerous appearances throughout the country, including, as he wrote, a lecture "in Philadelphia before a large audience of doctors at Dr. Wolffe's Heart Research Clinic where I also met some of the outstanding cardiologists from New York and Philadelphia."[75] Jokl was hired by Wolffe in March 1953, and moved his wife and two children to Norristown, Pennsylvania. He wrote to his former host Steinhaus: "My friend, Dr. Wolffe, who came to fetch me in Germany[,] is doing everything to make things pleasant for me." As an employee of the Valley Forge Heart Institute and Hospital, Jokl informed Steinhaus that he had accepted "the post of Director of Research and Head of the Department of Clinical Physiology."[76]

CORONARY HEART DISEASE AND PHYSICAL ACTIVITY EPIDEMIOLOGY

The early history of physical activity epidemiology began in the late 1940s with its roots in London, England. Here, Professor Jeremy Morris and his colleagues began to believe that coronary heart disease might be less common among those engaged in physically active work than among those doing sedentary work. In London, too, at about the same time, Richard Doll and Austin Bradford Hill began to study the relationship between smoking and lung cancer. Together, their research helped to define a new vision of public health that emphasized the role of lifestyle in chronic non-communicable disease. This concept had a profound impact on several of the founders and charter members of ACSM.[77]

Morris, like several of those to be instrumental in the founding of ACSM, was particularly interested in heart disease. He and others in England and the US noticed a curious epidemic in the 1940s—people had begun to die from heart attacks in unprecedented numbers. Accordingly, Morris set up a vast study to examine heart attack rates in people of different occupations. He remembered that "the very first results we got were from the London busmen" and "there was a striking difference in the heart attack rate." It was clear that "the drivers of these double-decker buses had substantially more [heart attacks], age for age, than the conductors." Morris realized that "the drivers were prototypically sedentary and the conductors were unavoidably active." From these data, which Morris did not publish for several years, he concluded that "exercise helps you live longer." His hypothesis was greeted with general disbelief with the majority of the skeptics asking: "What could exercise possibly have to do with heart attacks?"[78] As a result, Morris gave up smoking and took up running, becoming one of the earliest people to run regularly on Hampstead Heath.

Morris presented his research at the World Conference of Cardiology in Washington DC in 1954, where several of the ACSM founders and charter members were in attendance. Specifically, Morris met Henry L. Taylor there, an exercise physiologist who studied with charter member Ancel Keys at the Harvard Fatigue Laboratory. Taylor was a professor at the University of Minnesota at the time and worked with Keys in their Laboratory for Physiological Hygiene. Morris had shown that exercise helped prevent premature death, but did not understand how until Taylor sat him down in a Washington DC hotel room and, as Morris remembered, the "schoolboy taught me the physiology of exercise."[79]

Interestingly, at about this same time, a respected epidemiologist with the US Public Health Service, Ralph Paffenbarger, Jr., began to take an interest in cardiovascular disease, especially the possible role of physical inactivity. To this end, he had early conversations with Paul Dudley White, the famous Boston cardiologist who treated President Eisenhower after his heart attack, among others. Soon thereafter, Paffenbarger became an early investigator in the Framingham Heart Study and began research at the National Heart Institute. He and Morris became lifelong friends, and Paffenbarger quickly gained national notoriety by linking physical fitness with a reduced risk of chronic diseases. And, like Morris, Paffenbarger became a dedicated runner and early friend of several ACSM charter members.[80]

In conclusion, it has been shown that it was a few key cardiologists and physiologists who banded together in the early 1950s to form the ACSM. It was their interest and research in exercise, cardiovascular disease and youth fitness that brought them together. This is a distinct and unique heritage for the field of sports medicine because it differed greatly from the recognized definition of sports medicine as "the treatment of sport related injuries." ACSM's founders and charter members were not orthopedists or team physicians. Instead, they were MDs and PhDs working as cardiologists and physiologists who were concerned about national health and recognized the value of prevention and sound health behavior as it related to stress, smoking, nutrition and physical activity. They were also inherently interested in athletes as exemplars of the limits of human performance and physiological adaptation to a diversity of circumstances like altitude, fatigue, humidity and temperature. To them, keeping healthy people healthy and studying the fit rather than the sick were more central to their mission than treating the ill or injured. By the mid-1960s then, thanks to ACSM, it was apparent that the sporting body was not only worthy of medical and scientific inquiry, but that this study of the active body was also central to an overall understanding of health and public health more broadly.

NOTES

1. Berryman, *Out of Many, One.*
2. See "Federation of Sports Medicine," *Journal of Health, Physical Education, and Recreation* 25, no. 3 (1954) 26; and the program and proceedings for the 58th National Convention of AAHPER, 19–23 April 1954, New York.
3. Minutes of the Meeting of the Signers of the Certificate of Incorporation, American College of Sports Medicine, Washington DC, 2 February 1955; Minutes of the ACSM Administrative Council Meeting, 8 January 1955.
4. Ryan, "History of the Development"; Ryan, Smodlaka and Eriksson, "International Federation of Sports Medicine"; Hoberman, "Early Development."
5. Berryman, "Tradition"; Lewis, "Adoption"; Berryman, "Exercise Is Medicine."
6. Soare, "Two Theories"; Whorton, "Hygiene of the Wheel"; Raycroft, "History and Function."
7. Brooks, "Physiology of Exercise"; "Exercise Physiology Paradigm."
8. Montoye, "Raymond Pearl Memorial Lecture."
9. Byford, "On the Physiology of Exercise"; Flint, "Influence"; "On the Effects"; "Source of Muscular Power"; Hartwell, "On the Physiology of Exercise"; Lagrange, *Physiology of Bodily Exercise.* For additional details, see Park, "Athletes and Their Training."
10. Byford, "On the Physiology of Exercise," 32–33.
11. Park, "Emergence"; "Why Moralists?" For more information on Fitz, see Gerber, *Innovators and Institutions*, 302–307. In Germany, Zuntz and his collaborators were doing extensive experimentation on energy metabolism at rest and during exercise in the early 1900s. For additional information, see Chapman and Mitchell, "Physiology of Exercise"; and Buskirk, "Early History."

12. Quoted in Dill, "Historical Review," 39.
13. Hill, *Muscular Activity*; "Physiological Basis."
14. Dill, "Historical Review," 40. Also see Hill, "Revolution in Muscle Physiology."
15. Jokl, *Portraits from Memory*, 87; Dill, "Introduction"; Morehouse and Miller, *Physiology of Exercise*, 9.
16. Dill, "Historical Introduction"; Chapman and Mitchell, "Physiology of Exercise," 88–90; Dill, "Harvard Fatigue Laboratory"; Horvath and Horvath, *Harvard Fatigue Laboratory*; Horvath and Yousef, *Environmental Physiology*; Parascandola, "L.J. Henderson."
17. Dill, "Economy of Muscular Exercise"; *Life, Heat and Altitude*; "Applied Physiology." Bock did much of his early work at the Medical Laboratories of the Massachusetts General Hospital. See Bock, "On Some Aspects."
18. Dill, "Harvard Fatigue Laboratory," 165–170.
19. Ibid.
20. Buskirk, "Emergence of Exercise Physiology"; Dawson, *Physiology of Physical Education for Physical Educators*; Gould and Dye, *Exercise and Its Physiology*; Karpovich, *Physiology of Muscular Activity*; McCurdy, *Physiology of Exercise*; McCurdy and Lawson, *Physiology of Exercise*; Park, "Emergence," 29–35; Schneider, *Physiology of Muscular Activity*; Schneider, *Physiology of Muscular Activity* (2nd Ed.); Steinhaus, "Chronic Effects of Exercise."
21. Jokl, "On Indisposition"; Jokl and Cluver, "Physical Fitness"; Jokl, *Medical Aspects of Boxing*.
22. Brooks, "Exercise Physiology Paradigm," 232.
23. Van Dalen and Bennett, *World History*, 487.
24. White, "Lovelace Years," 11.
25. Hunsicker, "Survey of Laboratory Facilities," 422–423; Donnelly, "Laboratory Research," 232–234. Also, at the University of Minnesota, "Ancel Keys not only allowed but encouraged physical education majors to work with the faculty in the Laboratory for Physiological Hygiene"; see E.R. Buskirk to Jack W. Berryman, 30 October 1992. For an example of an early text evolving out of Brooklyn College's Department of Health and Physical Education, see Riedman, *Physiology of Work and Play*.
26. Hackensmith, *History of Physical Education*, 468.
27. Karpovich, "Heart of an Athlete," 12; "Textbook Fallacies," 33–37; Suzman and Jokl, "An Analysis of a Series," 206–214; Jokl and Suzman, "Mechanisms Involved."
28. Steinhaus, "Heart Size during Exercise," 40–41; "Heart—Immediately after Exercise," 40; "Heart Size Effects," 42–43.
29. Kisch, *Transactions*, 1:3; ibid., 2:3–4.
30. Mohr, *American Medical Directory*. Burgess Gordon became president of the American College of Chest Physicians, 1957–1958 and had been involved in research relating to exercise and circulation since the 1920s. See, for example, Gordon, Levine and Wilmaers, "Observations," 425; Levine et al., "Some Changes"; and Gordon et al., "Sugar Content." Gordon was also friends with McKenzie and was influenced by the classical Greek ideals of athletics. See, for example, Gordon, "Grecian Athletic Training." For much of his career, Gordon was at the Jefferson Hospital in Philadelphia.
31. Kisch, *Transactions*, 1:3; 2:3–4; *American College of Cardiology Bulletin* (March 1951), 1.
32. Geison, "Divided We Stand," 82–83; Howell, "Hearts and Minds," 248.
33. Buskirk, "Emergence of Exercise Physiology," 57.

34. Howell, "Soldier's Heart," 40–44; Wilson, *Beloved Physician*; Mair, *Sir James Mackenzie*; Garrison, *Introduction*, 687–688.
35. Mackenzie, "Discussion," 34.
36. Ibid., 35.
37. McKenzie, "Relation of Athletics."
38. Ibid., 195.
39. McKenzie, "Influence of Exercise," 69–74.
40. Whorton, "Athletes' Heart," 48.
41. McKenzie, "Athletes Do Not Die."
42. Wolffe, *R. Tait McKenzie*, 12.
43. Wolffe, "Cardiac Capacity," 762.
44. Ashbrook, "In Memoriam"; *National Cyclopedia of American Biography*, vol. 53, s.v. "Wolffe, Joseph Barnett," 257; Alice K. Hand (Administrator, Valley Forge Medical Center and Hospital) to Jack W. Berryman, 19 May 1989.
45. Wolffe called this instrument his "cardiovascular dynomometer" and had it manufactured by George P. Pilling and Sons Company of Philadelphia. It is described and pictured in Wolffe, "Cardiac Capacity," 763.
46. "Grover W. Mueller Retires," *Journal of Health, Physical Education, and Recreation* 32, no. 6 (1961): 79; "Grover Mueller Retires in August after 34 Years with Public School," *Philadelphia Evening Bulletin*, 12 May 1961, 30; "Grover W. Mueller, Biographical Data," 1 February 1961, ACSM Archives, Indianapolis, IN.
47. See "The Beloved Physician: A Eulogy of Memories," *Thermometer (Valley Forge Medical Center)* 4 (1967–1968): 3.
48. See "Testing Hearts of Athletes," *Philadelphia Evening Bulletin*, November 1944; "Hearts of Athletes Tested in Study Here," *Philadelphia Evening Bulletin*, August 1945; and "Is There Such a Thing as an 'Athlete's Heart'?" *Philadelphia Evening Bulletin*, 2 January 1946. Mueller Scrapbooks, ACSM Archives, Indianapolis, IN.
49. Wolffe and Mueller, "Heart of the Athlete," 17–22, 3–5; Wolffe et al., "Heart in the Athlete"; Wolffe and Digilio, "Heart in the Athlete," 8–9, 62–63. The steering committee for a national study of the heart and exercise sponsored by Phi Epsilon Kappa Fraternity was chaired by Grover W. Mueller. He was joined by charter members Arthur Esslinger, William Hughes, Charles McCloy and Elmer Mitchell. See "Steering Committee for Heart Study," *Physical Educator* 8, no. 4 (1951): 126.
50. Wolffe and Digilio, "Heart in the Athlete," 63.
51. Ibid.
52. "Grover W. Mueller, Biographical Data"; "A Record of Achievement," 1–2, ACSM Archives, Indianapolis, IN.
53. Alice K. Hand to Jack W. Berryman, 3 May 1989; "Wolffe, Joseph Barnett," *National Cyclopedia of American Biography*, vol. 53, s.v. 257. Also see Pollak, "American Society"; Wolffe, "Arteriosclerosis at Present"; and Clarkson, McMillan and McGill, Jr., "Origin of the Council."
54. See "Dr. Wolffe Honored for Health Aid," *Philadelphia Daily News*, 11 December 1948; and "Honored for Public Health Aid," *New York Times*, 12 December 1948, 78.
55. "A Record of Achievement," 23, ACSM Archives, Indianapolis, IN.; Joseph B. Wolffe to Howard B. Sprague, 23 May 1947, Sprague Papers, Francis A. Countway Library, Boston, MA. (I would like to thank W. Bruce Fye, historian for the ACC, for sending me a copy of this letter.)
56. Hyman, *Pioneering in Cardiology*, vol. 4, no. 4, 8. See also vol. 5, no. 4, 5–8; and vol. 6, no. 1, 5–8.

57. Ibid., vol. 3, no. 3, 7–8; no. 4, 6–8.
58. Ibid., vol. 3, no. 4, 6–8.
59. Ibid., vol. 3, no. 3, 8; Hyman and Parsonnet, *Failing Heart of Middle Life*. In 1939, Hyman devised the "Hyman-Optiz Index" as a measure of cardiac function at rest and after exercise.
60. Hyman and Parsonnet, *Failing Heart of Middle Life* .
61. Ibid.
62. Ibid.
63. "Albert Hyman, 79, Cardiologist, Dies," *New York Times*, 9 December 1972, 38; Larson, "Albert Hyman." Mueller assisted Wolffe and Hyman with the research for Wolffe et al., "Studies in Experimental Atheromatosis." See also Wolffe et al., "Liver in the Atheromatous Syndrome."
64. "Dr. Louis F. Bishop, 85, Dies; Leader in Field of Cardiology," *New York Times*, 4 June 1986, D-26. Bishop also took boxing and fencing lessons and lettered in fencing at Yale.
65. Bishop and Bishop, "Athletics and the Heart"; Bishop, "Racquet Games and Circulation"; "Preventing Heart Attacks"; "Exercise in the Treatment."
66. Bishop, *Birth of a Specialty*, 26, 33, 42, 54–55.
67. Bishop, "Soldier's Heart," *New York State Journal of Medicine*; "Soldier's Heart," *American Journal of Nursing*; *Birth of a Specialty*, 68–69, 120–121; Schuster, "Louis F. Bishop," 131–132; "Louis Faugeres Bishop—Curriculum Vitae," American College of Cardiology, Archives, Chicago, IL. In 1942, the American Board of Internal Medicine first accepted "Cardiovascular Disease" as a recognized specialty. Also see Bishop, "Cardiology as a Specialty," 1170–1174.
68. Kisch, *Transactions*, 1:3; 2:3–4; *American College of Cardiology Bulletin* (March 1951), 1. Graybiel and Paul D. White were the authors of *Electrocardiography in Practice*, published in 1941. Also see a description of their cardiac function tests in *Medical Clinics of North America* (May 1938): 773–784.
69. Grover W. Mueller to Joseph B. Wolffe, 8 May 1951, Mueller Papers, ACSM Archives, Indianapolis, IN.
70. Ibid.
71. Ibid.
72. Kisch, *Transactions*, 1:3, 11; 2:3–4, 32. See also *American College of Cardiology Bulletin* (January 1951): 1–2; ibid. (February 1951): 1–2; ibid. (March 1951): 1–2; and ibid. (May 1951): 1–2. The first volume of the *American Journal of Cardiology* appeared in January 1958, with charter members Graybiel as associate editor and Dill as editorial consultant.
73. "Ernst Jokl, Curriculum Vitae," ACSM Archives, Indianapolis, IN.
74. See series of letters in the Arthur Steinhaus Papers, Box 31, Folder 2, University of Tennessee Library, Knoxville.
75. Joseph B. Wolffe to Ernst Jokl, 12 May 1949, Steinhaus Papers, Box 31, Folder 2; and, Ernst Jokl to Charles H. McCloy, 7 February 1952, Steinhaus Papers, Box 31, Folder 2.
76. Ernst Jokl to Arthur Steinhaus, 13 April 1953, Steinhaus Papers, Box 31, Folder 2.
77. Morris and Doll were colleagues at the University College Hospital Medical School in London. Morris was professor of Social Medicine and Doll was director of the Medical Research Council Statistical Research Unit. Morris was also professor of Public Health at the London School of Hygiene and Tropical Medicine. Hill was professor of Medical Statistics at the University of London. In particular, see Morris et al., "Coronary Artery Disease"; and Doll and Hill, "Smoking and Carcinoma."

78. Paffenbarger et al., "History of Physical Activity"; Simon Kuper, "The Man Who Invented Exercise," *Financial Times*, 11 September 2009; "Professor Jeremy Morris, Who Has Died Aged 99, Pioneered the Scientific Study of How Exercise Helps to Prevent Heart Disease," *London Telegraph*, 2 November 2009.
79. Taylor had also worked earlier with other charter members Brouha and Dill. He earned his PhD from Harvard and, while at Minnesota, was the doctoral advisor for two ACSM luminaries, Elsworth Buskirk and Loring Rowell. See in particular, Taylor et al., "Effects of Bed Rest," 223. Also see Buskirk, "Early History"; Tipton, "Contemporary Historical Perspective." It is important to note that Henry Taylor was honored by ACSM in 1975 with its Citation Award and Honor Award in 1980.
80. Lee, Matthews and Blair, "Legacy"; Valerie J. Nelson, "Ralph S. Paffenbarger, Jr., 84; His Key Study Confirmed that Exercise Boosts Longevity," *Los Angeles Times*, 15 July 2007. Also see Dishman, Washburn and Heath, *Physical Activity Epidemiology*, 6–9. Jeremy Morris was honored by ACSM with its Honor Award in 1985, and Paffenbarger received the Citation Award in 1987. Together, Morris and Paffenbarger were the recipients of the first International Olympic Committee Prize for Sport Science in 1996. Paffenbarger donated his financial prize to ACSM.

BIBLIOGRAPHY

American College of Cardiology Bulletin (May 1951): 1–2.
———. (March 1951): 1–2.
———. (February 1951): 1–2.
———. (January 1951): 1–2.
Ashbrook, Willard P. "In Memoriam: Joseph B. Wolffe." Unpublished paper, 1966.
Berryman, Jack W. "Exercise Is Medicine: A Historical Perspective." *Current Sports Medicine Reports* 9, no. 4 (2010): 195–201.
———. *Out of Many, One: A History of the American College of Sports Medicine*. Champaign, IL: Human Kinetics, 1995.
———. "The Tradition of the 'Six Things Non-Natural': Exercise and Medicine from Hippocrates through Ante-Bellum America." *Exercise and Sport Sciences Reviews* 17 (1989): 515–559.
Bishop, Louis F. *The Birth of a Specialty: The Diary of an American Cardiologist, 1926–1972*. New York: Vantage Press, 1977.
———. "Cardiology as a Specialty." *New York State Journal of Medicine* 76, no. 7 (1976): 1170–1174.
———. "Soldier's Heart." *American Journal of Nursing* 42, no. 4 (1942): 377–380.
———. "Soldier's Heart. "*New York State Journal of Medicine* 41, no. 19 (1941): 1915–1921.
———. "Exercise in the Treatment of Chronic Cardiovascular Disease." *Archives of Physical Therapy* 19 (July, 1938): 415–418, 435.
———. "Preventing Heart Attacks." *Hygeia*, January 1935.
———. "Racquet Games and Circulation." *Sword and Racquet*, April 1932.
Bishop, Louis F., and Louis F. Bishop, Sr. "Athletics and the Heart." *Medical Review of Reviews* (October 1930).
Bock, A.V. "On Some Aspects of the Physiology of Muscular Exercise." *New England Journal of Medicine* 200, no. 13 (1929): 638–642.

Brooks, George. "The Exercise Physiology Paradigm in Contemporary Biology: To Molbiol or Not to Molbiol, That is the Question." *Quest* 39 (1987): 231–242.
———. "Physiology of Exercise." In *Perspectives on the Academic Discipline of Physical Education*, edited by George A. Brooks, 48–53. Champaign, IL: Human Kinetics Publishers, 1981.

Buskirk, Elsworth R. "Early History of Exercise Physiology in the United States." In *The History of Exercise and Sport Science*, edited by John D. Massengale and Richard A. Swanson, 367–396. Champaign, IL: Human Kinetics, 1997.
———. "The Emergence of Exercise Physiology." In *Perspectives on the Academic Discipline of Physical Education*, edited by George A. Brooks, 55–74. Champaign, IL: Human Kinetics Publishers, 1981.

Byford, William H. "On the Physiology of Exercise." *American Journal of the Medical Sciences* 30 (July 1855): 32–42.

Chapman, Carleton B., and Jere H. Mitchell. "The Physiology of Exercise." *Scientific American* 212 (May 1965): 88–96.

Clarkson, Thomas B., Gardner C. McMillan and Henry C. McGill, Jr. "The Origin of the Council on Arteriosclerosis." *Arteriosclerosis and Thrombosis* 12, no. 5 (1992): 543–547.

Dawson, Percy M. *The Physiology of Physical Education for Physical Educators.* Baltimore, MD: Williams and Wilkins, 1935.

Dill, D. Bruce. "Historical Review of Exercise Physiology Science." In *Science and Medicine of Exercise and Sport*, 2nd ed., edited by Warren Johnson and E.R. Buskirk, 37–41. New York: Harper and Row, 1974.
———. "The Harvard Fatigue Laboratory: Its Development, Contributions, and Demise." In *Physiology of Muscular Exercise*, edited by Carleton B. Chapman, 161–170. New York: American Heart Association, 1967.
———. "Historical Introduction: Personal Reminiscences." *Pediatrics* 32, no. 4 (October 1963): 653–655.
———. "Introduction." In *Physiology of Exercise*, Laurence E. Morehouse and Augustus T. Miller (9–10). St. Louis, MO: C.V. Mosby Co., 1948.
———. "Applied Physiology." *Annual Reviews of Physiology* 1 (1939): 551–576.
———. *Life, Heat and Altitude.* Cambridge, MA: Harvard University Press, 1938.
———. "The Economy of Muscular Exercise." *Physiological Reviews* 16 (1936): 263–291.

Dishman, Rod K., Richard A. Washburn and Gregory W. Heath. *Physical Activity Epidemiology.* Champaign, IL: Human Kinetics, 2004.

Doll, R., and A. Bradford Hill. "Smoking and Carcinoma of the Lung: Preliminary Report." *British Journal of Medicine* (September 1950): 739–748.

Donnelly, Richard J. "Laboratory Research in Physical Education." *Research Quarterly* 31, no. 2 (1960): 232–234.

"Dr. Louis F. Bishop, 85, Dies; Leader in Field of Cardiology," *New York Times*, 4 June 1986: D-26.

"Dr. Wolffe Honored for Health Aid," *Philadelphia Daily News*, 11 December 1948: n.p.

"Federation of Sports Medicine." *Journal of Health, Physical Education and Recreation* 25, no. 3 (1954): 26.

Flint, Austin. *Collected Essays and Articles on Physiology and Medicine.* 2 vols. New York: D. Appleton, 1903.
———. "The Source of Muscular Power as Deduced from Observations upon the Human Subject under Conditions of Rest and Exercise." *Journal of Anatomy and Physiology* 12, no. 1 (1877): 91–141.
———. "On the Effects of Severe and Protracted Muscular Exercise: With Special Reference to Its Influence Upon the Excretion of Nitrogen." *New York Medical Journal* (June 1871): 609–697.

————. "Influence of Excessive and Prolonged Muscular Exercise upon the Elimination of Effete Matters by the Kidneys; Based on an Analysis of the Urine Passed by Mr. Weston, while Walking One Hundred Miles in Twenty-One Hours and Thirty-Nine Minutes." *New York Medical Journal* 12 (October 1870): 280–289.

Garrison, Fielding H. *An Introduction to the History of Medicine*. Philadelphia: W.B. Saunders, 1963.

Geison, Gerald L. "Divided We Stand: Physiologists and Clinicians in the American Context." In *The Therapeutic Revolution: Essays in the Social History of American Medicine*, edited by Morris J. Vogel and Charles E. Rosenberg, 67–90. Philadelphia: University of Pennsylvania Press, 1979.

Gerber, Ellen W. *Innovators and Institutions in Physical Education*. Philadelphia: Lea and Febiger, 1971.

Gordon, Burgess. "Grecian Athletic Training in the Third Century (A.D.)." *Annals of Medical History* 7, no. 6 (1935), 513–518.

Gordon, Burgess, L.A. Kohn, S.A. Levine, Marcel Matton, W. de M. Scriver and W.B. Whiting. "Sugar Content of the Blood in Runners Following a Marathon Race: With Especial Reference to the Prevention of Hypoglycemia: Further Observations." *Journal of the American Medical Association* 85, no. 7 (1925): 508–509.

Gordon, Burgess, S.A. Levine and A. Wilmaers. "Observations on a Group of Marathon Runners with Special Reference to Circulation." *Archives of Internal Medicine* 33, no. 4 (1924): 425–434.

Graybiel, A. and Paul D. White. *Electrocardiography in Practice*. Philadelphia, PA: W.B. Saunders, 1941.

"Grover Mueller Retires in August after 34 Years with Public School," *Philadelphia Evening Bulletin*, 12 May 1961: 30.

"Grover W. Mueller Retires," *Journal of Health, Physical Education, and Recreation* 32, no. 6 (1961): 79.

"Grover W. Mueller, Biographical Data," 1 February 1961, ACSM Archives, Indianapolis, IN.

Gould, A.G. and J.A. Dye. *Exercise and Its Physiology*. New York, NY: A.S. Barnes, 1932.

Hackensmith, C.W. *History of Physical Education*. New York: Harper and Row, 1966.

Hartwell, Edward Mussey. "On the Physiology of Exercise." *Boston Medical and Surgical Journal* 116, no. 13 (1887): 297–302.

————. "On the Physiology of Exercise." *Boston Medical and Surgical Journal* 116, no. 14 (1887): 321–324.

Hill, A.V. "The Revolution in Muscle Physiology." *Physiological Reviews* 12, no. 1 (1932): 56–67.

————. *Muscular Activity*. Baltimore, MD: Williams and Wilkins, 1925.

————. "The Physiological Basis of Athletic Records." *Lancet* 206, no. 5323 (1925): 481–486.

Hoberman, John M. "The Early Development of Sports Medicine in Germany." In *Sport and Exercise Science: Essays in the History of Sports Medicine*, edited by Jack W. Berryman and Roberta J. Park, 233–282. Urbana: University of Illinois Press, 1992.

"Honored for Public Health Aid," *New York Times*, 12 December 1948: 78.

Horvath, Steven M., and Elizabeth C. Horvath. *The Harvard Fatigue Laboratory: Its History and Contributors*. Englewood Cliffs, NJ: Prentice Hall, 1973.

Horvath, Steven M., and Mohamed K. Yousef, eds. *Environmental Physiology: Aging, Heat and Altitude*. New York: Elsevier/NorthHolland, 1981.

Howell, Joel D. "Hearts and Minds: The Invention and Transformation of American Cardiology." In *Grand Rounds: One Hundred Years of Internal Medicine*, edited by Russel C. Maulitz and Diana Long, 243–275. Philadelphia: University of Pennsylvania Press, 1988.

———. "'Soldier's Heart': The Redefinition of Heart Disease and Speciality Formation in Early Twentieth-Century Great Britain." In *The Emergence of Modern Cardiology*, edited by W.F. Bynum, C. Lawrence and V. Nutton, 34–52. London: Wellcome Institute for the History of Medicine, 1985.

Hunsicker, Paul A. "A Survey of Laboratory Facilities in College Physical Education Departments." *Research Quarterly* 21, no. 4 (1950): 420–423.

Hyman, Albert S. *Pioneering in Cardiology: My First 50 Years.* Excerpted in *American College of Sports Medicine Newsletter* 3, no. 3 (1968): 7–8; 3, no. 4 (1968): 6–8; 4, no. 2 (1969): 6–8; 4, no. 4 (1969): 6–8; and 5, no. 1 (1970): 6–8.

Hyman, Albert S., and Aaron. E. Parsonnet. *The Failing Heart of Middle Life, The Myocardosis Syndrome, Coronary Thrombosis, and Angina Pectoris.* Philadelphia: F.A. Davis Co., 1932.

Jokl, E. *The Medical Aspects of Boxing.* Pretoria: Van Schaik, 1941.

———. "On Indisposition after Running: Athlete's Sickness and Vasomotor Collapse." *Research Quarterly* 12, no. 1 (1941): 3–11.

———. *Portraits from Memory.* Lexington, KY: Privately printed, 1990.

Jokl, E., and E.H. Cluver. "Physical Fitness." *Journal of the American Medical Association* 116, no. 24 (1941): 2383–2389.

Jokl, E., and M.M. Suzman. "Mechanisms Involved in Acute Fatal Non-Traumatic Collapse Associated with Physical Exertion." *American Heart Journal* 23, no. 6 (1942): 761–765.

Karpovich, Peter V. "Textbook Fallacies Regarding the Development of the Child's Heart." *Research Quarterly* 8, no. 3 (1937): 33–37.

———. "Heart of an Athlete." *Scholastic Coach* (February 1935): 12–28.

———. *Physiology of Muscular Activity.* Philadelphia, PA: W.B. Saunders, 1933.

Kisch, Bruno, ed. *Transactions of the American College of Cardiology*, vol. 2. New York: American College of Cardiology, 1952.

———. *Transactions of the American College of Cardiology*, vol. 1. New York: American College of Cardiology, 1951.

Kuper, Simon. "The Man Who Invented Exercise," *Financial Times*, 11 September 2009, n.p.

Lagrange, Fernand. *Physiology of Bodily Exercise.* New York: D. Appleton, 1898.

Larson, Leonard. "Albert Hyman, 1893–1972." *Medicine in Science and Sports* 5, no. 2 (1973): vii.

Lee, I-Min, Charles E. Matthews and Steven N. Blair. "The Legacy of Dr. Ralph Seal Paffenbarger, Jr.—Past, Present, and Future Contributions to Physical Activity Research." *President's Council on Physical Fitness and Sports Research Digest* 10, no. 1 (2009): 1–8.

Levine, Samuel A., Burgess Gordon and Clifford L. Derick. "Some Changes in the Chemical Constituents of the Blood Following a Marathon Race." *Journal of the American Medical Association* 82, no. 22 (1924): 1778–1779.

Lewis, Guy M. "Adoption of the Sports Program, 1906–1939: The Role of Accommodation in the Transformation of Physical Education." *Quest* 12, no. 1 (1969): 34–46.

Mackenzie, Sir James. *Principles of Diagnosis and Treatment in Heart Afflictions.* London: Henry Frowde, 1916.

———. "Discussion on the Soldier's Heart." *Proceedings of the Royal Society of Medicine* 9, no. 3 (1916): 27–36.

———. *Diseases of the Heart.* London: Henry Frowde, 1908.

———. *The Study of the Pulse.* London: Henry Frowde, 1902.

Mair, Alex. *Sir James Mackenzie, M.D., 1852–1925: General Practitioner.* London: Churchill Livingstone, 1973.

McCurdy, J.H. *The Physiology of Exercise, A Textbook for Students of Physical Education.* Philadelphia, PA: Lea and Febiger, 1928.

McCurdy, J.H. and L.A. Larson. *The Physiology of Exercise.* Philadelphia, PA: Lea and Febiger, 1939.

McKenzie, R. Tait. "Athletes Do Not Die Prematurely from Cardiac Diseases." *Medical Times* 40 (March 1912): 67.

———. "The Influence of Exercise on the Heart." *American Journal of the Medical Sciences* 145 (January 1912): 69–74.

———. "Relation of Athletics to Longevity." *Medical Examiner and Practitioner* 16 (1906): 195–199.

Mohr, Philip E., ed. *American Medical Directory 1956.* Chicago: American Medical Association, 1956.

Montoye, Henry J. "The Raymond Pearl Memorial Lecture, 1991: Health, Exercise, and Athletics: A Millennium of Observation—A Century of Research." *American Journal of Human Biology* 4, no. 1 (1992): 69–82.

Morehouse, Laurence E., and Augustus T. Miller. *Physiology of Exercise.* St. Louis, MO: C.V. Mosby Co., 1948.

Morris, J.N., J.A. Heady, P.A. Raffle, C.G. Roberts and J.W. Parks. "Coronary Artery Disease and Physical Activity of Work." *Lancet* 265 (1953): 1053–1057, 1111–1120.

National Cyclopedia of American Biography, vol. 53, s.v. 257. New York: J.T. White Publishing, 1971.

Nelson, Valerie J. "Ralph S. Paffenbarger, Jr., 84: His Key Study Confirmed that Exercise Boosts Longevity," *Los Angeles Times*, 15 July 2007: n.p.

Paffenbarger, Ralph S., Jr., Steven N. Blair and I-Min Lee. "A History of Physical Activity, Cardiovascular Health and Longevity: The Scientific Contributions of Jeremy N. Morris, DSc, DPH, FRCP." *International Journal of Epidemiology* 30 (2001): 1184–1192.

Parascandola, John. "L.J. Henderson and the Mutual Dependence of Variables from Physical Chemistry to Pareto." In *Science at Harvard University: Historical Perspectives*, edited by Clark A. Elliott and Margaret W. Rossitier, 167–190. Bethlehem, PA: Lehigh University Press, 1992.

Park, Roberta J. "Athletes and Their Training in Britain and America, 1800–1914." In *Sport and Exercise Science: Essays in the History of Sports Medicine*, edited by Jack W. Berryman and Roberta J. Park, 57–107. Urbana: University of Illinois Press, 1992.

Park, Roberta J. . "Why Moralists More than Scientists? Reflections on Origins and Consequences." *Academy Papers* 25 (1991): 12–18.

———. "The Emergence of the Academic Discipline of Physical Education in the United States." In *Perspectives on the Academic Discipline of Physical Education*, edited by George A. Brooks, 20–45. Champaign, IL: Human Kinetics Publishers, 1981.

Pollak, O.J. "The American Society for the Study of Arteriosclerosis." *Geriatrics* 2, no. 5 (1947): 291–292.

"Professor Jeremy Morris, Who Has Died Aged 99, Pioneered the Scientific Study of How Exercise Helps to Prevent Heart Disease," *London Telegraph*, 2 November 2009: n.p.

Raycroft, Joseph E. "The History and Function of the Athletic Team Doctor." *Journal-Lancet* 54, no. 9 (1934): 271–275, 279.

Riedman, Sarah R. *The Physiology Of Work and Play: A Textbook In Muscular Activity.* New York: Dryden Press, 1950.

Ryan, Alan J. "History of the Development of Sport Sciences and Medicine." In *Encyclopedia of Sport Sciences and Medicine*, edited by Leonard Larson, xxxiii–xlvii. New York: Macmillan, 1971.

Ryan, Alan J., Vojin Smodlaka and Edjar Eriksson. "The International Federation of Sports Medicine." *American Journal of Sports Medicine* 9, no. 2 (March/April 1981): 123–125.

Schneider, Edward C. *Physiology of Muscular Activity*. Philadelphia, PA: W.B. Saunders, 1931.

Schneider, Edward C. *Physiology of Muscular Activity (2nd Edition)*. Philadelphia, PA: W.B. Saunders, 1939.

Schuster, Karolyn. "Louis F. Bishop, Jr.: Sportsmedicine Pioneer." *Physician and Sportsmedicine* 9, no. 1 (1981): 131–132.

Soare, Warren G. "A History from 1820 to 1890 of Two Theories of Physical Training: The Collegiate Gymnastics Movement and the Rise of Intercollegiate Athletic Teams at Amherst, Harvard, Princeton, and Yale." EdD diss., Columbia University Teachers College, 1979.

Steinhaus, Arthur H. "Chronic Effects of Exercise." *Physiological Reviews* 13 (1933): 103–147.

———. "The Heart—Immediately After Exercise." *Journal of Health, Physical Education and Recreation* 2, no. 9 (1931): 40.

———. "The Heart Size During Exercise." *Journal of Health, Physical Education and Recreation* 2, no. 8 (1931): 40–41.

———. "The Heart Size Effects of Training." *Journal of Health, Physical Education and Recreation* 2, no. 10 (1931): 42–43.

Suzman, M.M., and Ernst F. Jokl. "An Analysis of a Series of Electrocardiograms Taken after Prolonged Intense Muscular Activity." *South African Journal of Medical Sciences* 1, no. 4 (1936): 206–214.

Taylor, Henry L., Austin Henschel, Josef Brožek and Ancel Keys. "Effects of Bed Rest on Cardiovascular Function and Work Performance." *Journal of Applied Physiology* 2, no. 5 (1949): 223–239.

"The Beloved Physician: A Eulogy of Memories," *Thermometer (Valley Forge Medical Center)* 4 (1967–1968): 3.

Tipton, Charles M. "A Contemporary Historical Perspective." *The History of Exercise and Sport Science*, edited by John Massengale and Richard Swanson, 396–438. Champaign, IL: Human Kinetics, 1997.

Van Dalen, Deobold B., and Bruce L. Bennett. *A World History of Physical Education*. Englewood Cliffs, NJ: Prentice Hall, 1971.

White, Clayton S. "The Lovelace Years." In *Oxygen Transport to Human Tissues: A Symposium in Honor Of Dr. U.C. Luft Held 25–27 June 1981 at the Veterans Administration Medical Center, Albuquerque, New Mexico, USA*, edited by Jack A. Loefpky and Marvin L. Riedesel, 3–12. New York: Elsevier/North-Holland, 1982.

Whorton, James C. "'Athlete's Heart': The Medical Debate over Athleticism, 1870–1920." *Journal of Sport History* 9, no. 1 (1982): 30–52.

———. "The Hygiene of the Wheel: An Episode in Victorian Sanitary Science." *Bulletin of the History of Medicine* 52, no. 1 (1978): 61–88.

Wilson, R. McNair. *The Beloved Physician*. New York: MacMillan, 1926.

Wolffe, Joseph B . *R. Tait McKenzie, M.D. (1867–1938): A Biographical Tribute Marking the Dedication of the R. Tait Mckenzie Gymnasium on the Grounds of the Valley Forge Medical Center and Heart Hospital*. Philadelphia, PA: Privately Printed, 1962.

———. "Arteriosclerosis at Present—A Melting Pot of Arteriopathies." *Geriatrics* 2, no. 5 (1947): 296–300.

————. "Cardiac Capacity Determined By Standardized Effort." *Archives of Internal Medicine* 38, no. 6 (1926): 761–769.

Wolffe, Joseph B., and Victor A. Digilio. "The Heart in the Athlete: A Study of the Effects of Vigorous Physical Activity on the Heart." *Journal of Health, Physical Education, and Recreation* 20, no. 1 (1949): 8–9, 62–63.

Wolffe, Joseph B., Victor A. Digilio, Max Schumann, A.D. Dale and A.W. Danish. "The Heart in the Athlete; Comparison of Actual and Predicted Cardiac and Aortic Measurements; Analysis of Measurements of Cardiac and Supracardiac Shadows." *Journal-Lancet* 68, no. 6 (1948): 228–232.

Wolffe, Joseph B., Albert S. Hyman, M.B. Plungian, A.D. Dale and G.E. McGinnis. "The Liver in the Atheromatous Syndrome." *Annals of Western Medicine and Surgery* 4, no. 11 (1950): 679–682.

Wolffe, Joseph B., Albert S. Hyman, M.B. Plungian, A.D. Dale, G.E. McGinnis and M.B. Walkow. "Studies in Experimental Atheromatosis: Atheromatosis and Hepato-Atherosis in Geese. Possible Reversibility and Clinical Implications." *Journal of Gerontology* 7, no. 1 (1952): 13–23.

Wolffe, Joseph B., and Grover W. Mueller, "The Heart of the Athlete." *Physical Educator* 6, no. 2 (1949): 3–5.

————. "The Heart of the Athlete." *Progressive Physical Educator* (May 1946): 17–22.

3 From Voluntarism to Specialization

Sports Medicine and the British Association of Sport and Medicine

Neil Carter

In 2005, sport and exercise medicine (SEM) was granted the status of a fully fledged medical specialty and was made available on the National Health Service (NHS) for injured recreational athletes. It was part of wider government strategies concerning national well-being and was an attempt to defuse a ticking public health time bomb posed by growing national levels of physical inactivity and obesity. The origins of this announcement can be traced back to the formation of the British Association of Sport and Medicine (BASM) in 1952.[1]

The story of BASM is also a history of sports medicine as a profession and a medical subdiscipline. In this sense, BASM comprises the cognitive component around which medical personnel have defined their profession. This consists of medical knowledge, the ethics that regulate relationships between practitioners and between practitioners and patients and institutional arrangements by which medicine perpetuates itself. Importantly, Gelfand has argued that one recurrent theme throughout the history of the medical profession has been the challenge in defining who is a member and who is not on the basis of these three criteria.[2] The pursuit of professional authority and expertise within BASM, like other medical organizations, has been a keenly contested area, which has resulted in disputes and power struggles among its members.

The aim of this chapter is to chart this process and the role of BASM, and place this relationship within its wider social context. At the center of BASM's development have essentially been three interrelated and overlapping issues. First, there has been a lack of clarity over the definition of sports medicine during the twentieth century. Second, the makeup of its membership has both reflected and reinforced these definitional uncertainties. Writing as late as 2007, John Lloyd Parry (president of BASEM, 2003–2005) could still state, "Debates about membership of sports medicine organizations continue to plague the discipline."[3] Third, and as a product of the first two, an overriding characteristic of BASM that has dominated its existence has been that it is a largely representative rather than a regulatory body. Professionalization generally, especially within medicine, tends to gravitate toward a process of specialization where entry is ring-fenced through strict qualifications. The specialization of sports medicine in Britain, however, has been subject to cultural traditions that have their roots in BASM.

Historians have argued that medicine in general is a social phenomenon in which ideas and practices are shaped by wider forces. In addition, medicine not only affects society, but it can also serve as a resource for claims of authority and expertise.[4] The story of BASM, therefore, not only provides an insight into the development of sports medicine as a medical subdiscipline, but it also highlights a wider process of professionalization. Harold Perkin has emphasized that a professional society is not just one dominated by professionals: professionalism itself permeates society from top to bottom. First, professional hierarchies extend to most occupations as they become subject to specialized training and also claim expertise beyond the common sense of the layman. Second, a professional social ideal, based on merit, embeds itself in society. Finally, professionals compete for income, power and status.[5] However, it has been argued "that sports medicine is both structurally and culturally distinct from the broader medical profession," thus highlighting that any process of professionalization is not fixed and has been subject to its own peculiarities.[6]

DEFINITION OF SPORTS MEDICINE

Before looking at BASM, it would be beneficial to understand what is meant by "sports medicine." As a practice, sports medicine can be dated back to Galen in Ancient Greece. In addition, from the late nineteenth century, coaches and trainers applied their own medical practices on athletes while football trainers, with their "magic sponges," were responsible for the treatment of injuries without any deference to doctors or medical organizations.

Defining "sports medicine" as a profession has been a modern concern. Nevertheless, the term has still been difficult to pin down, something that has reflected its development as a medical discipline and its professional status. Allan Ryan, for example, has noted that any definition is made complicated because of a "considerable overlapping of research interests and clinical practice among the different fields." As a result, sports medics have not been restricted to qualified doctors but have also included, among others, coaches, trainers, exercise physiologists and psychologists.[7] By 2004, there was still no consensus among sports medicine practitioners in the United Kingdom (nor in many other countries) as to what actually constituted a sports medicine specialist.[8]

The actual objectives of sports medicine have remained relatively consistent throughout the twentieth century. One definition has been: "the prevention, protection, and correction of injuries and preparation of an individual of physical activity in its full range of intensity."[9] Nevertheless, there has also been some dispute over the extent to which these objectives should be directed more toward elite athletes or the general population.

Some, for example, have seen it as an integral aspect of national fitness pro-grams. In the late 1950s, for example, the Canadian doctor Doris Plewes argued that sports medicine was about "the physical efficiency of normal people," not with athletes per se. Instead, any experiments on elite athletes should be for the benefit of the population as a whole.[10]

The debates over definition have also been echoed in the academy. Mike Cronin identified how much of the historiography of sports medicine had concentrated more on "the broad development of ideas that linked health and well-being with the pursuit of physical activity" rather than "as a prac-tice that treats injury."[11] In addition, with a greater emphasis placed on sporting national prestige during the Cold War era, the use of medical sci-ence to improve athletic performance was increasingly seen as a facet of sports medicine. In preparation for the 1968 Olympics, the British Olympic Association established the "Mexican Research Project" to investigate the effects of altitude on athletic performance and which "in the broader history of sports medicine . . . was part of a process of professionalization, requir-ing the establishment of recognized experts and specialized institutions."[12] Unsurprisingly, in 2006, even after the UK government had bestowed rec-ognition on sports medicine as a medical specialty, Paul McCrory, the edi-tor of the *British Journal of Sports Medicine* could still state:

> There is no universally accepted definition of sports and exercise medi-cine (SEM). The nature of the discipline has changed over time and continues to do so as SEM begins to clarify its scope more clearly and delineates itself from the traditional medical specialities.[13]

However, as McCrory also pointed out, the government now set the bound-aries of the discipline whereas previously an unregulated sports medicine landscape allowed for much flexibility in its definition.

Sports medicine's traditional lack of a professional identity, and hence definition, has been reflected in the burgeoning academic literature on the subject, which has generally concentrated on occupational groups such as club doctors and physiotherapists. This research has generally outlined how these groups, especially doctors, have been recruited on a largely informal basis until the twenty-first century and how they have lacked a professional identity. Doctors at British football and rugby clubs, for example, have been a combination of general practitioners (GPs) and fans of clubs. No professional structures have been in place.[14] The recruitment of trainers and physiotherapists has been more subject to market forces in which qualifications gained greater acceptance. However, even here, there was no formalized entry similar to the medical profession.[15] This lack of formal medical qualifications, allied to doubts over their methods for treatment of injuries, has elicited some criticism within medical circles in more recent years. On this issue, one GP, Malcolm Melrose, quite force-fully, stated:

I haven't been a doctor for forty years for nothing. I haven't dealt with sporting injuries for that long for nothing, and I know that at this moment we are misguided and misled. There is something basically structurally wrong with sports physios, their qualifications, their knowledge has to be addressed.[16]

Similarly, Waddington, Roderick and others have argued that the recruitment procedures in football for medical practitioners do not make for "good employment practice" when compared with the NHS's professional modus operandi.[17] Whatever the arguments over the professional status of these practitioners, it not only highlights how they lack "a coherent professional identity,"[18] but it also illuminates the difficulties to bring all these medics under one unifying umbrella organization such as BASM.

THE INSTITUTIONALIZATION OF SPORTS MEDICINE

During the twentieth century, sports medicine became increasingly institutionalized through the establishment of both national bodies and also international organizations. In part this process mirrored wider developments and debates within medicine. In Britain, since the 1858 Medical Act, the medical profession has attempted to extend its power and control over medicine generally through the marginalization and exclusion of what it has deemed are unorthodox and alternative practices. These unorthodox practices have included physiotherapy (which gained acceptance as a state-registered profession in 1960), osteopathy and homeopathy.[19] The establishment of specific medical organizations and associations, therefore, has represented attempts by doctors, in particular, to ring-fence their own specialties through the imposition of entry qualifications. Once established, these specialties have the opportunity to gain state recognition and funding. Within sports medicine, however, this particular process has been complicated due to the prominent role of nonmedics such as physical educators, trainers, coaches and sports scientists.

The growth of sports medicine had also been part of the new collectivist political will within Western nations that had promoted a greater intervention generally in health provision by the state from the early twentieth century.[20] However, attitudes to sports medicine differed from state to state and were largely dependent on the prevailing political culture within individual countries. As a consequence, some national governments, especially totalitarian regimes, which looked upon sport in terms of national prestige, were more sympathetic to sports medicine's demands.

Initially, in contrast to its European competitors, Britain lagged behind in the development of sports medicine. Germany had played the most prominent early role in the discipline's history. In 1912, for example, the first association of sports physicians had been founded in Thuringia following a Congress of the Scientific Investigation of Sports held at Oberhof.[21] After the First World War, other European countries began to follow Germany's lead. In 1922, the French Society of Sports Medicine published the first sports medicine journal. Sports medicine societies were also founded in the Netherlands (1922), Switzerland (1923), Poland (1937) and Finland (1939). The first Italian institute of sports medicine had been founded in 1929, and by 1935 its two thousand members had been placed in charge of sports medicine matters within state organizations.[22]

Another significant landmark was the establishment of the Association Medico-Sportive Internationale in 1928 at the St. Moritz Winter Olympics. It brought an international dimension as well as a forum for research within sports medicine. It was renamed the Fédération Internationale de Médecine Sportive (FIMS) five years later.[23] The organization grew rapidly, and at the 1936 congress, fifteen hundred physicians from forty nations attended.[24] Interestingly, an American College of Sports Medicine was only formed in 1954 and in 1960, the secretary-general of FIMS, Guiseppe La Cava, commented that continental medics were surprised that sports medicine was relatively unknown in Britain (and the US) when it was widely practiced in many European countries like Italy and France.[25]

THE ORIGINS OF BASM

BASM was formed in June 1952. It had been a response to the growing postwar interest in sports medicine in addition to the rise in international sporting competition brought about by the Cold War. An early forerunner to BASM had been the Research Board for the Correlation of Medical Science and Physical Education, which was set up in 1946. This board participated in the Congress on Physical Education during the London Olympics two years later and the actual medical committee for the Games would include future founder members of BASM, Adolphe Abrahams and Arthur Porritt.[26] In 1950, both the Amateur Athletics Association and the British Boxing Board of Control set up medical committees to monitor the health of their athletes.[27] However, the demand from sport for medical expertise was patchy. It was only in 1980, for example, that the Football Association formed a medical committee.

The beginnings of BASM were modest. There were six founder members, all doctors, and forty-eight members attended its first annual general meeting (AGM) in February 1953. Its initial aims, spelled out by its first president, Adolphe Abrahams, were ambitious and wide-ranging, which to a certain extent reflected the then elevated position of the medical profession within society. Abrahams wanted it to become the authoritative body on every medical aspect of athletics and exercise, to advise on all the general principles of athletic training and sports-related medical injuries and to conduct research into sports injuries.[28]

These original aims also highlight how BASM aspired to act as both an umbrella and the representative organization for medicine's relationship with sport. This was illustrated in the title of BASM. Rather than "sports medicine" it was the British Association of *Sport and Medicine*. Promoting "sports medicine" as a profession was probably not considered necessary, if it was considered at all. Instead, if the relationship between sport and medicine could be furthered it was to be through the professional cachet and social connections of those early members.

Moreover, as an association, BASM was part of the British voluntary tradition. It was an autonomous organization separate from the state and run on the unpaid efforts of its members—a state of affairs that has continued up to the present. Of course, much of sports medicine itself has been a voluntary activity with doctors giving up their free time to work at various sporting events. In this sense, BASM has reflected a political culture in Britain in which voluntary health and medical organizations have featured prominently. However, voluntarism is not neutral and has mirrored social power relations, something that has been evident in elitist sporting bodies such as the Marylebone Cricket Club and the Rugby Football Union. From the mid-twentieth century a mixed economy of welfare had emerged in which voluntary organizations became more reliant on state funding. This political culture, of course, also allowed for the future establishment of other sports medicine associations who were then able to act in the interests of their members.

BASM's first executive committee could be described as patrician and paternalistic. Whereas the early executive had an interest in sport, it also represented a form of "gentlemanly medicine" through its association with elite London hospitals, which dominated the medical profession. The executive contained two Knights of the Realm—Abrahams and Porritt—plus two high-ranking army officers, Brigadier Glyn Hughes and Lieutenant Colonel Milne. Some of these early figures were also part of the canon of sports medicine. This body of literature had been dominated by members of the Achilles Club (founded 1920), an athletics network of former students from Oxford and Cambridge Universities. They represented not only the amateur elite but also the ethic of amateurism and middle-class respectability. Their early body of work highlighted contemporary social attitudes toward the construction of the athletic body, something that continued to permeate ideas about sports medicine in Britain.

The two most high-profile figures in these early days were Adolphe Abrahams (1883–1967) and Arthur Porritt (1904–1994). Abrahams, the son of a Jewish immigrant from Lithuania, was the brother of Harold, who won the men's one-hundred meter at the 1924 Olympics. Adolphe was a useful runner and rower himself at university, and his initial foray into sports medicine was as the first honorary doctor for a UK athletics team at the 1912 Olympics. He later acted as the medical officer at a number of Olympics. Abrahams was a prolific writer on medicine and sport, and in particular was a prominent and influential figure in shaping prevailing discourses regarding women's sport. In 1936, writing about the effect of competitive athletics on girls and young women, for example, he remarked that the nervous systems of women were traditionally more susceptible than men, and that this could form an objection to women competing.[29]

Arthur Porritt was born in 1900, the son of a New Zealand GP. In 1923, he went to Oxford as a Rhodes Scholar to study medicine. (He returned to New Zealand in 1967 as its governor-general.) An all-around sportsman, he competed in the 1924 Olympics, where he won a bronze medal in the aforementioned one hundred meters.[30] He enjoyed a stellar medical career. He was surgeon to the royal family, and uniquely was elected president of the Royal College of Surgeons (1960–1963) and the British Medical Association (1960–1961) at the same time. Some of his other interests seem to fit the image of someone who was part of the upper echelons of British civil society. Not only was he the Red Cross commissioner for New Zealand in Britain, but he was also a prominent freemason who was appointed Grand Master of the Grand Lodge of New Zealand, undertaking much charity work. Porritt, like Abrahams, had also been part of the amateur elite that ran British sport. He was a member of the Achilles Club and was a vigorous defender of amateurism. He served on the Wolfenden Committee on Sport and, despite opposition from other committee members, he stated that he would refuse to sign the final report if the abolition of amateurism was recommended.[31] The amateur ethic was also reflected in his writing on training for athletics and general health, which placed an emphasis on moderation and style. In addition, he had been a pioneer in the adoption of drug testing, and saw it as a moral as much as a medical issue. As early as 1929, he had written, "Drugging is most definitely and absolutely to be deprecated. Apart altogether from the considerations of possible disqualification and not playing the game, the idea is medically unsound."[32]

THE EARLY MEMBERSHIP

The exclusive nature of BASM's early membership was reflected in its rules for joining, and this had an important impact on framing the prevailing culture of the association. BASM was initially only open to medical representatives nominated by national sporting bodies, qualified doctors with an interest in sport plus scientists with a similar interest who were eligible for honorary membership.[33] In addition, as many early members were Fellows of the Royal College of Physicians and Royal College of Surgeons, BASM's membership represented the interests of physical/orthopedic medicine. This clinical tradition would also continue to be at the center of future disputes concerning BASM's identity.

Early members were imbued with the voluntary tradition and most held honorary medical officer positions within sporting bodies. Horace Davies, for example, was not only a Fellow of the Royal College of Surgeons but had also been the medical officer for the Women's AAA and the English Schools Athletic Association.[34] Dr Frederick Basil Kiernander, a founder member of BASM, was also a fellow of the Royal College of Physicians. He served for several terms on the executive committee and was also a vice chairman then later a vice president. He had helped establish the Cheshire Homes for injured servicemen after the war and was also medical advisor to the Central Council of Physical Recreation (CCPR).[35]

During the 1950s, however, BASM struggled to attract many members. There were over one hundred members at the time of the first AGM but this had only risen to 130 by 1959. Its restrictive membership policy based on medical qualifications contrasted with the evolution of sports medicine in America, which had had a strong input from physical educators (see Berryman's contribution in this collection). It illustrated that sports medicine in Britain was a wide, unregulated field and that BASM's influence over the field was limited at best. Moreover, between March 1960 and December 1962 only one executive meeting was held. In addition, other sports medics, like football club doctors and physiotherapists, who were independent of BASM, felt little loyalty to it or a need to defer to it on medical matters.

This early stunted development did not go unnoticed. In 1961, it was commented about BASM, "Although a sports medicine association was formed in this country some years ago, it has never appeared to have got down to any worthwhile activity."[36] Dr. D.J. Cussen, then the honorary secretary, grudgingly admitted that there had been considerable advances made in other countries whereas BASM's work had been "helpful" but not spectacular.[37] Later, in 1964, it was still commented that whereas many countries had established research institutes to study athletes, little was done in Britain.[38]

Writing in the *Lancet*, J.D.G. Troup identified some of the causes behind sports medicine's growing pains as a discipline in Britain. He acknowledged that medicine only provided a supervisory role for sport in Britain and that there was little expert advice forthcoming on the injuries of athletes.[39] The Wolfenden Committee had noted that there was a lack of work in the area of sports medicine. In addition, what research that had taken place was largely uncoordinated regarding organizations like BASM, the CCPR, the Medical Research Council (MRC) and the medical officers of sports' governing bodies. Wolfenden anticipated that the proposed Sports Council would stimulate an increase in research into medical and scientific matters related to sport.[40]

Efforts were made to expand BASM's membership from the early 1960s. In 1962, a special class of membership was established that was open to students of medicine, physiotherapy and physical education.[41] The subsequent rise in numbers also reflected wider changes in the nature of the postwar medical profession, which was less gentlemanly and more meritocratic due to the expansion of the NHS. In addition, to become more inclusive, in 1965 it was decided that representatives of other prominent bodies with an interest in sport would be invited onto the BASM executive committee. These were the British Olympic Association, the Physical Education Association (PEA), the Institute of Sports Medicine (ISM) and the Fitness and Training Section of the Ergonomics Research Society.[42]

By 1968, BASM's membership was more egalitarian and reflected the multidisciplinarity and complexity of sports medicine. Of its 441 members, about 45 percent were either doctors or fellows of the royal colleges. Other groups included those from a physical education background (20 percent) and physiotherapy (8 percent). Women made up approximately 10 percent of the membership. Another group—about 30 percent—consisted of members with no definable medical background. It also contained important figures from the sporting world, including the athletic coaches Geoff Dyson, Ron Pickering, Frank Dick and Wilf Paish. The England team doctors, Neil Phillips and Alan Bass, as well as the FA chairman, Andrew Stephens, who was also a GP, represented football. Former England manager, Walter Winterbottom represented the CCPR.[43]

Like most voluntary associations, the survival and success of BASM was dependent on a small number of dedicated members who gave up much of their free time to meet its administrative demands. From the early 1960s until the late 1980s, much of this burden fell on Henry Robson. Robson, a doctor, had worked as a lecturer in medicine at Loughborough College (later university) before becoming a local GP. He had joined BASM in 1960 and became the honorary treasurer two years later. In 1967, he became editor of the fledgling *BASM Bulletin*, which morphed into the *British Journal of Sports Medicine* in 1968, and he held that position until 1986. He edited and produced each issue. Some of the early sports medicine meetings in Loughborough were held in his house with BASM members put up in his rooms and in tents in his garden; others would stay in caravans and camper vans parked on the driveway. To save on catering costs, Robson cooked chicken curry in a large vat. It was estimated that Robson devoted up to thirty-five hours per week in the cause of BASM.[44]

THE ACTIVITIES OF BASM

What did BASM actually do? Initially, it held a series of lectures on the medical aspects of sport, such as boxing and athletic injuries and their treatment. In 1960, Nobel Prize winner A.V. Hill gave a lecture on "Human Athletic Performance." In general, though, relatively few members attended. In addition, there was little money available to undertake research projects. Exceptions to this general rule included the formation, in 1958, by BASM, along with the British Olympic Association (BOA) and the MRC, of a Medical Advisory Committee for the preparation of athletes going to the Rome Olympics. In 1965, BASM also received a grant from the BOA to set up an Olympic Medical Archive based on examinations of athletes.

As a further indication of BASM's fledgling professional status, a journal, the *British Journal of Sports Medicine*, was first published in December 1968. Its precursor, the association's *Bulletin*, had a flimsy physical appearance and gave the impression of a struggling organization. The first edition of the *Bulletin* had been devoted to PE and had been published in conjunction with the PEA.

One important, and later controversial, development was the establishment of the ISM in 1965, jointly sponsored by BASM, the BOA and the PEA.[45] The ISM had initially been founded as a specialist postgraduate medical institution for the promotion of sports medicine knowledge through research and education. BASM as a membership organization that aspired to charity status was unable to establish an academic institute on legal grounds, and it was felt at the time that the ISM would act as BASM's academic arm to give it greater credibility within medicine as a whole. However, due to internal politics, it was alleged that it became "the personal fiefdom" of its chairman, Peter Sebastian.[46] Initially, BASM had four representatives on the ISM's board of management but this representation ceased after three to four years when Sebastian disassociated the ISM from BASM.[47] It had been during this period that the Sports Council had been established and offered the promise of money for sports medicine research from government funds.[48] BASM cut its links with the ISM in 1974.[49] It was later claimed that because of this split, the ISM was used as an excuse by the Sports Council, stretching into the late 1980s, for not recognizing BASM as *the* representative sports medicine organization in Britain.[50] With this potential source of funding restricted, tensions heightened within the executive over BASM's future direction and attempts to convert sports medicine into a specialty.

THE FRAGMENTATION OF SPORTS MEDICINE

During the 1970s and 1980s, attempts to convert sports medicine into a medical specialty became part of the micro-politics of BASM. Of course, every organization is subject to politics, self-interest and competing factions of varying degrees of intensity; however, a closer look at the internal debates of BASM also illuminates the wider tensions regarding attempts to professionalize sports medicine in Britain.

During the 1970s, the status of sports medicine had been given a boost by government legislation, which had been aimed at raising the status of the GP. Although GPs made up the vast bulk of doctors in medicine's traditionally strict tripartite structure, their status was regarded as inferior to physicians and surgeons. The 1968 Todd Report and the Health Services and Public Health Act from the same year promoted the GP's role and professional status through providing, and making compulsory, their attendance at postgraduate courses. The act also provided for any expenses incurred. As many doctors had an interest in sport, they chose sports medicine and in

1975 BASM organized its first residential sports medicine course at Lough-borough, which was sponsored by FIMS.[51]

In addition, sports medicine was expanding across the country through the setting up of regional BASMs and their own training courses. In 1964, BASM Scotland was established; Wales followed in 1978, and the North West began holding BASM conferences in the mid-1960s. However, there were some complaints that "the London boys were in control."[52] In 1972, highlighting the growing demand for sports medicine services, physiothera-pists had formed their own separate body, the Association of Chartered Physiotherapists in Sports Medicine (ACPSM), which was affiliated to the Chartered Society of Physiotherapists. Although many would be both mem-bers of BASM and the ACPSM, the latter was concerned with the profes-sional credentials of physiotherapists, which had only been accepted in the NHS in 1960. It signaled the first real split in BASM's attempts to remain as the umbrella organization for sports medicine.

Despite the potential for expansion, by the late 1970s BASM experi-enced a serious fracture over its future direction that revolved around a dispute between two of its most important officials: John Williams and Peter Sperryn. In talking about the dispute, Ian Adams, a future chairman of BASM, explained that "there was nothing but trouble for a good few years. I opted completely out of that side of sports medicine, i.e., BASM. It was just a battleground [in the 1970s]."[53]

Initially, Williams and Sperryn had worked closely together and wrote *Sports Medicine* (1976), an important text for the discipline. Williams was a British pioneer. He had edited *Sports Medicine* (1962), the first English-language book to carry the phrase, and was secretary of BASM from 1962 to 1973. He specialized in soft tissue injury and rehabilitation, and his colleague, Dan Tunstall-Pedoe, described him as "*the* sports medicine authority in Britain" for years. Sperryn had trained in physical medicine and rehabilitation. He had met Williams at Stoke Mandeville Hospital in Aylesbury and it was Williams who "got him into" sports medicine. Sper-ryn joined BASM in 1964 and succeeded Williams as its secretary, staying in that post until 1983.[54]

However, despite sharing a passion to develop sports medicine's pro-fessional credentials, each had distinct ideas on BASM's future direction. Williams's approach could be described as "top-down"; Sperryn's as "bot-tom-up." Williams felt that academic respectability for sports medicine could only come about with a strongly doctor-led organization, and he was keen for BASM to have different categories of membership. Writing in the *BJSM* in 1978, he had argued that "in recent years, it has become more and more apparent that BASM is seriously disadvantaged by its lack of differen-tiation amongst its members."[55]

Sperryn, on the other hand, very much wanted BASM to retain its multi-disciplinary identity and role as an umbrella organization for sports medi-cine. As a result, he supported the membership rights of physiotherapists and other nondoctors. In 1977, he had claimed, "BASM can serve sports medicine well by attracting members from widely different backgrounds initially and then helping them to channel more specifically their own professional interests which would naturally be expected to culminate in special interest organizations."[56] Sperryn had held a number of positions working as a sports doctor, such as at the World Student Games and for the British Amateur Athletics Board. He was also the sports medicine editor for *Medical News*, a GP newspaper, and his regular column reflected his sympathies for the daily grind of sports medicine practitioners, including physiotherapists.[57] By contrast, Williams was intent on establishing and maintaining high academic standards. He was frustrated with practitioners who only dabbled in sports medicine and felt that they thought of BASM as principally a club for ex-sporting doctors who saw no need for a greater recognition of sports medicine. These different approaches were at the center of a row between them over who had the right to stage a FIMS-sponsored training course.[58] The fracture within BASM that came out of this dispute later led to Williams withdrawing from active involvement in the organization.[59]

These anxieties within BASM's executive were carried over into the 1980s. To a certain extent, this was reflected in a cultural shift in the ethos among sports medicine practitioners, as well as GPs more generally, away from voluntarism to one of professionalism. Whereas doctors had usually taken on positions within sport for nothing or just a minimal fee, some were increasingly aware of the value of their services. As the club doctor at Nottingham Forest from 1976 to 1984, Michael Hutson, for example, claimed he earned around £4,000–5,000 per year. He also received "a reasonable return" for his services to Nottinghamshire County Cricket Club.[60] In addition, British sport was in the process of shaking off the mud of amateurism from its boots. In 1962, the gentleman-player distinction in cricket had been abolished, and in 1981, athletics went professional. Moreover, through its deregulatory economic policies, the Thatcher Conservative government created an environment for the growth of commercial opportunities within British sport, and as sporting competition became more intense a demand for specialist medical services began to grow. Sports medicine also began to attract sponsorship, especially from pharmaceutical companies, which increased the commercial possibilities within the discipline. In addition, different medical philosophies within BASM also began to emerge with some who believed that only the overuse injuries of Olympic athletes were sports injuries whereas those who treated injuries sustained in contact sport felt that these should be given a higher priority.[61]

These developments provided the background to the formation of the British Association of Trauma in Sport (BATS) in 1980. It was a splinter group from BASM that reflected the growing frustrations of doctors within sports medicine. These had first manifested in 1979 with the publication of a free monthly sports medical review *Medisport*, launched by John Davies and John Williams. It was hoped that *Medisport* would complement the *British Journal of Sports Medicine*.[62] Initially, it was only delivered to BASM members who were doctors, which caused disquiet among the nonmedical members. The formation of BATS was announced in December 1980 in rather covert fashion and included two members of the BASM committee, Patrick England and John Davies. England claimed that the reason behind its formation was "to fill a vacuum because BASM had no teeth or capacity to provide sports medicine to the injured athlete. The object [of BATS] was to provide primary care of all sorts to injured athletes."[63]

Although it was claimed that BATS was not in competition with BASM, it was argued that BASM was wrongly structured, i.e., it was not aligned enough to the needs of sport doctors. BATS, it was claimed, was "a completely professional body" and aimed to push harder for the recognition of sports medicine as a specialty.[64] Advocates argued that BATS represented a groundswell of opinion among doctors in BASM who felt that they were not represented on issues such as payment for attendance at events and full professional recognition through the Royal Colleges. It was vehemently denied that there was any financial motive behind its formation, although an insurance broking company, CT Bowrings, initially sponsored BATS. It was later discovered that the four officers of BATS, Davies, England, Greg McLatchie and Dr. L. Walkden, were also the medical advisors to Sportcare, a soft tissue injury insurance that was promoted by Bowrings.[65] The splinter group caused great resentment within BASM. At one BASM meeting some BATS members had stood up and taken their jackets off to reveal T-shirts with a bat on them.[66] By 1982 BATS had attracted 190 members, but it was ultimately unable to fulfill its original aims and was wound up in 1985.

Like BATS, other disciplines established their own representative bodies, as the ACPSM had in 1972, to complement—some people were members of both—and to act in de facto opposition to BASM. From the 1980s, there were a number of these medical splinter groups from the sports medicine umbrella.[67] In addition to pressures from the doctors, sports science was gaining an increasing influence within sports politics and further weakened BASM's central role in sports medicine. Sports science articles had made up a considerable proportion of those published in the *British Journal of Sports Medicine*. This influence had been recognized within BASM and, as a consequence, in 1977 there was an unsuccessful attempt to change BASM's name to the British Association of Sports Science and Medicine. In 1977, the Society of Sports Scientists had also been founded, and its two founding members, doctors Vaughan Thomas and John Kane, also members of BASM, proposed the name change at that year's AGM. Thomas argued that the change in name should reflect "the changing nature of sports medicine towards a wider base than clinical medicine" and that this would make it "representative of wider interests than purely clinical ones."[68] The motion was defeated thirty to two.

Part of BASM's problems regarding the professional status of sports medicine stemmed from the perceived low standing of the journal.[69] It further reinforced those concerns that BASM, in academic terms, was too lightweight, hence its frustrations over the disassociation from the ISM and the subsequent cold shoulder of the Sports Council when it came to handing out grants as well as bestowing professional respectability. As a compromise—from BASM's perspective—an informal standing liaison committee of sports sciences and medical organizations was formed in 1983 to meet twice a year under the aegis of the Sports Council.[70] A further attempt to change BASM's name to include the word *science* was also defeated in 1984.[71] In that year the sports scientists went their own way and formed the British Association of Sports Sciences.[72]

Later in 1987, the British Olympic Medical Centre, the first sports science and sports medicine facility in the UK, was opened near Harrow. It catered to elite athletes and was founded by Mark Harries and Craig Sharp, who had been a member and on the committee of BASM but described himself as a founder of UK sports science.[73] Although Tunstall-Pedoe was on the board and there was much collaboration between medics and scientists within sport, this charitable trust of the BOA marked another significant moment in the development of sports science as a specialty in itself and further diminished BASM's position.[74]

In response to these pressures from doctors and scientists, there had been a number of attempts during the early 1980s, led by Peter Sperryn, for BASM to adopt a federal structure, based on that of the ACSM. The aim here was to cater for the growing friction among its diverse membership and to allow smaller specialist groups a greater voice.[75] The ACSM had three divisions—clinical, scientific and physical education—each had a degree of autonomy and elected their own vice president on an annual basis, and the president of the ACSM was drawn from this group. Peter Sperryn noted that "multi-disciplinism clearly works," although even here a group of US orthopedic surgeons had split to form their own sports medicine organization.[76] However, one probable reason for the relative success of the ACSM was that the vast majority of its members were nonclinicians (numbering about eight thousand compared to one thousand doctors), whereas doctors made up the largest group in BASM, and it was assumed by them that a doctor would always be chairman.[77] This group subsequently dominated the organization.[78]

The time, therefore, had passed for a federal structure in British sports medicine. There were now too many well-structured and firmly established professional bodies that represented the interests of these disciplines and their members, despite a large proportion making up the BASM membership.[79] Both in 1982 and 1984, attempts to establish a federal structure with a medical practitioners' subcommittee failed because each group was reluctant to submerge its own identity.[80] In addition, there was reluctance among sporting bodies to utilize medicine, which did not help in forming a closer relationship between sport and medicine and prevented sports medicine gaining wider recognition. Partly because of this stagnation, BASM's membership fell. In 1984, BASM's membership had numbered 1,375, with doctors making up 47 percent (644).[81] Membership dropped to around eight hundred by 1987.[82]

EDUCATIONAL INITIATIVES

While BASM tried to come to terms with its inability to act as the representative organization for the discipline, there was still a large demand among sports medicine practitioners for training and education courses. A series of educational developments, culminating in the establishment of the Intercollegiate Academic Board of Sport and Exercise Medicine (IABSEM) in 1998, were vital in giving the subdiscipline greater respectability within the medical profession more generally.

Moreover, important changes in the sporting world expedited a greater demand, and hence more opportunities, for sports medicine and sports science. First, sport was transformed through the money it began to receive from satellite television. Second, the UK government began to invest in sport, both in terms of trying to improve the nation's health and for reasons of national sporting prestige. The profile of sports medicine was also raised through the widely reported injuries to footballers such as Paul Gascoigne and David Beckham, who had become part of a celebrity culture due to sport's symbiotic relationship with the media. In addition, because of a boom in the fitness industry, there was now a greater demand for sports medicine among the general public, highlighted by products such as sprays and bandages as well as the proliferation of sports injury clinics. Importantly, on a professional level, educational developments led to the emergence of two increasingly distinct groups within sports medicine: first, those practitioners working in the NHS who had an interest in sports medicine; second, those, especially doctors, who worked privately in sports medicine, had their own clinics and whose sole source of income was the discipline.

An early sports medicine qualification had been the London Hospital diploma in sports medicine. It was established in 1981 by John King FRCS and was a three-year part-time course that enrolled a maximum of forty GPs. Later in 1986, the London Sports Medicine Institute (LSMI) was set up, with Dan Tunstall-Pedoe as its medical director.[83] The LSMI was taken over by the Sports Council in 1992 and became the National Sports Medicine Institute. However, it was closed down in 1997 due the withdrawal of UK Sport funding.

Many of the GPs who took the London Hospitals diploma went on to take other courses. These included the Society of Apothecaries' diploma in sports medicine, which was established in 1989. Another diploma was offered by the Scottish Royal Colleges Board for Sports Medicine. This board had been set up in 1986, mainly through the efforts of Donald

McLeod (president of BASM/BASEM, 1995–2002), and gave the discipline greater credibility.[84] Initially these courses only catered to a relatively small number of sports medicine specialists. Higher degrees in sports medicine later became available, initially in Nottingham and Glasgow. In 1994 the Royal Society of Medicine's sports medicine section was established with Roger Bannister as the first president. By 2005, there were eight master's degrees in SEM.

FROM BASM TO BASEM

In 1999, to take into account the formation of the intercollegiate board, BASM's name changed to the British Association of Sport and Exercise Medicine.[85] Accompanying this name change to incorporate exercise medicine, there were also changes in membership regulations. Now only doctors could have full membership rights whereas, unless they were already full members, those from the allied professions were offered only associate membership (previously they had enjoyed equal rights with doctors).[86]

The name change also marked a change in outlook, probably borne out of necessity. The medical care of elite athletes was firmly the responsibility of the governing bodies of sport and backed up by UK Sport. In this sense, BASEM had little input bar its representation on various committees. With a growing emphasis on promoting exercise for the population, the change to "sport and exercise medicine" seemed inevitable. It also marked a shift from BASM's traditional wide-ranging aims of having responsibility for the care of elite athletes. The scientific scope of sports medicine was also changing and now extended to other specialties such as cardiology, respiratory medicine, gynecology, rheumatology and neurology. Moreover, there were growing calls for the use of evidence-based medicine (EBM) in research to further improve the status of sports medicine within the medical profession as well as with sporting bodies.[87]

Despite the membership changes in favor of doctors, there continued to be tensions among this group. In 2001, there were 760 members of BASEM, with 517 doctors (approximately 65 percent of the membership); physiotherapists numbered 123 (16 percent); and the rest comprised sports scientists, chiropodists, educators, osteopaths (who had been banned thirty years previously), dental and veterinary surgeons and students.[88] For those working in the private sector, however, the lack of specialist recognition caused problems over insurance. Because of government legislation, to qualify as a consultant a new specialist qualification—Certificates of Completion of Specialist Training (CCSTs)—had been introduced as a mandatory requirement from 1997. Insurance companies like BUPA and PPP now required that doctors work six years full-time to gain this recognition (or ten years part-time). Norwich Union would not insure anyone working in sports medicine or in musculoskeletal medicine, which threatened the financial future of those working in this area.[89]

In 2001, BASEM polled its members on whether they should become a doctors-only organization or remain multidisciplinary. The executive had advocated that BASEM remain multidisciplinary. However, Malcolm Read and Nick Webborn put the case for BASEM to become a doctors-only group: the "Association for Doctors with an Interest in Sport and Exercise Medicine." They argued that there had been a drift away to other more specialist sports medicine organizations like BASES and the ACPSM. Moreover, it was claimed that BASEM could not speak for all groups and lacked focus; all similar to arguments that had been raised twenty years previously over BATS.[90]

Subsequently, in 2001, following the failure and frustrations of not becoming a doctors-only organization another group broke away: the United Kingdom Association of Doctors in Sport (UKADIS). The formation of UKADIS grew from a motivation for career development, and also importantly for representation for doctors. Its mandate was to "increase the momentum behind establishing SEM as a bona fide career choice for doctors with agreed high standards of practice and education, good professional support." By 2005, it had two hundred members and a number of its members were on the editorial board of the *Clinical Journal of Sports Medicine*.[91]

CONCLUSION

UKADIS opened up a few old wounds; however, it was short-lived due to the recognition of SEM as a medical specialty, and in 2005 it re-amalgamated with BASEM and quickly became subsumed.[92] Membership of BASEM had risen to twelve hundred in 2009.[93] However, what UKADIS had further demonstrated was an almost inexorable impulse within sports medicine toward specialization. Medicine in general had always been the most "professionalized" of occupations through its emphasis on education and research. Although this process may have been inexorable, the acceptance of SEM as a medical specialty was not inevitable in 2005; instead, its approval by the state can be seen in light of wider medical developments. By the end of the twentieth century, public confidence in doctors generally and the competence of modern medicine had begun to decline due partly to the challenge from alternative medicine and an expansion in consumer choice (see, for instance, the contributions of Pike and Atkinson in this collection). Alternative therapies challenged the biomedical orthodoxy of the medical profession with a more holistic approach to healing. In response, in trying to gain the public's confidence, there has been an intensification of professionalization within orthodox medicine; something, ironically, that has been copied by alternative therapies.[94] Sports medicine, therefore, as part of orthodox medicine, has sought this recognition.

Sports medicine itself though was also subject to the cultural traditions of BASM that shaped its micro-politics. The strong belief within BASM that sports medicine should remain a multidisciplinary organization was not only a reflection of the importance of individual personalities within any organization, but it was a tradition that stemmed from its origins. Although even in the 1950s it was felt that doctors should be in the vanguard, they still thought that they would represent all of medicine in its relationship with sport. However, it proved to be difficult to achieve a balance between the desire to professionalize and to keep other sports medicine practitioners under the same umbrella due to the changing motivations of doctors who became more career-minded. There was also a growing demand for more professional sports medicine services within sport as commercialization, and competition intensified. For some, what had started out as a hobby in a voluntary capacity had turned into a specialist vocation. Of course, specialization in sports medicine has not been total. Whereas SEM has become a specialty for which a small number of doctors are able to gain status as a consultant, most sports medicine practitioners in Britain continue to struggle for a professional identity.

NOTES

1. The BASM changed its title to the British Association of Sport and Exercise Medicine in 1999.
2. Gelfand, "History," 1119.
3. Quoted in Reynolds and Tansey, *Development of Sports Medicine* (hereafter, *Witness Seminar*), xxxvi.
4. Brunton, "Introduction."
5. Perkin, *Rise of Professional Society.*
6. Malcolm, "Unprofessional Practice?" 382.
7. Ryan, "Sports Medicine," 3, 13.
8. Thompson et al., "Defining the Sports Medicine Specialist."
9. Kent, *Sports Science and Medicine,* 419–20.
10. Safai, "Critical Analysis," 326.
11. Cronin, "Not Taking the Medicine," 24.
12. Heggie, "Only the British," 213.
13. McCrory, "What Is Sports," 955–957.
14. Carter, "Mixing Business with Leisure?"; Malcolm, "Unprofessional Practice?"
15. Carter, "Rise and Fall."
16. Interview with Malcolm Melrose.
17. Waddington, "Jobs for the Boys," ; Waddington, Roderick and Parker, *Managing Injuries*; Waddington, Roderick and Naik, "Methods of Appointment," 48.
18. Malcolm, "Unprofessional Practice?" 381.
19. Saks, "Introduction"; *Orthodox and Alternative Medicine.*
20. Porter, *Health, Civilization and the State.*
21. Anon., *Lancet*, 5 October 1912, 977; Hollmann, "Sports Medicine."
22. Gori, *Italian Fascism.*
23. Ergen et al., "Sports Medicine."
24. La Cava, "Sports Medicine," ; "International Federation."
25. Anon., *Lancet*, 19 November 1960, 1144.

26. *Manchester Guardian*, 2 August 1956, 8.
27. The athletics' medical committee also included Porritt and Abrahams.
28. BASM AGM, 27 February 1953. The following year BASM was accepted as an associate member of FIMS.
29. Abrahams, "Athletics," 225; Anon., *Lancet*, 10 April 1937, 899–890.
30. He was an advisor for the 1981 film *Chariots of Fire* about the 1924 Olympics, but in the film he was referred to as Tom Watson.
31. Wolfenden Committee on Sport, Draft Report, 8 July 1960.
32. Lowe and Porritt, *Athletics*, 108–109.
33. BASM Executive Committee Minutes, 23 June 1952.
34. Anon., *British Journal of Sports Medicine*, November 1971.
35. Anon., "Obituary," *British Journal of Sports Medicine*, June 1982, 121.
36. Adamson, "Sports Medicine," 7.
37. Cussen, "By Way of Reply," 4.
38. Anon., *British Medical Journal*, 3 October 1964, 834.
39. Anon., *Lancet*, 24 September 1960, 699.
40. *Sport and the Community*.
41. BASM Executive Committee Minutes, December 1962.
42. Ibid., 5 February 1965.
43. Anon., *BASM Bulletin*, 1968, 96–104.
44. Interview with Elizabeth Robson; Robson, "Dr. Henry Evans Robson"; Sperryn et al., "Obituary," 136–136.
45. BASM Minutes, AGM, 19 October 1965.
46. Interview with Ian Adams.
47. *Witness Seminar*, 25–30; Anon., *British Journal of Sports Medicine*, December 1975; Robson, "Obituary," 241.
48. An advisory Sports Council was first established in 1965 and it gained its Royal Charter in 1972.
49. Anon., *British Journal of Sports Medicine*, December 1975.
50. Tunstall-Pedoe, "Obituary."
51. Carter, "Mixing Business with Leisure?"; *Witness Seminar*.
52. Interview with Ian Adams.
53. Ibid.
54. Tunstall-Pedoe, "Obituary," 220–222; *Witness Seminar*, 21–22, 25, 128–129.
55. Anon., *British Journal of Sports Medicine*, September 1978, 157.
56. Sperryn, "Secretary's Column," 242.
57. *Witness Seminar*.
58. BASM, Executive Committee Minutes, 27 October 1980.
59. Tunstall-Pedoe, "Obituary."
60. *Witness Seminar*, 48.
61. Ibid.
62. BASM, Executive Committee Minutes, 31 January 1979.
63. Ibid., 12 January 1981.
64. Ibid.
65. Sperryn, "Unity or Fragmentation."
66. Interview with Elizabeth Robson.
67. These included the British Institute of Musculoskeletal Medicine (1992), formed from the merger of the Institute of Orthopaedic Medicine and the British Association of Manipulative Medicine, and the British Association of Manipulative Medicine (1993).
68. BASM, AGM, 25 May 1977.
69. BASM, Executive Committee Minutes, 28 November 1979.
70. Sperryn, "Honorary Secretary's Column."
71. BASM, AGM, 14 October 1984.

72. BASS combined the Biomechanics Study Group, the British Society of Sports Psychology and the Society of Sports Sciences. In 1993, it was renamed the British Association of Sport and Exercise Sciences (BASES).

73. *Witness Seminar.*

74. *Witness Seminar,* passim.

75. Sperryn, "Personal Letter."

76. Sperryn, "Honorary Secretary's Column," 288.

77. BASM Executive Committee Minutes, 18 January 1982.

78. In 1983, Sperryn resigned as secretary to fight for election as chairman on the grounds that some members of the committee were obstructive to his plans to reform BASM. He narrowly lost to Dan Tunstall-Pedoe.

79. BASM, AGM Secretary's Report, 1984.

80. BASM, Executive Committee Minutes, 10 November 1982. The organizations were: Institute of Sports Medicine, British Society of Sports Psychology, Society of Sports Scientists and ACPSM. BASM, AGM Secretary's Report, 1984. The proposed groups were: chartered physiotherapists, sports scientists, psychologists and podiatrists.

81. Robson, "Editorial," 3. Other groups included: physiotherapists—260; remedial gymnasts—55; chiropodists—87; other clinical professions—35; physical education and sports sciences—266; and administrators—28.

82. "Honorary Treasurer's Report for the year 1987," *British Journal of Sports Medicine,* n.d. The dramatic fall had been partly due to BASM's change to an incorporated (as opposed to an unincorporated) association, which had meant members transferring their standing orders from the old to the new. Only seven hundred did, with one hundred new members joining.

83. *Witness Seminar.*

84. The establishment of the IABSEM brought the Scottish royal colleges exam and the apothecaries' diploma under its wing, and so there was only a single diploma.

85. BASM, Executive Minutes, 1 December 1999.

86. *Witness Seminar.*

87. McCrory, "Evidence-Based Sports Medicine."

88. By contrast, the ACPSM had twelve hundred, almost exclusively physiotherapists and the osteopaths' group, OSCA had 250 members. "The Future of BASEM: Opinion Poll of BASEM Members," BASEM Archives, in possession of author.

89. *Witness Seminar.*

90. "The Future of BASEM: Opinion Poll of BASEM Members," BASEM Archives.

91. Meeuwisse, "Welcome, UKADIS."

92. *BASEM Today* 7 (Winter 2006).

93. *Witness Seminar.*

94. Saks, "Medicine and the Counter Culture."

BIBLIOGRAPHY

Primary

BASEM Today
Interviews: Malcolm Melrose (18 July 2005); Ian Adams (22 August 2005); Elizabeth Robson (19 August 2009).
Manchester Guardian

74   *Neil Carter*

Records of British Association of Sport and Medicine, Wellcome Trust Library, London.
Records of Wolfenden Committee on Sport, Sport England.

Secondary

Abrahams, Adolphe. "Athletics." In *The British Encyclopaedia of Medical Practice*, vol. 2, edited by Humphrey Rolleston, 220–225. London: Butterworth, 1936.
Adamson, G.T. "Sports Medicine and the Athlete." *Coaching Newsletter* (January 1961): 7.
Anon. *BASM Bulletin*, 3 no. 2, (1968): 96–104.
———. *British Journal of Sports Medicine* 6, no. 1 (November 1971): 26.
———. *British Journal of Sports Medicine* 12, no. 3 (September 1978): 157.
———. "Obituary." *British Journal of Sports Medicine* 16, no. 2 (June 1982): 121.
———. *British Medical Journal* (October 1964): 834.
———. *Lancet*, 5 October 1912, 977.
———. *Lancet*, 10 April 1937, 899–90.
———.*Lancet*, 24 September 1960, 699.
———. *Lancet*, 19 November 1960, 1144.Brunton, Deborah. "Introduction." In *Medicine Transformed: Health, Disease and Society in Europe 1800–1930*, edited by D. Brunton, xi-xviii. Manchester: Manchester University Press, 2004.
Carter, Neil. "Mixing Business with Leisure? The Football Club Doctor, Sports Medicine and the Voluntary Tradition." *Sport in History* 29, no. 1 (March 2009): 69–91.
———. "The Rise and Fall of the Magic Sponge." *Social History of Medicine* 23, no. 2 (August 2010): 261–279.
Cronin, Mike. "Not Taking the Medicine: Sportsmen and Doctors in Late Nineteenth-Century Britain." *Journal of Sport History* 34, no. 1 (Spring 2007): 23–35.
Cussen, D.J. "By Way of Reply." *Coaching Newsletter* (April 1961): 4.
Ergen, E., F. Pigozzi, N. Bachl and H.H. Dickhuth. "Sports Medicine: A European Perspective. Historical Roots, Definitions and Scope." *Journal of Sports Medicine and Physical Fitness* 46, no. 2 (June 2006): 167–175.
Gelfand, Toby. "The History of the Medical Profession." In *The Companion Encyclopaedia of the History of Medicine*, edited by W.F. Bynum and R. Porter, 11119–1149. London: Routledge, 1993.
Gori, Gigliola. *Italian Fascism and the Female Body: Sport, Submissive Women and Strong Mothers*. London: Routledge, 2004.
Heggie, Vanessa. "'Only the British Appear to Be Making a Fuss': The Science of Success and the Myth of Amateurism at the Mexico Olympiad, 1968." *Sport in History* 28, no. 2 (June 2008): 213–235.
Hollmann, W. "Sports Medicine in the Federal Republic of Germany." *British Journal of Sports Medicine* 23, no. 3 (1989): 142–144.
Kent, M., ed. *The Oxford Dictionary of Sports Science and Medicine*. Oxford: Oxford University Press, 1994.
La Cava, Guiseppe. "The International Federation for Sports Medicine." *Journal of the American Medical Association* 162 (November 1956): 1109–1111.
———. "Sports Medicine in Modern Times: A Short Historical Survey." *Journal of Sports Medicine and Physical Fitness* 13, no. 3 (July–September 1973): 155–158.
Lowe, Douglas, and Arthur Porritt. *Athletics*. London: Longmans, 1929.

Malcolm, Dominic. "Unprofessional Practice? The Status and Power of Sport Physicians." *Sociology of Sport Journal* 23 (2006): 376–395.

McCrory, Paul. "Evidence-Based Sports Medicine." *British Journal of Sports Medicine* 35 (2001): 79–80.

———. "What Is Sports and Exercise Medicine?" *British Journal of Sports Medicine* 40 (2006): 955–957.

Meeuwisse, Willem H. "Welcome, UKADIS." *Clinical Journal of Sport Medicine* 13, no. 4 (2003): 199.

Perkin, Harold. *The Rise of Professional Society: England since 1880*. London: Routledge, 1989.

Porter, Dorothy. *Health, Civilization and the State: A History of Public Health from Ancient to Modern Times*. London: Routledge, 1999.

Reynolds, L.A., and E.M. Tansey, eds. *The Development of Sports Medicine in Twentieth-Century Britain: The Transcript of a Witness Seminar Held by the Wellcome Trust Centre for the History of Medicine at UCL, London, on 29 June 2007*. London: Wellcome Trust Centre, University of London, 2009.

Robson, Elizabeth. "Dr. Henry Evans Robson, 1922 to 1992: The Workhorse of the Sports Medicine Pioneers." Unpublished paper, 2009.

Robson, Henry, "Editorial." *British Journal of Sports Medicine* 19, no. 1 (March 1985): 3.

———. "Obituary: William Eldon Tucker." *British Journal of Sports Medicine* 25, no. 4 (1991): 241.

Ryan, Allan J. "Sports Medicine in the World Today." In *Sports Medicine*, edited by A.J. Ryan and F.L. Allman, Jr. , 3–12. London: Academic Press, 1989.

Safai, Parissa. "A Critical Analysis of the Development of Sport Medicine in Canada." *International Review for the Sociology of Sport* 42 (2007): 321–341.

Saks, Mike. "Introduction." In *Alternative Medicine in Britain*, edited by M. Saks, 1–21. Oxford: Clarendon Press, 1992.

———. "Medicine and the Counter Culture." In *Medicine in the Twentieth Century*, edited by R. Cooter and J. Pickstone , 113–124. Amsterdam: Harwood, 2000).

———. *Orthodox and Alternative Medicine: Politics, Professionalization and Health Care*. London: Continuum, 2003.

Sperryn, Peter. "Honorary Secretary's Column." *British Journal of Sports Medicine* 15, no. 4 (March 1983): 1.

———. "Honorary Secretary's Report." *British Journal of Sports Medicine* 9, no. 4 (December 1975): 203.

———. "A Personal Letter from the Retiring Honorary Secretary." *British Journal of Sports Medicine* 17, no. 3 (September 1983): 217.

———. "Secretary's Column." *British Journal of Sports Medicine* 11, no. 2 (June 1977): 242.

———. "Unity or Fragmentation." *British Journal of Sports Medicine* 15, no. 2 (June 1981): 116.

Sperryn, Peter, Harry Thomason, Dan S. Tunstall-Pedoe and John G.P. Williams. "Obituary: Henry Evans Robson." *British Journal of Sports Medicine* 26, no. 3 (1992): 136–137.

Sport and the Community: The Report of the Wolfenden Committee on Sport. London: Council of Physical Recreation, 1960.

Thompson, B., D. MacAuley, O. McNally and S. O'Neill. "Defining the Sports Medicine Specialist in the United Kingdom: A Delphi Study." *British Journal of Sports Medicine* 38 (2004): 214–218.

Troup, J.D.G. "Sports Medicine." *Lancet*, 24 September 1960, 699–700.

Tunstall-Pedoe, Dan. "Obituary: Dr. John G.P. Williams." *British Journal of Sports Medicine* 29, no. 4 (1995): 220–222.

Waddington, Ivan. "Jobs for the Boys: A Study of the Employment of Club Doctors and Physiotherapists in English Professional Football." *Soccer and Society* 3 (2000): 51–64.

Waddington, I., M. Roderick and R. Naik. "Methods of Appointment and Qualifications of Club Doctors and Physiotherapists in English Professional Football: Some Problems and Issues." *British Journal of Sports Medicine* 35 (2001): 48–53.

Waddington, I., M. Roderick and G. Parker. *Managing Injuries in Professional Football: A Study of the Roles of the Club Doctor and Physiotherapists.* Leicester: Leicester University Press, 1999.

Williams, John G.P. "Challenge!" *British Journal of Sports Medicine* 12, no. 3 (September 1978): 157.

4 From Rehabilitation Patients to Rehabilitating Athletes

Searching for a History of Sports Medicine for Athletes with Disabilities[1]

Fred Mason

Throughout the Western world, elite-level athletes rely on sports medicine physicians and allied professionals as integral parts of the team that supports their training and competition. The relationship between athletes and sports medicine professionals strongly developed in the last half of the twentieth century, with the 1960s through the 1980s standing as a significant time period for sports medicine as a specialty, concomitant with major developments in sport in terms of professionalization, commercialization and politicization. Similarly, elite athletes with disabilities expect access to sports medicine professionals, at least at major championships. The relationship between sports medicine and disability sport has grown significantly, albeit in a later period than with mainstream elite sport, mirroring trends in disability sport since the 1980s.[2]

A growing body of historical literature has documented the rise of elite sport for athletes with disabilities in some detail. For example, Steve Bailey's recent history of the Paralympic Movement covered significant events and personalities over the last fifty years, benefiting greatly from access to official Paralympic and Olympic sources.[3] Most historical work dealing with disability sport provides detailed treatment of its "origins" in rehabilitative medicine immediately following World War II.[4] However, relatively little information is extant on *sports medicine* for disability sport, especially from a historical perspective. This chapter is an attempt[5] at addressing this gap, in sketching a history of sports medicine for elite athletes with disabilities through considering trends in sports medicine research, relative to developments in disability sport.

To construct this history, I primarily drew on literature in sports medicine (and related fields like physiotherapy and athletic training) that discussed sport for athletes with disabilities.[6] I also spoke to or conducted e-mail conversations with a number of individuals involved in sports medicine and disability, including leading researchers and medical officers of national Paralympic committees.[7] Working in an international context downplays or misses national or more local developments, but is arguably more appropriate for a work fairly exploratory in nature. This study is most interested in the interests of physicians and researchers, in seeing how knowledge and opinion in sports medicine was constructed about disability sport and how these related to changes in the wider sporting context.[8]

Determining exactly what is and is not "sports medicine" is tricky, given the late establishment of the field as an official medical specialty and the differing health-related and paramedical professions involved. Jack Berryman's history of the American College of Sports Medicine (ACSM) describes the long-term involvement of cardiologists, physiatrists, orthopedists, physiologists and physicals educators. As Patricia Vertinsky has noted, you could almost say that it is "anything that relates to sports or physical welfare that interests those who are interested in sports medicine."[9] Following Mathias, who argues that "modern" sports medicine is "prescriptive and much more ambitious with respect to maximizing athletic performance,"[10] for my purposes, I considered anything related to the care and prevention of injuries, or the management of the health of athletes related to performance, to be relevant sports medicine. Thus, I included material from allied fields such as athletic training, but ruled out literature concerned with measuring physiological aspects of performance, as such material does not relate to pain or injury.[11] Given the focus on disability sport, I also delimited to material on *sport* for athletes with disabilities, rather than exercise or fitness activities.[12]

Ultimately then, this chapter draws on the literature available on sports medicine for athletes with disabilities and disability sport in general, and information gathered from key informants involved from about the 1970s to the present.[13] I will sketch how, similar to sports medicine's incorporation in mainstream sports from the 1960s, sports medicine encompassed, interacted with and influenced elite sport for athletes with disabilities in an international context.

PERIODIZING SPORTS MEDICINE AND DISABILITY SPORT

Both sports medicine and disability sport possess longer histories than many presume. Jack Berryman traces medical concern for and use of exercise as therapy back to ancient times, with Hippocrates and Galen.[14] Some of the gymnastics movements promoted in the late nineteenth century on a global basis could be taken as a precursor to sports medicine. However, developments specifically tied to sport and sport-related injuries are an early twentieth-century phenomenon.

In the 1920s and 1930s, physicians involved with sports and exercise programs began to seek association, especially in Germany and other European countries. The International Federation of Sports Medicine (FIMS) was established in 1928 in Amsterdam, and held meetings at least biannually.[15] At the same time, exercise physiologists and other sports scientists began to explore the athletic body as a research question. As Hoberman argues in *Mortal Engines*, scientists and physicians initially approached the athlete more as a unique experiment in human nature, rather than worrying about sport performance and ways to maintain or enhance it, hallmarks of more recent sports medicine and allied fields.

The ACSM was formed in 1954, taking a broad view of exercise, fitness, sport and human movement as its mandate. Douglas Jackson argues that the ACSM has always been concerned more with muscle and cardiovascular physiology, leading to the breakaway/establishment of the American Orthopaedic Society's Committee on Sports Medicine in the late 1960s to early 1970s.[16] The 1950s through 1970s represented a period of establishment of professional associations in different countries, and by a number of allied professions such as the National Athletic Trainers Association (NATA) in the US in the early 1950s. From the late 1960s, the "team approach" commonly now in place began to take root, with specialists such as orthopedists, physiotherapists, nutritionists and trainers increasingly working together.[17]

Ivan Waddington links the rapid growth of sports medicine from the 1950s to increasing medicalization of life and to social trends that politicized and commercialized sport. Waddington argues that physicians medicalized the athletic body, so that routine medical supervision of athletes was assumed necessary.[18] Athletes' bodies also became more "valuable," in both political and economic senses, throughout the Cold War period. With the notion of competing social systems through international sport, the surveillance and care of athletes' bodies took on ideological dimensions. Further, with the commercialization of sport and increasing material rewards, athletes and teams began to increasingly seek medical attention.[19] Added to this, the running, aerobics and fitness booms led to more widespread participation, injury and advice-seeking in sports and exercise. All of these factors led to demand for and expansion of sports medicine practice over the latter part of the twentieth century.

Michael Cronin indicates the steady growth of athletes consuming sports medicine from the 1950s and accelerating after the 1970s. Using the Canadian example, Teetzel describes how sports medicine professionals increasingly became an integral part of Olympic teams from the 1972 Games in Munich. By the 1980s, sports medicine was well established on the sporting and medical scene. A number of sports medicine journals were in publication by the early 1980s, and the field held official status as a medical specialty in numerous countries, with the American Board of Medical Specialty recognition coming late, in 1989.[20]

Elite sport for athletes with disabilities thus arose in a context where sports medicine was reasonably well institutionalized. The received version of disability sport history links it almost entirely to the post–World War II era. Whereas that period is most significant in the "origins" of sport for the disabled, developments date back much further. Some histories of adapted physical education point to sporting activities in institutions for children with hearing or visual impairments.[21] Deaf sport arose early in the 1900s, in part as a consequence of the institutionalization process, with "the Deaf" emerging as a social group considering themselves a linguistic minority as much as people with a disability. The Comité International des Sports des Sourds (CISS) held its first competitions in 1924, and has been holding "Deaflympics" since 1949.[22]

In terms of rehabilitation medicine, sport made up part of a battery of manipulative and physical therapies used to treat disabled veterans of the First World War in a number of countries. Although there was preference for work therapies, which the term *rehabilitation* meant at the time, physicians incorporated sport as part of the exercise regimen for the sake of interest.[23] However, with the Depression of the 1930s and the slow reduction of the special social status of Great War veterans, these early efforts were largely forgotten by the Second World War.

The most important post–World War II rehabilitative programs for the history of the Paralympics was Dr. Ludwig Guttmann's work at the Stoke Mandeville Hospital in Aylesbury, England, during the late 1940s and 1950s. Guttmann was one of the first physicians to try to really treat people with spinal cord injuries, who had previously been viewed as hopeless cases. Guttmann used sport for rehabilitative purposes, and he served as a driving force behind rehabilitation and wheelchair sport for a number of decades.[24]

Sports competitions for people using wheelchairs grew out of his rehabilitative work, with the organization of the first Stoke Mandeville Games in 1948. These games became annual and added more sports and competitors over time, becoming international in 1952 with the addition of Dutch ex-servicemen. The International Stoke Mandeville Games Federation (ISMGF) was established in 1952 and became the global sport body for wheelchair sport. By 1960, the International Stoke Mandeville Games had grown into a multisport event of 350 athletes from twenty-two countries. The 1960 games, held in Rome in the former Olympic facilities and called "the Olympiad for the Disabled," are considered the first "Paralympics."[25]

Even in the immediate postwar era, competing visions of what forms disability sport should take existed. The Stoke Mandeville Games, specifically for those with "spinal paralysis," maintained a rehabilitative, and consequently medical, vision. In the US, competitively focused wheelchair sports emerged from Veterans Administration hospitals in the early 1950s, since it was sport run by the participants themselves. The National Wheelchair Basketball Association was established in 1950, followed by the National Wheelchair Athletics Association in 1957. Athletes affiliated with these associations brought their competitive orientation to Stoke Mandeville starting in 1960.[26]

Sport associations for people with other types of disabilities formed over the next two decades on a disability-by-disability basis. The World Federation for Ex-Servicemen created the International Sport Organization for the Disabled (ISOD) in Paris in 1964. ISOD historically served as the international governing body for sport programs for amputees, dwarf athletes, athletes with cerebral palsy and the group known as "les autres" (individuals with other physical and locomotor disabilities who did not fit into other classification schemes). Cerebral palsy athletes split away in 1968, when the International Cerebral Palsy Society formed a subcommittee on sport and leisure. Over time, the committee's activities expanded, and it became a separate entity in 1978, the Cerebral Palsy-International Sport and Recreation Association (CP-ISRA). Other associations currently part of the Paralympic Movement were created in the 1980s—the International Blind Sports Association in 1981 and the currently named International Sports Federation for People with an Intellectual Disability (INAS-FID) in 1986.[27]

Scholars trying to periodize the development of the Paralympic Games describe the "first stage" as 1960–1976, when the Games continually expanded in size, but did not include any athletes other than "the spinal Paralysed."[28] The 1976 "Torontolympiad for the Disabled" was the first in which ISOD athletes competed (amputee, blind and les autres), and a Winter Paralympics began in 1976 with alpine and Nordic skiing.[29] Given the variety of groups now associated with the movement, and the ongoing expansion of the games, the "second period" of the disability sports movement (1976–1988) was quite fractured.

The first umbrella organization of international disability sport governing bodies was formed in 1983—the International Coordinating Committee of World Sports Organizations for the Disabled, known as the ICC for short. However, member organizations disliked the structure of the ICC, and the depth of infighting in part led to the 1984 Summer Paralympics being split into two.[30] The member federations of the ICC voted to change its format and create a new organization, the International Paralympic Committee (IPC), in 1989.

In 1988, the Paralympic Games entered a third stage, which resembles the current context. The Seoul Olympic Organizing Committee offered to host the Paralympic Games, shortly after the Olympic Games, in the former Olympic facilities. The Barcelona Olympic Organizing Committee followed suit. These committees acted largely independently of the International Olympic Committee (IOC), which slowly came to negotiate with, then promote, the IPC and the Paralympic Games over the 1990s.[31] This third stage, from 1988 on, witnessed expansion of the games, increasing public and media attention, and a shift from a participatory sports movement to one focused on elite sports performance. As we will see, sports medicine became an important part of training and competing in disability sport from the 1990s on.

This brief history is meant to serve as an introduction on how disability sport moved from being a form of medical rehabilitation in the 1950s to elite, international sport in the 2000s. We could uncritically take this as a natural "evolution." However, this movement has been accompanied by gains and losses and a deepening of power relationships in disability sport. It is beyond the scope of the chapter here to go into detail on any of the problems facing the Paralympic Movement but a brief mention of some is warranted, especially as many have been impacted or caused by the move to elite sport and medical involvement in it. International sport is known to cause issues with medal-hunting, national rivalries and the specter of doping. International disability sport has proved no different in those regards. Inequities due to technology are especially pronounced in disability sport, with wheelchair and prosthesis design explaining part of why the Western world dominates the medal tables. As well, the move away from inclusion and toward commercialization has meant the compression of functional classification categories, with athletes with more severe impairments, especially cerebral palsy competitors, being pushed out of the marquee stadium events.[32]

For good and ill, disability sport has transitioned to professionalized elite sport. Now that we have sketched the historical landscape of sports medicine's move toward specialization and disability sport's move to elite competition, it remains to explore how these two have come together as change occurred. Similar to sports medicine's relation to mainstream sport in a slightly earlier period, it reacted to, interacted with and influenced developments in disability sport from the 1970s on.

SPORTS (MEDICINE) FOR REHABILITATION—THE 1970S

The earliest instance found of disability sport appearing in a publication specifically on sports medicine was a book chapter written by Ludwig Guttmann in 1962. This chapter did not really focus on medicine, per se. Instead, Guttmann discusses the history of sport for the disabled, gives approximately two pages to "physiological" and "psychological aspects" and describes the ISMGF for the majority of the chapter.[33]

Guttmann clearly indicates his concern for things other than competitive sport in this early work. After discussing archery records as a means to show similar performance to able-bodied archers, he states:

> It must be emphasized that, important as athletic performance and the number of records broken may be, the Stoke Mandeville Games have a greater significance than that. They have become an annual reunion of men, women and young adults stricken by one of the most tragic disablements which can ever beset mankind. Through international sport, they have come to know, understand and appreciate one another and, moreover, these Games have become the cradle of hope for thousands of others who still dwell in darkness and despair.[34]

Guttmann demonstrated a focus on rehabilitation, rather than sport for sport's sake, throughout his career. This is clearly shown in his many writings across the 1970s, in both medical and sporting publications.[35] As one example, in an article in the *Journal of the Royal Society of Health* in 1973, Guttmann sets out the "object of sport for the disabled" as curative, recreational, and a factor in the "psychological readjustment" and "social reintegration" of the disabled.[36] Such sentiments strike a chord much more with current visions of therapeutic recreation than competitive sport.

In 1976 Guttmann compiled much of his work and writing in what is now considered a classic text, his *Textbook of Sport for the Disabled*. This book encompassed most of the major groups of people with physical disabilities participating in sport, including people with spinal cord injuries, amputations, hearing and visual impairments and cerebral palsy . Yet, although it covered history, rules, athlete classification and records, the notion of rehabilitation and reintegration undergirded all the writing and stood out in the "aims of sport" for all the groups.[37] Guttmann remained steadfast in his rehabilitative focus for sport, to the point of intransigence. Even as disability sport achieved its "take-off" phase in the mid-1970s, as Steve Bailey notes, "Guttmann never seemed to give up his stance as a medical expert first and foremost—with all athletes treated as patients."[38] This is quite important given his role as a major administrator in disability sport. With one of the "founding fathers" so rehabilitation oriented, and wider social conception of people with disabilities at the time, it is not surprising that rehabilitation from traumatic injury, rather than from sports injuries, represented the main stance among sports medicine physicians for athletes with disabilities across the 1970s.

An article appearing in the relatively new journal the *Physician and Sportsmedicine* in 1974 indicates the uncertain approach with an interesting mix of criticism of negative social attitudes, discussion of the need for greater exposure of disability sport and advocacy for more doctors in the US prescribing sport for their patients with disabilities. "Contributions" in medical classification of athletes with disabilities are detailed, but academic and disability sports administrator Tim Nugent (of the National Wheelchair Basketball Association) is quoted as saying, "We can't expect them (physicians) to depart from their first professional responsibilities and do more than recognize this as an integral part of rehabilitation and lend their support."[39]

Other "special reports" appeared in the same journal in 1976, one on blind sports in general and the other on the 1976 Toronto Olympiad. Both of these attempt to lay the landscape of the types of disability sports under discussion and raise awareness in the audience. The work of the medical team at the Torontolympiad is highlighted in Ryan's article whereas, in a completely opposite vein, Ross discusses how sport can rouse the blind out of a life of state-supported "relative comfort" and dependence.[40]

One of the more strident versions of sports for the disabled being solely for rehabilitation appeared in the IOC's *Basic Book of Sports Medicine* in 1978. The author, P.N. Sperryn, was a leading sports medicine physician of the time (see Carter's contribution to this collection). He starts by noting: "This subject [Sport and Disability] may be considered under two headings: firstly, the use of exercise and sport in the rehabilitation of patients suffering from a wide range of disabilities, and secondly, the use of recreational exercise and physical pursuits for those suffering from permanent handicap."[41] Having thus established the rehabilitative/recreational aspects of sport, he subsequently dealt with sport as competition at great length. This is worth quoting extensively:

> It is sad that some of the protagonists of the sports movement for the disabled have exaggerated the "normality" of the disabled sportsman without allowing for the natural anatomical limitations imposed by disability or for the necessary addition of the stress and disappointment of sports failure to the pre-existing burden of the severely disabled person. Rather than break the spirit of a disabled person who simply cannot compete adequately, it may be that recreational pursuits are often preferable. This should not, however, exclude the use of sports in the rehabilitation program.[42]

Rather than impugning the individual author here, this should be taken as evidence of commonly held opinions, in both the medical field and the society at large, about people with disabilities and their potential. However, this particular book was published under the IOC's Olympic Solidarity program, meaning that it was intended as an "official" document meant to be sent to emerging national Olympic committees and fledgling sports associations. It constituted a powerful view.

Looking at the context of the mid to late 1970s, the continuing prevalence of the rehabilitation perspective in sports medicine is quite understandable. Sports medicine as a subfield was still quite diverse and had not yet gone so far down the performance enhancement route. Disability sport was itself just transitioning into a more competitive orientation, post the 1976 Torontolympiad. Further, many of the physicians involved in the medical classification of athletes at competitions or in providing their medical care had come through orthopedic or physical medicine involvement with people with disabilities, so their background would heavily influence their orientation. This would remain true throughout the 1980s, and many who would assume positions of power in the disability sport movement would come from the rehabilitation setting.[43]

In the late 1970s, disability sport began to move toward a competitive sporting model. In 1976, the first Winter Paralympics was held in Sweden. In 1978, the United States Olympic Committee, reacting to the new Amateur Sports Act, established a Committee on Sports for the Disabled (COSD), which would eventually become the national Paralympic Committee. Similar developments occurred in other countries. Cerebral palsy athletes competed at the Summer Paralympics for the first time in 1980.[44]

Reflecting some of this change, research in the areas of physiology and biomechanics of disability sport grew, especially related to wheelchair athletes, across the 1970s.[45] The first specialized research center for athletes with disabilities was established at the University of Alberta in 1978, and they held the first international research conference on disability sport in 1979.[46] In 1980, the "First International Medical Congress on Sports for the Disabled" was held in Oslo, Norway.[47] Indicating a bit more of a competitive sport focus in sports medicine for athletes with disabilities, a 1979 article by Jackson and Fredrickson went into detail on medical care at the previous Paralympics. The article starts with some history and discussion of general information and ends with a section on the "benefits of sport." The middle portion describes, for the first time in sports medicine literature, the setup of treatment facilities and the types of cases commonly seen at major competitions with multiple disability groups.[48] This focus on sport-related medicine, rather than rehabilitation, would continue to blossom in the next decade.

THE DESCRIPTIVE DECADE—THE 1980S

Mirroring developments in disability sport across the 1980s, which moved increasingly toward an elite sporting model, people involved in sports medicine for athletes with disabilities began to take interests in training, performance and injuries. The issue of medical classification systems served as subject of much debate, and little extant evidence of a rehabilitative orientation appeared in sports medicine writing as compared to previously. Many authors instead turned to describing common injuries and ways of providing appropriate medical service.

One of the first serious attempts to review the knowledge on disability sport, coauthored by eight physicians and sport scientists, considered wheelchair racing. The longest and most extensive article until then, it covered disability sport history, explained classification systems and discussed various aspects of physiology and training. The authors insisted: "Medical personnel interested in wheelchair sports must balance their interest in health and injury prevention against the importance of allowing disabled athletes to take risks and push themselves to their limits, just as able-bodied athletes are permitted to do."[49] They then went into particular problems for wheelchair athletes, including temperature regulation issues and shoulder joint stress, taking these not as signs of weakness or nonathleticism, but unique aspects of the athletes' physiology due to their impairments.

In 1981, the magazine *Sports 'N Spokes* published a series of articles now considered "classic" in the field. Physical therapist Kathleen Curtis wrote a four-part article delving into physiology, training, stretching and sports medicine (injury causes and prevention) for wheelchair athletes.[50] As part of this, she reported on a questionnaire distributed to over twelve hundred athletes that asked about sport participation and injury history. This represents the first published attempt at tracking athletic injuries in athletes with disabilities.

Two clear trends in sports medicine writing on disability sport in the 1980s are the efforts at providing an informational overview and at explaining athlete classification for other physicians, associated professions and those involved in sport.[51] Both of these express the sense that more attention to disability sport was needed. Describing medical classification is an effort at explaining one of the more unique and confusing aspects of disability sport, one particularly relevant to a medical audience as classification exams typically took place (then as now) with a three-person team of a physician, an associated professional like a physiotherapist and a sports scientist.[52]

International attention for athletes with disabilities increased as a result of wheelchair-racing exhibition events held at the Olympic Games in Los Angeles in 1984. The Pre-Olympic Scientific Congress, held in Oregon prior to those Games, included a section on "Sport and Disabled Athletes." Inclusion in the Congress leant legitimacy to disability sport and research associated with it, and the resulting book, with nineteen papers presented at the Congress and nine papers added to provide comprehensive coverage, was the first legitimate book on the international sports movement for athletes with disabilities. One section covered classification with four papers, and Curtis and Dillon reported more fully on the survey of wheelchair athletic injuries mentioned in the preceding.[53]

Other notable work at the end of the decade came from athletic therapist Brent Mangus and Canadian exercise scientist Roy Shephard. Drawing on his practice split between wheelchair athletes and athletes with intellectual disabilities, Mangus wrote two articles that described typical injuries seen in wheelchair athletes and ways to manage them. Both served as articles trying to raise awareness, but offered some depth for the first time. He made note that "rehabilitation physicians" often stop at "functional use of the injured part," so athletes needed physicians specialized in athletic injuries.[54]

Shephard's work represents a certain amount of maturity for disability sport and related research. He wrote an extensive review on "Sports Medicine and the Wheelchair Athlete" in 1988, which included basic medical considerations and problems and classification issues, as well as physiology, psychosocial considerations and the biomechanics of wheelchair propulsion.[55] The fact that enough research literature existed to write such a review speaks to the growth of sports medicine and exercise physiology interest in disability sport. Drawing on this work, and expanding it to include other disability groups, Shephard wrote the book *Fitness for Special Populations* in 1990. Despite the title, the book was heavily sport focused, and its publication by commercial press Human Kinetics suggests enough market demand for such a title.

When it came to the sports medicine literature on athletes with disabilities, the 1980s could be call the "descriptive decade." Although in some cases offering very specific information on the care and treatment of injured athletes, much of the available literature was essentially descriptive, based on personal experience or conducting reviews. In the 1990s, as disability sport really transitioned into elite competition, sports medicine research took to surveying patterns of injuries and unique forms of performance enhancement.

TRACKING AND TREATING INJURIES TO ELITE ATHLETES—THE 1990S

Perusal of the shelves of several university libraries indicates growth in the publication of textbooks in sports medicine in this decade, understandable in light of the firm establishment and expansion of the field as a medical specialty and growth in the associated paramedical fields. Significantly, many of these books included chapters on sport for athletes with disabilities. Some focused primarily on physiological and training aspects, reflecting the background of the scholars authoring them.[56] However, many included specific sections on the care and treatment of injuries, in addition to sections on physiology and medical classification systems.[57] Kathleen Curtis (by now long interested and well published on injuries) and Gailey's textbook chapter dealt almost entirely with prevention, care and treatment of injuries to athletes with disabilities, perhaps reflecting their physical therapy experience.[58] Finally, Harmer's chapter in a book on the epidemiology of sports injuries benefited from earlier studies in describing and tracking injuries, providing a comprehensive overview of the state of the knowledge at the time.[59]

The first of the Vista conferences was held in 1993 at the Rick Hansen Centre in Edmonton.[60] Aside from precedence as the first, the 1993 conference holds historical importance as the establishment of the IPC's Sport Science Committee came directly from it.[61] In the late 1990s and early 2000s, the IPC Sport Science Committee began to sponsor major research projects at the Paralympic Games, such as the recently published study of "boosting" practices among wheelchair athletes.[62]

Boosting came to light in the 1990s as an issue that transcended sports science and medicine boundaries. Now collectively decided to be a banned "doping" practice, boosting is the intentional inducing of autonomic dysreflexia in wheelchair athletes with spinal injuries above the T6 vertebra. The blocking of sympathetic nervous responses due to the injury means that a dramatic increase in blood flow and blood pressure can be induced by actions such as overtightening leg straps, inflicting self-injury in the lower body or clamping a catheter to cause bladder distension.[63] It can apparently improve racing performance up to 12 percent, but the response is not controllable and can lead to hemorrhaging and stroke. The first instance mention of intentional dysreflexia in the medical literature seems to have appeared in 1989, but the issue really came to light at the Vista 93 conference. Robert Burnham presented a paper on clinical aspects, and athlete Serge Raymond suggested that most athletes who could do this, in fact were.[64] Boosting has been the subject of debate and investigation since then.[65] This practice certainly signals the transition to elite disability sport that occurred in the 1990s, along with the problems arising.

Similar to articles that promoted and advocated for disability sport to sports medicine physicians in the late 1970s and 1980s, a selection of articles in the 1990s promoted the involvement of other related professions.[66] Some of these overviews were quite wide-ranging, covering common types of injuries, ways to treat immediately and more long term, in the sense of rehabilitating athletes back to their sport, a notable change over previous approaches.[67] Whereas some of this can be read as efforts to increase the client base for particular professions, there is recognition of the *athlete* part of "athlete with a disability."

The best demonstration of sports medicine's recognition of disability sport as elite-level sport, and its deepening involvement, is the large amount of work done on surveying and tracking patterns of injuries for different groups of athlete with disabilities across the 1990s.[68] Although much of the work represented "ground-clearing" studies that surveyed athletes on injuries they incurred and whether they sought treatment, some of it involved control groups and experimental conditions.[69] A major study, tracking over thirteen hundred athletes over an extended time frame, resulted in the creation of the Athletes with Disabilities Injury Registry, a sample drawn on for further research.[70] This particular study documented that one in ten athletes were injured over a two-year period, and that they did not seek medical consultation 15 percent of the time.

ONGOING MEDICAL INVOLVEMENT—THE 2000S

Arguably, the Paralympic Games entered a fourth stage in the 2000s. Cooperative agreements signed between the IOC and IPC integrated organizing committees for the Games and, later, the marketing efforts of the associations. On the field, sports truly professionalized, with record setting and national rivalries taking center stage.[71]

The 2000s are too current to really be able to assess in any true historical sense; there is not enough distance to allow determination of what events and people had significant impact. However, as we have done for previous decades, we can suggest the major trends in the sports medicine literature. Many of the same concerns and types of writing are evident. Although I have argued that the "sport" elements came to the fore in the 1990s, there are still a number of advocacy/overview-type articles in the

2000s.[72] The attention paid by associated professions remained—Christine Stopka wrote a series of articles for athletic trainers in the early part of the decade.[73] There were ongoing efforts in injury tracking, as well.[74] Even with the studies published, Yves Vanlandewijck remarked in 2006: "A relative paucity still exists in published research on the injury patterns and risk factors for injury among elite athletes with disabilities."[75] The IPC's Sport Science Committee has an ongoing project of injury surveillance.

A growing interest in child athletes with disabilities emerged in the 2000s.[76] This perhaps indicates a "trickle-down" from elite sport, or growing opportunities (and growing injury rates) for children with disabilities. Attention to athletes with disabilities other than spinal cord injuries also grew in the sports medicine literature, a positive trend.[77] If one considers all sports medicine literature of the three previous decades as a whole, it is clear that wheelchair athletes received the vast amount of attention. This ties into the historical legacy of wheelchair sport organizing first. It also speaks to hierarchies within disability sport, where wheelchair athletes map best onto the wider society's concept of "athlete," and thus receive disproportionate attention, media, medical and otherwise.[78]

CONCLUSION

Looking across the time period from the late 1960s through to the present, there is a clear movement from a firm rehabilitation orientation to physicians and other professionals recognizing and advocating for sporting aspects to a legitimate sports medicine for athletes with disabilities marked by tracking injuries and treating athletes. The development of a sports medicine in disability sport was initially hampered by the traditional therapeutic orientation and medical perception of people with disabilities. This is understandable, given that until even the early 1990s, many of the medical personnel involved possessed backgrounds in fields like physical medicine, orthopedics or neurology.

Disability sport expanded in the 1970s, with athletes with different types of disabilities coming together in multisport, multidisability competitions. In the late 1980s, the Paralympic Games became a major international competition similar in stature to its current state. Within sports medicine in the 1980s, there were efforts to describe the changing situation and bring attention to the specific conditions and concerns for athletes with disabilities. The first conferences on international disability sport took place, and by the end of the decade, enough work had been done in sport science and sport medicine to warrant significant reviews. The 1990s saw surveying and tracking injury as the major concern, and the related professions taking a promotional, information-sharing stance.

Sport is still part of a battery of therapeutic methods drawn on in enabling people with newly acquired disabilities to adjust to their impairments, so the rehabilitative element remains relevant. However, the elite level, in place since the early 1990s, is truly international-level competition, with the priority on performance, success and medal counts. Sports medicine is part of the process at the international level, at least at major championship games.[79] Getting to this point has been a slow process of growth, with sports medicine professionals seeming to react to and interact with developments in disability sport, rather than necessarily being at the forefront of change. Having said that, there were certain sport medicine professions that stressed the competitive sport aspects, with the participants being fully considered athletes, very early on as disability sport developed. Sports medicine has been an essential part over the last forty years in the shift from rehabilitating patients through sport to rehabilitating injured athletes in elite disability sport. As disability sport continues to develop and change, sports medicine concerns and practices will be fundamental elements in future historical change.

NOTES

1. This research was in part funded by a partnered grant for the History of Medicine from the Canadian Institutes of Health Research and Associated Medical Services (CIHR-AMS 91240).
2. Following common usage and "people-first language," I use the terms *athletes with disabilities* to describe participants and *disability sport* to describe the practice. See DePauw and Gavron, *Disability Sport*, 7–8. The latter term has come in for some criticism, aside from being grammatically unwieldy. David Howe points out that in most instances, it really still is sport organized by able-bodied people for athletes with a disability. He advocates the older term *sport for the disabled* to denote aspects of social power and sport's place in the "disability industry." See Howe, *Cultural Politics*, 1.
3. Bailey, *Athlete First*. More critical works assessing the current status of disability sport also include good histories of recent events. Brittain's *The Paralympic Games Explained* and Thomas and Smith's *Disability, Sport and Society* offer useful historical summaries of events in disability sport, in a writing style aimed at undergraduates. Howe's *Cultural Politics of the Paralympic Movement* also includes a historical chapter and unique perspectives in lived history told from the point of view of an anthropologist/athlete/administrator in disability sport.
4. For example, see DePauw and Gavron, *Disability Sport*, 38–43; Guttmann, "Development of Sport," 111; Webborn, "Fifty Years," 138–139.
5. The use of the word *attempt* is purposive given that much of this is such recent history, since (as will be discussed) the 1970s on. One issue with contemporary history is the question of whether we have enough distance to make a reliable assessment of the historical significance of events, their causes and effects. However, like many working in contemporary historical timeframes, I argue that this work represents a "first pass" at writing on the topic, with the expectation that later scholars will access more and different sources and offer subsequent reinterpretations (see Woodward, "Study of Contemporary History," 2–6). This is part of the process of historical scholarship, with contemporary history making initial contributions. Thanks to David Charters

of the history department at the University of New Brunswick, who works in military and strategic studies, for conversation and guidance on writing contemporary history.

6. Literature was identified through searches in SportDiscus, PubMed and MedLine databases, as well as snowballing from article references. Thanks to research assistant Scott Hill for his work on this, and to the document delivery department at the Harriet Irving Library, UNB, for their great service.

7. Interviews and discussions were held with seven key informants, all who held high-profile positions in national Paralympic committees or who contributed significantly to the sports medicine literature on disability sport. Given their ongoing work in the field, they will remain anonymous.

8. There are obvious affinities here for the Foucauldian idea of knowledge as discourse. As discussed in a leading cultural studies dictionary, "various social practices and institutions (for example, those of education, politics, religion and the law) are constituted by and situated within various forms of discourse (that is, ways of speaking about the world of social experience). A discourse, on this view, is a means of producing and organizing meaning within a social context" (Peter Sedgwick, "Discourse," in *Key Concepts in Cultural Theory*, ed. Andrew Edgar and Peter Sedgwick [London: Routledge, 2002], 117). This social constructionist idea of discourse underlines this paper, but I would not go so far to say that it is methodologically a discourse analysis.

9. Vertinsky, "Commentary," 87. Berryman's *Out of Many, One* is a detailed institutional history of the ACSM up until 1992.

10. Mathias, "Competing Demands," 196.

11. Although there are links between physiological measures of performance and sports medicine, I wanted to focus on injury management because currently, and over the last few decades, sport has been marked by an acceptance and normalization of risk, pain and injury. There is a strong sociological literature on sport, pain and injury. Readers would do well to start with two edited collections that cover many topic areas and include a number of key scholars working on them: Young, *Sporting Bodies, Damaged Selves* and Loland, Skirstad and Waddington, *Pain and Injury in Sport*. There is also a growing sociological literature on sports medicine and how physicians and professionals working within it must negotiate competing demands. See, for example, Malcolm, "Medical Uncertainty," 191–210; Pike, "Doctors Just Say," 201–219; Safai, "Healing the Body," 127–146; Theberge, "It's Not about Health," 176–194.

12. Some material, of course, crosses over from exercise to sport and back, because some physicians and academics conduct research in both branches. One final delimitation—this chapter does not deal with athletes with intellectual disabilities, other than in the context of the Paralympic Movement. Although there have been sports medicine professionals interested in Special Olympians, the issues and the movement itself are so different as to require a separate study.

13. The choice to draw on published literature likely means a disconnect between the trends identified here and the everyday practice of sports medicine physicians. However, very few sports medicine physicians regularly deal with elite athletes with disabilities unless they have links to a specific training program, even still. Survey research by Henehan and colleagues found that "exposure to disabled athletes" was one area of sports medicine fellowships rated as poor. See Henehan, Shiple and Coppola, "Nonsurgical Sports Medicine," 288–290.

14. Berryman, "Exercise and the Medical Tradition," 1–7.
15. Ryan, "History," xxxvii–xxxix.
16. Jackson, "History of Sports Medicine," 255. On the origins and early context of the ACSM, see Berryman, *Out of Many, One*, 39–74.
17. On international associations, see Ryan, "History," xl–xlv. On the team approach, see Wappes, "30 Years," 15.
18. Waddington, "Development of Sports Medicine," 179–181.
19. Ibid., 181–185.
20. Cronin, "Not Taking the Medicine," 26–27; Teetzel, "Sports, Medicine," 79–81. On official establishment of specialties, see Minigh, *Sports Medicine*, 19–21.
21. Sherrill and DePauw, "Adapted Physical Education," 40, 55.
22. Burch, "Reading between the Signs,'" 214–235. On the basic history of deaf sport, see the official CISS website, http://www.deaflympics.com/about (accessed 5 July 2010).
23. On sport as therapy, Mason, "R. Tait McKenzie's Medical Work," 45–70; Mason, "Sport in the Service." On work therapies and rehabilitation, see Reznick "Work-Therapy," 183–205.
24. Brittain's historical chapter is more analytical on Guttmann (*Paralympic Games Explained*, 8–11) than many of the more celebratory works, such as Lomi, Geroulanos and Kekatos, "Sir Ludwig Guttmann;" Scruton, "Sir Ludwig Guttmann," 52. Bailey, *Athlete First*, 15–18, 32–33, also offers a more evaluative stance.
25. There is some debate over the original meaning of the term *Paralympics*, coined at some point between 1964 and 1968. The debate centers on whether it meant "paraplegic Olympics" (as the general public often still thinks), or, as officially it stands now, "parallel Olympics," or in connection with them. Bailey, *Athlete First*, 6–7, and Brittain, *Paralympic Games Explained*, 15–16, both take on the origins of Paralympic terminology.
26. Stan Labanowich tracked US involvement in wheelchair sports and argues it offered a "twin track" to developments at Stoke Mandeville. Labanowich, "Physically Disabled in Sports," 34–37. Also see his PhD dissertation on wheelchair basketball in 1975.
27. DePauw and Gavron, *Disability Sport*, 39, 42–43; Doll-Tepper, "Disability Sport" 178–179. One of the more detailed versions of the rise and change of International Organizations of Sport for the Disabled (IOSDs) is Steadward and Foster, "History of Disability Sport," 471–496.
28. Steadward and Petersen, *Paralympics*, 29–34; Prystupa, Prystupa and Bolach, "Developmental Trends," 78–79. This article attempts some unusual and interesting quantitative analyses of developmental trends in the Paralympics.
29. At the time of the 1976 Games, Guttmann was president of both ISMGF and ISOD, helping somewhat with this transition. David Grieg made the 1976 Torontolympiad the focus of his master's thesis. His work analyzes a key moment in Canadian and world disability sport, and offers one of the more complete pictures of issues surrounding a particular set of Games. See Greig, "South African Apartheid and the 1976 Totontolympiad."
30. Stoke Mandeville in Aylesbury had the games for athletes with spinal cord injuries, and New York hosted the games for athletes with visual impairments, amputations and cerebral palsy. See Steadward and Peterson, *Paralympics*, 34. The wheelchair competitions were originally slated for the University of Illinois at Champaign, but funding fell through four months out. See Gold and Gold, "Access for All," 137.

31. On the often contentious history between the IOC and the IPC, see Mason, "Creating Image," 113–122. Also see Kell, Kell and Price et al., "Two Games"; Legg et al., "Examining the Inclusion," 244–258.

32. For good overviews of the many issues in disability sport, see DePauw and Gavron, *Disability Sport*, 241–256; Brittain, *Paralympic Games Explained*, 91–122 (106–122 on the place of women and athletes with severe disabilities). An edited collection by Gilbert and Schrantz, *The Paralympic Games: Empowerment or Sideshow?*, has several chapters that deal with problematic aspects, including the Paralympics and the media. In Howe's *Cultural Politics and the Paralympic Games*, his chapter on "The Politics of Sporting Disablement" (82–98) provides an excellent assessment of issues with medical classification. One of the more political and pointed critiques comes from Danielle Peers, "Governing Bodies."

33. Guttmann, "Sport and the Disabled," 367–391.

34. Ibid., 382.

35. For example, Guttmann, "Significance of Sport," 195–197; "Reflection," 225–240; Guttmann, "Value of Sport," 16–20, 45; Guttmann, "Development of Sport," 179–182.

36. Guttmann, "Sport and Recreation," 208–212, 217.

37. Guttmann, *Textbook of Sport*.

38. Bailey, *Athlete First*, 32. Guttmann had a particularly autocratic style as well, which served him well in establishing sport for the disabled, but annoyed many once disability sport expanded and democratized. See Bailey, *Athlete First*, 32–33; Howe, *Cultural Politics*, 35–36.

39. Shapira, "Is Medicine Catching Up," 57.

40. Ryan, "Another Olympics, Another Flame," 137; Ross, "Blind Break through Old Barriers," 98. On how ideas of sports medicine and rehabilitation were often considered one and the same, see Ghosh, "Sports Medicine," 275–276.

41. Sperryn, "Sport and Disability," 334.

42. Ibid., 336–337.

43. As one example, see the self-published biography of John Grant, who came from a neurosurgery background through wheelchair sport to chair the 2000 Sydney Paralympic Committee (*Different Theatres*).

44. Legg et al., "Historical Overview," 34.

45. DePauw, "Sport for Individuals," 81–82; Doll-Tepper and DePauw, "Theory and Practice," 3.

46. See Steadward, *Proceedings*. This research institute has gone through a number of name changes. Originally, it was the Research and Training Centre for Athletes with Disabilities. After the "Man in Motion" tour it was renamed the Rick Hansen Centre in 1988. In 2000, it was renamed the Steadward Centre for Personal and Physical Achievement, after the center's founder Robert W. Steadward, who, among other things, was the first IPC president.

47. Natvig, *Proceedings*. Papers included areas topics from physiology and biomechanics to doping in sport. Unfortunately, despite the best efforts of librarians and used book sellers, I have been unable to obtain a copy of these proceedings at time of writing.

48. Jackson and Fredrickson, "Sports for the Physically Disabled," 294–295. Frederickson was director of the field hospital at the 1976 Games; Jackson, originally an orthopedic surgeon, served as chairman of the Games. He was a major force in disability sport in Canada from the late 1960s until his recent death in January 2010.

49. Corcoran et al., "Sports Medicine," 699. Other articles around the same time also stressed the sporting similarities between athletes with disabilities and able-bodied athletes. See Jackson and Davis, "Value of Sports," 305; Shephard, "Exercise for the Disabled," 111.
50. Curtis, "Wheelchair Sportsmedicine," parts I–IV.
51. Stewart, "Handicapped in Sports," 183–190, is a good example of an overview article. Work that combines overview with a focus on classification includes: Schaeffer and Proffer, "Sports Medicine," 239–245; Jackson and Davis, "Value of Sports," 301–315. One entirely on classification is McCann, "Classification," S167–S170. Throughout the rest of this chapter, references will list articles on topics under discussion. None of these references is meant to be exhaustive, but instead indicative of the literature available.
52. Classification is meant to provide a level playing field, where athletes with similar impairments compete against each other. The historical legacy of disability sport organizing by disability group is that different groups operate under different classification systems, sometimes in the same sport. Although this is a medical issue, I am not going to deal with classification in much detail, because frankly, a history of changes in the classification systems is properly the object of its own study. It is still a massive debate, with implications in the new commercial era, for who belongs and gets to compete. One of the more recent (2006) Vista conferences (a semiregular, international multidisciplinary conference now sponsored by the IPC) focused entirely on classification issues. For good overviews on classification and its problems, see Howe, *Cultural Politics*, 82–98; Howe and Jones, "Classification," 29–46; Jones and Howe, "Conceptual Boundaries," 133–146; Wu and Williams, "Paralympic Swimming Performance," 251–270; Wu, Williams and Sherrill, "Classifiers as Agents," 421–436.
53. The proceedings, published as an edited book, are Sherill, *Sport and Disabled Athletes* (see Curtis and Dillon, "Survey," 211–216, in this collection).
54. Mangus, "Sports Injuries," 308. The other article was Mangus, "Medical Care," 90–95.
55. Shephard, "Sports Medicine," 226–247.
56. Bernhardt, "Physically Challenged Athlete," 242–251; Shephard, "Sports Medicine," 41–62; Shephard and Davis, "Sports and Recreation," 544–562.
57. Booth, "Athletes with Disabilities," 634–646; Fallon, "Disabled Athlete," 488–511; Ferrara and Palutsis, "Athletes with Different Abilities," 817–827; McCann, "Disabled Athlete," 174–197.
58. Curtis and Gailey, "Athlete with a Disability," 959–980.
59. Harmer, "Disability Sports," 161–174.
60. Steadward, R.D., E.R. Nelson and G.D. Wheeler, *Vista '93—The Outlook. Proceedings from Vista '93* (Edmonton, AB: Rick Hansen Centre, 1993). The discussions in sessions were also published as *The Outlook Companion*. These will serve as useful historical documents of the time period in disability sport.
61. Bailey, *Athlete First*, 155.
62. Bhambani et al., *Boosting in Athletes*.
63. Burnham, Wheeler and Bhambani, "Intentional Induction," 1–10; Webborn, "'Boosting' Performance," 74–75.
64. The earliest instance I could find was in an article aimed at family physicians who might have to deal with an athlete with a disability. See Schaeffer and Proffer, "Sports Medicine," 243–244. Burnham, "Intentional Induction," 224–241; Raymond, "Boosting," 242–249.
65. For example, Bhambani et al., *Boosting in Athletes*; Schmid et al., "Catecholamines Response," 2–7.

66. Buckley, "Physios," 20–21; Reynolds et al., "Paralympics—Barcelona 1992," 14–17; Salvary, "Sports Massage Therapist," 28–30; Webborn, "Role of a Medical Officer," 13–14.
67. See Stopka, "Sports Medical Concerns," 24–31. *Athletic Therapy Today* devoted a special injury to athletes with disabilities in 1997. See Buckley, "Medical Considerations," 5.
68. Burnham, Higgins and Steadward, "Wheelchair Basketball Injuries," 43–49; Ferrara and Davis, "Relationship," 115–120; Ferrara et al., "Injury Experience," 55–60; Hoeberigs, Debets-Eggen and Debets, "Sports Medical Experience," 418–421; Kegel and Malchow, "Incidence of Injury," 50–54; McCormack et al., "Injury Profiles," 35–40. In an article on the "state of the art" in 1999, Ferrara identified twelve studies across the decade, which does not include some of the ones noted above. See Ferrara, "Injuries to Athletes," 257–266.
69. Burnham et al., "Acute Median Nerve Dysfunction," 513–518; Burnham and Steadward, "Upper Extremity Peripheral Nerve Entrapments," 519–524.
70. Ferrara and Buckley, "Athletes with Disabilities," 50–60. Results are published more fully in Ferrara and Peterson, "Longitudinal Study," 221–224.
71. Howe, *Cultural Politics*, 7–10; 32–33.
72. Curiously, much of this seems to be in British journals. See Crompton, "Spreading the Massage," 6–7; Mitchell, "Assessing and Managing," 6–9; Nyland, "Paralympic Movement," 243–245; Pheasey, "Sport Science," 6–9.
73. Matthews White, "Sports Medicine," 46–57. Stopka's series: "Athletic Therapy for Athletes with Disabilities" (March 2003): 37–39; (May 2003): 23–25; (July 2003): 30–31.
74. Examples of this research include: Ferrara, "Injuries to Athletes," 137–143; Groah and Lanig, "Neuromusculoskeletal Syndromes," 201–208; Nyland et al., "Soft Tissue Injuries," 368–373; Ramirez et al., "Sports Injuries," 690–696.
75. Vanlandewijck, "Sport Science," xx.
76. Lai, Stanish and Staniah, "Young Athlete," 793–819; Patel and Greydanus, "Pediatric Athlete," 803–837; Wilson, "Exercise and Sports," 907–923.
77. Carroll, Leiser and Paisley, "Cerebral Palsy," 319–322; Naugle, Stopka and Brennan, "Common Medical Conditions," 18–20; Webster et al., "Sports and Recreation," S38–S44.
78. On hierarchies within disability and disability sport, see DePauw, "(In)Visibility of DisAbility," 421–424.
79. David Howe discusses how many athletes with disabilities do not have access to sports medicine outside of major competitions. Howe, "Role of Injury," 215–216. In the context of other work, several athletes on the Canadian wheelchair basketball teams complained to me about their lack of access to sports medicine outside of competition, with one discussing how regular doctors still have difficulty seeing her as an athlete in training with injuries, rather than a patient with complications.

BIBLIOGRAPHY

Bailey, Steve. *Athlete First: A History of the Paralympic Movement.* Chichester, England: Wiley, 2008.
Beaver, David P. "The Athlete with a Disability." In *Sports Medicine*, edited by A.J. Ryan and F.L. Allman, 429–446. San Diego: Academic Press, 1989.
Bernhardt, D. "The Physically Challenged Athlete." In *ACSM's Guidelines for the Team Physician*, edited by R.C. Cantu and L.J. Micheli, 242–251. Philadelphia: Lea and Febiger, 1991.

Berryman, Jack W. "Exercise and the Medical Tradition from Hippocrates through Antebellum America." In *Sport and Exercise Science: Essays in the History of Sports Medicine*, edited by J.W. Berryman and R.J. Park, 1–56. Urbana: University of Illinois Press, 1992.

———. *Out of Many, One: A History of the American College of Sports Medicine*. Champaign, IL: Human Kinetics, 1996.

Bhambani, Y., J. McTavish, S. Warren, W. Thompson, A. Webborn, et al. *Boosting in Athletes with High Level Spinal Cord Injuries: Incidence, Knowledge and Attitudes in Paralympic Sport*. Report to World Anti-Doping Agency by IPC Sport Science Committee, April 2009.

Booth, Darren W. "Athletes with Disabilities." In *Oxford Textbook of Sports Medicine*, edited by M. Harries, C. Williams, W.D. Stanish and L.J. Micheli, 634–652. New York: Oxford University Press, 1994.

Brittain, Ian. *The Paralympic Games Explained*. London: Routledge, 2010.

Buckley, Jane. "Physios—Vital for Disabled Sport." *SportHealth* 13, no. 4 (1995): 20–21.

Buckley, W.E. "Medical Considerations for Disabled Athletes: Theme Introduction." *Athletic Therapy Today* 2, no. 1 (1997): 5.

Burch, Susan. "Reading between the Signs: Defending Deaf Culture in Early Twentieth Century America." In *The New Disability History: American Perspectives*, edited by P.K. Longmore and L. Umansky, 214–235. New York: New York University Press, 2001.

Burnham, Robert. "Intentional Induction of Autonomic Dysreflexia Among Quadriplegic Athletes for Performance Enhancement: Efficacy, Safety and Mechanism of Action." In *Vista '93—The Outlook. Proceedings from Vista '93*, edited by R.D. Steadward, E.R. Nelson and G.D. Wheeler, 224–241. Edmonton, AB: Rick Hansen Centre, 1993.

Burnham, R.S, M. Chan, C. Hazlett, J. Laskin and R.D. Steadward. "Acute Median Nerve Dysfunction from Wheelchair Propulsion: The Development of a Model and Study of the Effect of Hand Protection." *Archives of Physical Medicine and Rehabilitation* 75, no. 5 (1994): 513–518.

Burnham, R.S., J. Higgins and R.D. Steadward. "Wheelchair Basketball Injuries." *Palaestra* 10 (1994): 43–49.

Burnham, R.S., and R.D. Steadward. "Upper Extremity Peripheral Nerve Entrapments Among Wheelchair Athletes: Prevalence, Location and Risk Factors." *Archives of Physical Medicine and Rehabilitation* 75 (1994): 519–524.

Burnham, R.S., G. Wheeler and Y. Bhambani. "Intentional Induction of Autonomic Dysreflexia among Quadriplegic Athletes for Performance Enhancement: Efficacy, Safety and Mechanism of Action." *Clinical Journal of Sports Medicine* 4 (1994): 1–10.

Burnham, R.S., G. Wheeler, M. Riding and R. Steadward. "The Implications of Boosting for Performance Enhancement." *Athletic Therapy Today* 2, no. 1 (1997): 36–39.

Carroll, K.L., J. Leiser and T.S. Paisley. "Cerebral Palsy: Physical Activity and Sport." *Current Sports Medicine Reports* 5 (2006): 319–322.

Corcoran, P.J., R.F. Goldman, E.F. Hoerner, C. Kling, H.G. Knuttgen, B. Marquis, B.C. McCann and A.B. Rossier. "Sports Medicine and the Physiology of Wheelchair Marathon Racing." *Orthopedic Clinics of North America* 11, no 14 (1980): 697–716.

Crompton, Katherine. "Spreading the Massage at the Paralympics." *SportEX Dynamics* 4 (April 2005): 6–7.

Cronin, Mike. "Not Taking the Medicine: Sportsmen and Doctors in Late Nineteenth-Century Britain." *Journal of Sport History* 34, no. 1 (2007): 23–35.

Curtis, Kathleen A. "Wheelchair Sportsmedicine: Part I: Basics of Exercise Physiology." *Sports 'N Spokes* 7, no. 1 (1981): 26–28.

———. "Wheelchair Sportsmedicine: Part II: Training." *Sports 'N Spokes* 7, no. 2 (1981): 16–19.

———. "Wheelchair Sportsmedicine: Part III: Stretching Routines." *Sports 'N Spokes* 7, no. 3 (1981): 16–18.

———. "Wheelchair Sportsmedicine: Part IV: Athletic Injuries." *Sports 'N Spokes* 8, no. 1 (1982): 20–24.

Curtis, K.A., and D.A. Dillon. "Survey of Wheelchair Athletic Injuries—Common Patterns and Prevention." In *Sport and Disabled Athletes*, edited by C. Sherill, 211–216. Champaign, IL: Human Kinetics, 1986.

Curtis, K.A., and R.S. Gailey. "The Athlete with a Disability." In *Athletic Injuries and Rehabilitation*, edited by J.E. Zachazewski David J. Magee, and William S. Quillen, 959–980. Philadelphia: W.B. Saunders, 1996.

DePauw, Karen P. "The (In)Visibility of DisAbility: Cultural Contexts and 'Sporting Bodies.'" *Quest* 49 (1997): 416–430.

———. "Sport for Individuals with Disabilities: Research Opportunities." *Adapted Physical Activity Quarterly* 5 (1988): 80–89.

DePauw, K.P., and S.J. Gavron. *Disability Sport*. 2nd ed. Champaign, IL: Human Kinetics, 2005.

Doll-Tepper, Gudrun. "Disability Sport." In *The International Politics of Sport in the Twentieth Century*, edited by J. Riordan and A. Krüger, 177–190. London: E & FN Spon, 1999.

———. "The Winter Paralympics: Past, Present, and Future." In *The Winter Olympics: From Chamonix to Salt Lake City*, edited by L. Gerlach, 281–303. Salt Lake City: University of Utah Press, 2004.

Doll-Tepper, G., and K.P. DePauw. "Theory and Practice of Adapted Physical Activity: Research Perspectives." *Sport Science Review* 5, no. 1 (1996): 1–11.

Ergen, E., F. Pigozzi, N. Bachl and H.H. Dickhuth. "Sports Medicine: A European Perspective. Historical Roots, Definitions and Scope." *Journal of Sports Medicine and Physical Fitness* 46, no. 2 (2006): 167–175.

Fallon, K.E. "The Disabled Athlete." In *Textbook of Science and Medicine in Sport*, edited by J. Bloomfield, P.A. Fricker and K.D. Fitch, 488–511. Champaign, IL: Human Kinetics, 1992.

Ferrara, M.S. "Injuries to Athletes with Disabilities: The State of the Art." In *New Horizons in Sport for Athletes with Disabilities: Proceedings of the International Vista '99 Conference*, vol. 1, edited by G. Doll-Tepper, M. Kröner and W. Sonnenschein, 257–266. Aachen: Meyer and Meyer.

Ferrara, M.S., and W.E. Buckley. "Athletes with Disabilities Injury Registry." *Adapted Physical Activity Quarterly* 13 (1996): 50–60.

Ferrara, M.S., W.E. Buckley, D.G. Messner and J. Benedict. "The Injury Experience and Training History of the Competitive Skier with a Disability." *American Journal of Sports Medicine* 20, no. 1 (1992): 55–60.

Ferrara, M.S., W.E. Buckley and C.L. Peterson. "Epidemiology of Sports Injuries for Athletes with Disabilities." *Athletic Therapy Today* 2, no. 1 (1997): 30–33.

Ferrara, M.S., and R.D. Davis. "Relationship of Sport Classification and Gender to Injury for the Athlete with Cerebral Palsy." *Sports Medicine, Training and Rehabilitation* 5 (1994): 115–120.

Ferrara, M.S., and G.R. Palutsis. "Athletes with Different Abilities." In *Athletic Training and Sports Medicine*, edited by Chad Starkey and Glen Johnson, 675–686. Rosemount, IL: American Academy of Orthopaedic Surgeons, 1999.

Ferrara, M.S., G.R Palutsis, S. Snouse and R.W. Davis. "A Longitudinal Study of Injuries to Athletes with Disabilities." *International Journal of Sports Medicine* 21 (2000): 221–224.

Ferrara, M.S., and C.L. Peterson. "A Longitudinal Study of Injuries to Athletes with Disabilities: Identifying Injury Patterns." *Sports Medicine* 30, no. 2 (2000): 221–224.

Ghosh, Aloke. "Sports Medicine for the Disabled and the Handicapped." *Journal of the Indian Medical Association* 64, no. 1 (1975): 275–276.

Gilbert, Keith, and Otto J. Schantz (Eds.). *The Paralympic Games: Empowerment or Sideshow?* Maidenhead, UK: Meyer & Meyer, 2008.

Gold, J.R., and M.M. Gold. "Access for All: The Rise of the Paralympic Games." *Journal of the Royal Society for the Promotion of Health* 127, no. 3 (2007): 133–141.

Grant, John. *Different Theatres: From Neurosurgery to Sport for People with Disabilities.* Self-published. Australia, 2005.

Greig, David A. "South African Apartheid and the 1976 Totontolympiad: A Historical Analysis of Influential Actions and Events Affecting the 5th Paralympic Games." Master's thesis, University of Windsor, 2005.

Groah, S.L., and I.S. Lanig. "Neuromusculoskeletal Syndromes in Wheelchair Athletes." *Seminars in Neurology* 20, no. 2 (2000): 201–208.

Guttmann, Ludwig. "Development of Sport for the Spinal Paralysed (II)." *Olympic Review* 111 (March 1977): 179–182.

———. "Reflection on the 1976 Toronto Olympiad for the Physically Disabled." *Paraplegia* 14 (1976): 225–240.

———. "Significance of Sport in Rehabilitation of Spinal Paraplegics and Tetraplegics." *Journal of the American Medical Association* 236, no.2 (July 12, 1976): 195–197.

———. "Sport and the Disabled." In *Sports Medicine*, edited by J.G.P. Williams, 367–391. Baltimore, MD: Williams and Wilkins, 1962.

———. "Sport and Recreation for the Mentally and Physically Handicapped." *Journal of the Royal Society of Health* 4 (1973): 208–212, 217.

———. *Textbook of Sport for the Disabled.* Aylebury, UK: HM and M, 1976.

———. "The Value of Sport for the Severely Physically Handicapped." *Olympic Review* 111 (January 1977): 16–20, 45.

Harmer, Peter A. "Disability Sports." In *Epidemiology of Sports Injuries*, edited by D.J. Caine, C.G. Caine and K.J. Lindner, 161–174. Champaign, IL: Human Kinetics, 1996.

Henehan, M., B. Shiple and G. Coppola. "Nonsurgical Sports Medicine Training in the United States: A Survey of Sports Medicine Fellowship Graduates." *Clinical Journal of Sport Medicine* 13, no. 5 (2003): 285–291.

Hoberman, John M. *Mortal Engines: The Science of Performance and the Dehumanization of Sport.* New York: Free Press, 1992.

Hoeberigs, J.H., H.B.L. Debets-Eggen and P.M.L. Debets. "Sports Medical Experience from the International Flower Marathon for Disabled Wheelers." *American Journal of Sports Medicine* 18, no. 2 (1990): 418–421.

Howe, P. David. *The Cultural Politics of the Paralympic Movement.* London: Routledge, 2008.

———. "The Role of Injury in the Organization of Paralympic Sport." In *Pain and Injury in Sport: Social and Ethical Analysis*, edited by S. Loland, B. Skirstad and I. Waddington, 211–226. London: Routledge, 2006.

Howe, P.D., and C. Jones. "Classification of Disabled Athletes: (Dis)Empowering the Paralympic Practice Community." *Sociology of Sport Journal* 23 (2006): 29–46.

Jackson, Douglas W. "The History of Sports Medicine. Part 2." *American Journal of Sports Medicine* 12, no. 4 (1984): 255–257.

Jackson, R.W., and G.D. Davis, "The Value of Sports and Recreation for the Physically Disabled." *Orthopedic Clinics of North America* 14, no. 2 (1983): 301–315.

Jackson, R.W., and A. Fredrickson. "Sports for the Physically Disabled." *American Journal of Sports Medicine* 7, no. 5 (1979): 293–296.
Jones, C., and P.D. Howe. "The Conceptual Boundaries of Sport for the Disabled: Classification and Athletic Performance." *Journal of the Philosophy of Sport* 32 (2005): 133–146.
Kegel, B., and D. Malchow. "Incidence of Injury in Amputees Playing Soccer." *Palaestra* 10 (1994): 50–54.
Kell, P., M. Kell and N. Price. "Two Games and One Movement?: The Paralympics and Olympic Movement." In *Learning and the Learner: Exploring Learning in New Times*, edited by P. Kell, W. Vialle, D. Konze and G. Vogl, 65–78. Wollongong: University of Wollongong. http://ro.uow.edu.au/edupapers/37/ (accessed 5 July 2010).
Knaus, Ronald L. "Physiological and Psychological Benefits of Exercise for Athletes with Disabilities: An Interview with George Murray." *Journal of Osteopathic Sports Medicine* 1, no. 4 (1987): 7–9.
Labanowich, Stan. "The Physically Disabled in Sports: Tracing the Influence of Two Tracks of a Common Movement." *Sports 'N Spokes* 12, no. 6 (1987): 33–38, 40, 42.
———. "Wheelchair Basketball: A History of the National Association and an Analysis of the Structure and Organization of the Teams." PhD dissertation, University of Illinois at Urban-Champaign, 1975.
Lai, A.M., W.D, Stanish and H.I. Staniah. "The Young Athlete with Physical Challenges." *Clinics in Sports Medicine* 19, no. 4 (2000): 798–819.
Landry, Fernand. *Paralympic Games and Social Integration*. Barcelona: Centre d'Estudis Olimpics UAB, 2010. http://olympicstudies.uab.es/pdf/wp041_eng.pdf (accessed 5 July 2010).
Legg, D., C. Emes, D. Stewart and R.W. Steadward. "Historical Overview of the Paralympics, Special Olympics, and Deaflmpics." *Palaestra* 20, no. 1 (2004): 30–35, 56.
Legg, D., T. Fay, M.A. Hums and E. Wolff. "Examining the Inclusion of Wheelchair Exhibition Events within the Olympic Games 1984–2004." *European Sport Management Quarterly* 9, no. 3 (2009), 243–258.
Loland, S., B. Skirstad and I. Waddington, eds. *Pain and Injury in Sport: Social and Ethical Analysis*. London: Routledge, 2006.
Lomi, C., S. Geroulanos and E. Kekatos. "Sir Ludwig Guttmann—'The de Coubertin of the Paralysed.'" *Acta Orthopaedica et Traumatologica Hellenica* 55, no. 1 (2010). http://www.acta-ortho.gr/v55t1_6.html (accessed 5 July 2010).
Madorsky, J.G.B., and K.A. Curtis. "Wheelchair Sports Medicine." *American Journal of Sports Medicine* 12, no. 2 (1984): 128–132.
Malcolm, Dominic. "Medical Uncertainty and Clinician–Athlete Relations: The Management of Concussion Injuries in Rugby Union." *Sociology of Sport Journal* 26 (2009): 191–210.
Mangus, Brent C. "Medical Care for Wheelchair Athletes." *Adapted Physical Activity Quarterly* 5 (1988): 90–95.
———. "Sports Injuries, the Disabled Athlete, and the Athletic Trainer." *Athletic Training* 22, no. 4 (1987): 305–310.
Mason, Fred. "Creating Image and Gaining Control: The Development of the Cooperation Agreements between the International Olympic Committee and the International Paralympic Committee." In *The Global Nexus Engaged: Past, Present, Future Interdisciplinary Olympic Studies*, edited by K.B. Wamsley, R.K. Barney and S.G. Martyn, 113–122. London: International Centre for Olympic Studies, University of Western Ontario, 2002.
———. "R. Tait McKenzie's Medical Work, and Early Physical Activity Programs for People with Disabilities." *Sport History Review* 39 (2008), 45–70.

————. "Sport in the Service of Restoration: Sport as Physical Therapy during the First World War." In *Actas X Congreso Internacional de Historia del Deporte*, edited by Jose Aquelsolo. Seville: Universidad Pablo de Olavide, 2005. http://www.cafyd.com/HistDeporte/htm/pdf/1–6.pdf (accessed 5 July 2010).

Mathias, Michael B. "The Competing Demands of Sport and Health: An Essay on the History of Ethics in Sports Medicine." *Clinics in Sports Medicine* 23, no. 2 (2004): 195–214.

Matthews White, Joan M. "Sports Medicine and Disability Sport." *Athletic Therapy Today* 9, no.1 (2004): 46–47.

McCann, B.C. "Classification of the Locomotor Disabled for Competitive Sports: Theory and Practice." *International Journal of Sports Medicine* 5 (1984): S167–S170.

————. "The Disabled Athlete." In *Prevention of Athletic Injuries: The Role of the Sports Medicine Team*, edited by F.O. Mueller and A.J. Ryan,174–197. Philadelphia: F.A. Davis, 1991.

————. "Sports for the Disabled: The Evolution from Rehabilitation to Competitive Sport." *British Journal of Sports Medicine* 30, no. 4 (1996): 279–280.

McCormack, D.A.R., D.C Reid, R.D. Steadward and D.G. Syrotiuk. "Injury Profiles in Wheelchair Athletes: Results of a Retrospective Survey." *Clinical Journal of Sport Medicine* 1 (1991): 35–40.

Miller, Stuart L. "Medical Aspects of Paralympic Sport." *SportEX Medicine* 42 (October 2009): 13–20.

Minigh, Jennifer L. *Sports Medicine*. Westport, CT: Greenwood Press, 2007.

Mitchell, Linda. "Assessing and Managing and Athlete with a Disability." *SportEX Medicine* 32 (April 2007): 6–9.

Natvig, Harald, ed. *Proceedings of the First International Medical Conference on Sport for the Disabled*. Oslo: Royal Ministry of Church and Education, State Office for Youth and Sports, 1980.

Naugle, K., C. Stopka and J. Brennan. "Common Medical Conditions in Athletes with Spina Bifida." *Athletic Therapy Today* 12, no. 1 (2007): 18–20.

Nyland, John. "The Paralympic Movement: Addition by Subtraction." *Journal of Orthopaedic and Sports Physical Therapy* 39, no. 4 (2009): 243–245.

Nyland, J., S.L. Snouse, M. Anderson, T. Kelly and J.C. Sterling. "Soft Tissue Injuries to USA Paralympians at the 1996 Summer Games." *Archives of Physical Medicine and Rehabilitation* 81 (2000): 368–373.

Patel, D.R., and D.E. Greydanus, "The Pediatric Athlete with Disabilities." *Pediatric Clinics of North America* 49 (2003): 803–837.

Peers, Danielle L. "Governing Bodies: A Foucaultian Critique of Paralympic Power Relations." MA Thesis, University of Alberta, 2009.

Pheasey, Clare. "Sport Science And Medicine Support For British Paralympic Swimmers." *SportEX Medicine* 25 (2005): 6–9.

Pike, Elizabeth C.J. "Doctors Just Say 'Rest and Take Ibuprofen': A Critical Examination of the Role of 'Non-Orthodox' Health Care in Women's Sport." *International Review for the Sociology of Sport* 40, no. 2 (2005): 201–219.

Prystupa, E., T Prystupa and E. Bolach. "Developmental Trends in Sports for the Disabled: The Case of Summer Paralympics." *Human Movement* 7, no. 1 (2006): 77–83.

Ramirez, M, J. Yang, L. Bourque, J. Javien, S. Kashani, M.A. Limbos and C. Peek-Asa. "Sports Injuries to High School Athletes with Disabilities." *Pediatrics* 123, no. 2 (2008): 690–696.

Raymond, Serge. "Boosting." In *Vista '93—The Outlook. Proceedings from Vista '93*, edited by R.D. Steadward, E.R. Nelson and G.D. Wheeler, 242–249. Edmonton, AB: Rick Hansen Centre, 1993.

Reynolds, J., A. Stirk, A. Thomas and F. Geary. "Paralympics—Barcelona 1992." *British Journal of Sport Medicine* 28, no. 1 (1994): 14–17.

Reznick, Jeffrey S. "Work-Therapy and the Disabled British Soldier in Great Britain during the First World War: The Case of Shepherd's Bush Military Hospital, London." In *Disabled Veterans in History*, edited by D.A. Gerber, 185–203. Ann Arbor: University of Michigan Press, 2000.

Ross, John. "Blind Break through Old Barriers to Sports." *Physician and Sportsmedicine* 5, no. 3 (1977): 98–102, 104.

Ryan, Allan J. "Another Olympics, Another Flame; Different Athletes, Different Game." *Physician and Sportsmedicine* 4, no. 10 (1976): 133, 135, 137.

———. "Examining the Disabled Individual." In *Sports Medicine*, edited by A.J. Ryan and F.L. Allman, 417–445. New York: Academic Press, 1974.

———. "History of the Development of Sport Sciences and Medicine." In *Encyclopedia of Sports Sciences and Medicine*, edited by L.A. Larson and D.E Hermann, xxxiii–xlvii. New York: MacMillan, 1971.

———. "Sportsmedicine History." *Physician and Sportsmedicine* 6, no. 10 (1978): 77–82.

Safai, Parissa. "The Demise of the Sport Medicine and Science Council of Canada." *Sport History Review* 36 (2005): 91–114.

———. "Healing the Body in a Culture of Risk: Examining the Negotiation of Treatment Between Sports Medicine Clinicians and Injured Athletes in Canadian Intercollegiate Sport." *Sociology of Sport Journal* 20 (2003): 127–146.

Salvary, Chris. "A Sports Massage Therapist at the IPC World Athletics Championships." *SportCare Journal* 2, no. 2 (1995): 28–30.

Schaeffer, R.S., and D.S. Proffer. "Sports Medicine for Wheelchair Athletes." *American Family Physician* 39, no. 5 (1989): 239–245.

Schmid, A., A. Schmidt-Trucksäß, M. Huonker, D. König, I. Eisenbarth, et al. "Catecholamines Response of High Performance Wheelchair Athletes at Rest and during Exercise with Autonomic Dysreflexia." *International Journal of Sports Medicine* 22 (2001): 2–7.

Scruton, Joan. "Sir Ludwig Guttmann: Creator of a World Sports Movement for the Paralyzed and Other Disabled." *Paraplegia* 17 (1979): 52–55.

Sedgwick, Peter. "Discourse." In *Key Concepts in Cultural Theory*, edited by A. Edgar and P. Sedgwick, 116–119. London: Routledge, 2002.

Shapira, Will. "Is Medicine Catching Up with the Wheelchair Athlete?" *Physician and Sportsmedicine* 2, no. 7 (1974): 54–57.

Shephard, Roy J. *Fitness in Special Populations*. Champaign, IL: Human Kinetics, 1990.

———. "Exercise for the Disabled: The Paraplegic." In *Current Therapy in Sports Medicine, 1985–1986*, edited by R.P. Welsh and R.J. Shephard, 110–111. Toronto: B.C. Decker, 1985.

———. "Sports Medicine and the Wheelchair Athlete." In *Sports and Exercise Medicine*, edited by S.C. Wood and R.C. Roach, 41–62. New York, Marcel Dekker, 1994.

———. "Sports Medicine and the Wheelchair Athlete." *Sports Medicine* 5, no. 4 (1988): 226–247.

Shephard, R.J., and G. M. Davis. "Sports and Recreation for the Physically Disabled." In *Sports Medicine*, 2nd ed., edited by R.H Strauss, 544–562. Philadelphia: W.B. Saunders, 1991.

Sherrill, Claudine, ed. *Sport and Disabled Athletes: The 1984 Olympic Scientific Conference Proceedings*, vol. 9. Champaign, IL: Human Kinetics, 1986.

Sherrill, C., and K. DePauw. "Adapted Physical Education." In *The History of Exercise and Sport Science*, edited by J.D. Massengale and R.A. Swanson, 39–109. Champaign, IL: Human Kinetics, 1997.

Sperryn, P.N. "Sport and Disability." In *Basic Book of Sports Medicine*, 333–337. Lausanne: Olympic Solidarity/IOC, 1978.

Steadward, Robert D. "Integration and Sport in the Paralympic Movement." *Sport Science Review 5*, no. 1 (1996): 26–42.

———. "The Paralympic Movement: A Championship Future." In *International Olympic Academy Annual Proceedings 2000*, 82–90. Lausanne: IOC, 2000.

———, ed. *Proceedings—First International Conference on Sport and Training of the Physically Challenged Athlete*. Edmonton: University of Alberta, 1979.

Steadward, R., and S. Foster. "History of Disability Sport." In *Adapted Physical Activity*, edited by R. Steadward, G. Wheeler and J. Watkinson, 471–496. Edmonton, AB: University of Alberta Press, 2003.

Steadward, R.D., E.R. Nelson and G.D. Wheeler, eds. *Vista '93—The Outlook. Proceedings from Vista '93*. Edmonton, AB: Rick Hansen Centre, 1993.

Steadward, R., and C. Peterson, *Paralympics: Where Heroes Come*. Edmonton, AB: One Shot Holdings, 1999.

Stewart, Marcus J. "The Handicapped in Sports." *Clinics in Sports Medicine 2*, no. 1 (1983): 183–190.

Stopka, Christine. "Athletic Therapy for Athletes with Disabilities, Part 1: Introduction and Overview." *Athletic Therapy Today 8*, no. 2 (2003): 37–39.

———. "Athletic Therapy for Athletes with Disabilities, Part 2: Special Conditions." *Athletic Therapy Today 8*, no. 3 (2003): 23–25.

———. "Athletic Therapy for Athletes with Disabilities Part 3: Rehabilitation Tips." *Athletic Therapy Today 8*, no. 4 (2003): 30–31.

———. "Sports Medical Concerns for Conditioning Athletes with Disabilities." *Strength and Conditioning 20*, no. 1 (1998): 24–31.

Teetzel, Sarah. "Sports, Medicine, and the Emergence of Sports Medicine in the Olympic Games: The Canadian Example." *Journal of Sport History 34*, no. 1 (2007): 75–86.

Theberge, Nancy. "'It's Not about Health, It's about Performance.' Sport Medicine, Health, and the Culture of Risk in Canadian Sport." In *Physical Culture, Power and the Body*, edited by J. Hargreaves and P. Vertinsky, 176–194. London: Routledge, 2007.

Thomas, N., and A. Smith. *Disability, Sport and Society: An Introduction*. London: Routledge, 2009.

Vanlandewijck, Yves. "Sport Science in the Paralympic Movement." *Journal of Rehabilitation Research and Development 43*, no. 7 (2006): xvii–xxiv.

Vertinsky, Patricia. "Commentary: What Is Sports Medicine?" *Journal of Sport History 34*, no. 1 (2007): 87–95.

Waddington, Ivan. "The Development of Sports Medicine." *Sociology of Sport Journal 13* (1996): 176–196.

Wappes, James R. "30 Years of Sports Medicine—and *Sportsmedicine*." *Physician and Sportsmedicine 31*, no. 1 (2003): 15–16, 18.

Webborn, A.D.J. "'Boosting' Performance in Disability Sport." *British Journal of Sports Medicine 33*, no. 2 (1999): 74–75.

Webborn, A.D.J. "Fifty Years of Competitive Sport for Athletes with Disabilties: 1948–1998." *British Journal of Sports Medicine 33* (1999), 138–139.

Webborn, Nick. "Role of a Medical Officer for the British Paralympic Association." *Physiotherapy in Sport 18*, no. 2 (1995): 13–14.

Webster, J.B., C.E. Levy, P.R. Bryant and P.E. Prusakowski. "Sports and Recreation for Persons with Limb Deficiency." *Archives of Physical Medicine and Rehabilitation 82*, no. 1 (2001): S38–S44.

Wilson, Pamela E. "Exercise and Sports for Children Who Have Disabilities." *Physical Medicine Clinics of North America 13* (2002): 907–923.

Woodward, Llewellyn. "The Study of Contemporary History." *Journal of Contemporary History* 1, no. 1 (1966): 1–13.

Wu, S.K, and T. Williams. "Paralympic Swimming Performance, Impairment and the Functional Classification System." *Adapted Physical Activity Quarterly* 16, no. 3 (1999): 251–270.

Wu, S.K., T. Williams and C. Sherrill. "Classifiers as Agents of Social Control in Disability Swimming." *Adapted Physical Activity Quarterly* 17 (2000): 421–436.

Young, Kevin. *Sporting Bodies, Damaged Selves: Sociological Studies of Sports-Related Injury*. Amsterdam: Elsevier, 2004.

Part II

Sports Medicine Organized

5 Women Professional Athletes' Injury Care

The Case of Women's Football[1]

Joseph A. Kotarba

The purpose of this chapter is to report on a preliminary study of work-related injuries among professional female athletes in the US. The number of women participating in professional sports, as well as the number of professional sports and leagues dedicated to women, has increased over the past twenty years. Women now participate in professional football, softball, golf, volleyball, basketball, bowling, tennis, boxing and other traditionally male sports. There is a substantial literature examining health, risk of injury, prevalence of injury and health care delivery to amateur male athletes, and a growing literature on these issues relevant to amateur female athletes. There is also a nascent literature on these issues relevant to professional male athletes, yet very little research has been conducted on professional female athletes' injury experiences, especially from a public health perspective.

One of the major barriers to developing this line of research is conceptualization. Researchers have focused on the *custodial* relationships between amateur athletes and their organizational environments. As students or club members, amateur athletes are dependent upon their schools, clubs or parents for health and injury care. In this study, I have conceptualized the relationship between professional female athletes and their organizational environments as *contractual*, that is, as a work relationship. Health and injury care, at least as related to job performance, is a condition of employment. Thus, the factors that shape health and injury care to factory and office workers—such as job description, social class of the worker and gender—can be examined in the work experience of the professional athlete. An aim of this chapter is to better draw out the policy implications of understanding health and injury among groups like professional female athletes by observing these behaviors in the organizational environments within which they occur.

Social psychology, largely in terms of symbolic interaction, has informed the disciplinary framework for this study.[2] The primary conceptual framework has been self-identity, specifically how a person's self-identity affects health and risk of injury, and consequently how illness, injury and access to health care affect one's sense of self-identity. In my early research on the chronic pain experience, I examined the relationship between pain and injury and self-identity among professional athletes.[3] I focused exclusively on team sports, and the athletes/respondents were all men. I found that athletes who were unsure about their status on the team (as a result of nonguaranteed contracts) or their ability to perform were most likely to disguise injuries and hide pain problems from coaches, managers, team physicians and team trainers for fear of losing their jobs. These athletes commonly consulted alternative healers on their own and at their own expense to manage pain and injury problems beyond the purview of team personnel. Retired athletes who succumbed to chronic arthritic and degenerative joint pain felt that their suffering was an unfortunate reminder that their previous self-identity as professional athlete was spoiled. In a comparative study, I found the same phenomenon among NASA astronauts at Johnson Space Center, whose strong desire to be assigned to a mission in space led them to overcome if not hide health problems (e.g., vision problems) that would detract from their expected identity of physical and psychological perfection.[4]

I began to consider the experiences of women in this line of research through a study of the wellness movement. Self-identity was a major factor in the decision to join preventive care and fitness programs (e.g., aerobics classes and cardiovascular monitoring) offered at work by employers, often on company time. Body image emerged as a key factor in the decision to enroll, since many women who felt they were fat or out of shape decided not to join because, ironically, they felt that the aerobics class was "really" intended for the "young and skinny" women who looked good in their tight Danskins and warm-up socks. The men who were potential class members seemed in general less susceptible to body image issues.[5]

I have recently come to see the value of extending my research to include organizational and community variables when approaching the study of women professional athletes; a major reason for this is the simple fact that women are increasingly involved in professional team sports. The literature on professional women athletes and their injuries is overwhelmingly devoted to individual participation; for example, dance,[6] figure skating,[7] downhill skiing[8] and horse riding.[9] There is likely one main reason why very little has written on women's professional team sports and injuries: they are a recent, albeit growing, phenomenon that is still overshadowed by the enormous world of men's professional team sports.[10]

A public health approach to understanding the place injuries and injury management have in women professional team sports is appropriate. A major reason for this claim is that the discipline and profession of public health posit *community* as a prominent concept in understanding the complete context health and illness behavior. As DiClemente, Crosby and Kegler, and others, have noted, public health is still very much community health, although the number and types of communities have increased historically.[11] There are two common(sense) definitions for community: a geographical area with defined boundaries and governance, or more generally and to the point, a group with shared characteristics and, interests, values and norms.[12] In this chapter, I will report on a comparative, ethnographic study of health and injury risk and care delivered to female professional athletes in terms of formal/medical care resources and informal/community care resources. The study examined how the various *communities* to which the women belong provide resources to help them manage injuries. I also examined the effectiveness of this care from the perspectives of the athletes and their injury care providers, for the purpose of improving the quality and availability of this care.

The driver of this study was the belief that the quality and availability of injury care varied to the degree the team/organization and league generated policy for, committed financing to, and regulated health and injury care for the athletes. The organizational structure of health and injury care is complemented by the culture of injury care present in the various communities relevant to the female athletes. The research questions included:

- What are the athletes' social-demographic-cultural-performance profiles?
- What are the typical and exceptional career patterns in each sport?
- What are the injuries common to each sport, and what are the risks of incurring these injuries?
- What health care is provided by the work organization/team, and by whom (e.g., team physician and team trainer)?
- What health care services are provided by the athletes themselves?
- What is the nature of the local culture(s) informing health and injury management?
- What are the strengths and shortcoming in the effectiveness of existing health and injury care systems?
- How can we improve health and injury care to professional female athletes?

METHODOLOGY

To answer these questions, I conducted a qualitative study of athletes and health/injury care providers in five cities in Region VI in the US, as identified by the Centers for Disease Control, the grant provider for this study. This was a comparative study involving eight teams and six team sports: the Houston Pinks and New Orleans Spice professional football teams; the Houston Comets and San Antonio Silver Stars professional basketball teams; the Oklahoma Outrage professional soccer team; the Houston Wranglers professional tennis team; the Houston Thunder professional softball team; and the Austin Rollergirls Roller Derby team. To establish comparative analysis, we also studied six female athletes who participated in individual professional sports: professional rodeo barrel racing, dance, boxing and golf.

I designed this study as a collaborative team field research project. The team was composed of graduate students and organized around a special problems graduate seminar. In all, we conducted observations at twelve events in five Region VI cities: Houston, San Antonio, Austin, Dallas and Oklahoma City. We conducted interviews with athletes (n = 35); coaches (n = 11); trainers, team physicians and exercise physiologists (n = 10); and team managers and owners (n = 4). We conducted the semi-structured interviews in the cities where the teams were located. The interviews lasted approximately one to two hours each, and were audio tape-recorded. We abided by all relevant human subjects considerations. We also conducted a site visit of each team's health care or training facility and videotaped practices and competitions where possible. All names used in this study and in the present report are pseudonyms.

We used thematic analysis to examine the qualitative data obtained through our interviews.[13] A major feature of the analysis was to create a typology of relevant community memberships, including both the resources and barriers they afforded professional female athletes. In this report, I will present an in-depth, case study examination of one team, the Houston Pinks professional football team. The two categories in our typology to be discussed are: the community of supportive team and the community of women.

CASE STUDY: PROFESSIONAL FOOTBALL

A brief discussion of the history and state of women's professional football in the US can provide insight into the broader sports context within which these women participate—including the gender inequities that they experience as women participating in a nontraditional, male-dominated sport—and has implications for their health and injury care. Women have participated in football since the early twentieth century, and, today, the only differences in the rules of the game for men and women are that female footballers use a smaller football and they kick from the thirty-yard line instead of the forty.

Women's football in the early years was designed primarily as entertainment for men. According to Mitchi Collete, a women's football historian, the first football game ever played by women happened circa 1896 in New York City.[14] One Saturday night at Sulzer's Harlem River Park, a pleasure club called Les Jolts Jarcon held a masked ball in the casino. The primary attraction was a football game between two teams of girls wearing the colors of Yale and Princeton. During play, the women tackled each other and fell into a heap: "There was a wild scramble and the crowd of men looking on, excited by the struggle, closed in with a rush."[15] Several decades later, circa 1925, it was recorded that at the San Diego State Teacher's College, two girls' football teams were assembled from the gymnasium classes. They played only one game but still made headlines in the *New York Times*.[16] The following year, several NFL teams like the Frankford Yellow Jackets fielded women's teams for the purpose of half-time entertainment. Then in the early 1930s, two Toledo-based women's tackle football teams played exhibition games against each other in a barnstorming tour through the Midwest. The women wore uniforms they gathered from a little league football team and were coached by men. Opposition to women playing football was strong, and the two Toledo teams disbanded when the US First Lady, Mrs. Herbert Hoover, accused the male coaches of exploiting "womanhood."[17]

By the 1960s, the sport for women started to become far more organized such that over the next four to five decades, numerous teams and leagues all over the US were established. Although conceived of as a gimmick, circa 1965, talent agent Sid Friedman started a women's semiprofessional tackle football league called the Women's Professional Football League (WPFL). In 1970, Patricia Palinkas was the first woman to play in a professional football game. She had a contract with the Orlando Panthers to hold the football for point-after touchdown kicks.[18] In 1976, a new league, called the National Women's Football League (NWFL), formed; within two years of its inception, it had enough teams to split into three divisions (Eastern, Southern and Western). In 1978, the Western States Women's Professional Football League was developed after the California-based franchises broke away from the NWFL (the restructuring largely the result of travel costs of intersectional play). The entire southern division of the NWFL quickly followed suit. Between the mid-1970s and the early 1980s, the NWFL had decreased in its number of teams by half, leaving them with only six. Five years later, in 1988, the NWFL had broken down even further because there was a separation among players who wanted to play tackle football and those who wanted to play flag-touch.

For several years during the 1980s, much of the excitement of women's football had begun to fade, but, in 1998, the WPFL was able to regenerate itself and has become the longest-operating women's professional sports league in the nation. Today, the league consists of eighteen teams, three of which began play in 2006. In August of 2000, the National Women's Football Association (NWFA) was formed by a sports and entertainment entrepreneur Catherine Masters. The association began with only two teams, but by the end of the 2004 season, the NWFA had fielded thirty-seven teams. And, as of early 2006, the league has landed an agreement with a Hollywood production company. The Independent Women's Football League (IWFL) was also formed in 2000, founded by a small group of women "dedicated to making the sport a household name."[19] Their primary mission has been to promote a positive, safe and fun environment for women to play tackle football. There are twenty-four teams in the league. The most recent addition to women's professional football is the Women's Football League, which began play in 2002. Twelve teams represent the league and will most likely expand with the growing notoriety of women's professional football.

Of the existing leagues, the WPFL is known to be the most competitive. When the league was initially founded, athletes came from sports like basketball, rugby and soccer. Today, the league is recruiting more women from established flag football teams, and women try out each year to play on a team either in the American Conference or the National Conference. Since the WPFL gained momentum in 1999, only three different teams have held the championship title: Houston Pinks, Northern Ice and Dallas Diamonds.

The focus of this chapter is on the Houston Pinks, founded in 1999. Currently, the team is owned by its head coach, and approximately sixty players make up the roster. In the mid-1970s, it cost about $10,000 to keep a women's football team in the league. Today the cost has risen to $30,000 and is borne chiefly by the head coach. Each player must locate sponsors to help raise $1,000 to be a part of the team. The money is mostly used to help cover travel costs. Houston Pinks players have recently gained limited access to a local sport facility, known as PLEX, to train in the off-season. This facility also services NFL players. As one player remarked of the head coach:

> He's put us in with the professionals so we can have that feeling. Before, we weren't professionals—we were working out in the backfields of the school with ants and mosquitoes biting us and no lights. Now we have posters, calendars, media, 5k runs—I love the coach!

Overall, the Pinks are a low-budget business operation. Attendance is approximately two hundred to three hundred for each home game, and many fans attend as "guests." We would thus expect to find health and injury care to also be low budget.

THE RISK TO WOMEN FROM PLAYING FOOTBALL

DeHaven and Lintner state that for both sexes, contact sports cause more injuries than noncontact sports do, and strains and sprains are the most common injuries in both men and women.[20] Fortunately, players on the Pinks have not experienced many major injuries, but minor ones occur all the time. Jane, the team owner, noted that the most severe injuries she had seen were knee injuries, torn ligaments, meniscus tears and dislocated shoulders; she also knew of a few broken ribs and mild concussions. Mr. Cook, a team volunteer, who had been with the team for three years, also mentioned the same kinds of common injuries: sprained ankles, sprained knees, dislocated shoulders, bruises and fractures. There are no official team data on incidence and severity of injuries.

To a large extent, the injuries were related to player position. For example, Julie, a linebacker and fast-food restaurant manager, had numerous problems with her lower back—and complications that have arisen from her lower back injuries—as a result of her position as tackle on the team:

Most of the issues are with my lower back though. And recently, all the pressure I had experienced over the years, I've had some trouble with my bladder. I had surgery to repair my bladder. A lot of squatting and positioning would cause my bladder to do its own thing. That's something I've had a lot of work done on. With my back, I see a chiropractor and do a lot of core strengthening. After five years of having problems with my bladder, I've begun talking to more people, and found out I could fix it. But lower back injuries are very common. It's all the pounds of gear. Because this is a part-time job and not how we make a living, we don't spend all the hours in the gym strengthening those more important parts, so you see a lot of low back pains and neck strains. Last year, there were a few ACL injuries because of all the turning and the quick cuts in some of those positions. In my position, you see more of the lower back injuries.

A good example of a common injury is an ACL knee injury. Boden, Griffin and Garrett assume that at least one-third of ACL-deficient patients require surgery,[21] at about $17,000 per reconstruction—a high cost for the most of the players at Houston Pinks. An ex-player, Janet, played for the first four years of the team but then had to have surgery on her knee and her foot. After an absence of two years, she returned to the Pinks and came to the tryouts. Her son, who came to support and watch her, told the story of her injury:

> In the game against Dallas three years (Pinks lost) ago she broke her foot in the last quarter but didn't know, so she kept playing on it. She also tore ligaments in her knee and had to get knee surgery. She has a two-inch screw in her foot. She took three years off, rehabilitated it and got the okay (from the sports doctor) to come try out. The broken foot is not a normal injury for the players but things getting torn because not stretching enough and things bending the wrong way. . . . The difference between men and women? We think it's the same injuries, the same game—ball's a little smaller, that's it. It's a lot of fun to watch. Talk about someone with a lot of heart—she's coming back with a screw in her foot.

Another commonly cited comparison with men is that both play football and put up with risk and incidence of injuries because "we like to hit."

THE COMMUNITIES OF CARING

The general finding of the broader study is that the quality and availability of health and injury care for female athletes are lower than that provided for men. Another important distinction is that the range of professional health and injury care options among women is much narrower than those afforded men. A useful analytical strategy for sorting out the varieties of health and injury care is *social class*. In both the social sciences and in common parlance, *social class* refers to the social position in society shared by people who have the same economic resources and potentials. We ordinarily think of three classes: the upper class, composed of people with great wealth largely accumulated by property ownership and inheritance; the middle class, composed of professional people and others with high-paying salaried jobs; and the working class, composed of people who work hard for hourly wages. Although these definitions are clearly oversimplified, they are useful in separating the status of professional athletes by gender and the quality of health and injury care afforded them. Male professional team sports have three classes: upper class (e.g., the National Football League), the middle class (e.g., professional soccer) and working class (e.g., local professional wrestling and rodeo).[22] The quality of health and injury care relates very closely to the economic value of the player to the team. In contrast, there are only two "social classes" in the female sports studied: *middle class*, as exemplified by the (now-defunct) Houston Comets basketball team, and *working class*, as exemplified by all other team sports examined in the larger study, including women's football and the Houston Pinks. Women who compete in individual sports—golf, dance, barrel racing and gymnastics—are in economic and occupational terms proprietors, providing their own health and injury care. More affluent individual sports (golf and tennis)—especially with corporate endorsements—allow for high-quality care (e.g., personal trainers and medical specialists).

The role of *community* appears more relevant to female than male athletes. Since female professional team sports are middle class or lower in status, their participants do not routinely have access to the high-quality care afforded their male counterparts. Therefore, these female athletes depend much more heavily on their immediate, nonmedical communities for health and injury care. There are, in fact, three communities—*the intimate community of family, the supportive community of women* and *the informal community of teammates*—that provide this care. These communities provide fairly holistic (cognitive, affective and evaluative) support during times of distress related to participation in professional football. In the remainder of this chapter, I will explain the nature of working-class health and injury care delivered to the Pinks by the team. I will then describe the supplementary health and injury care provided by the women's supportive communities.

WORKING-CLASS HEALTH CARE
PROVIDED BY THE TEAM

All the players understood the limited nature of health and injury care provided by the team. Mary, a defensive back and office secretary, explained how their care is different than other women's sports, especially those subsidized by men's sports teams:

> It's all about having the services available and accessible to you. Most women's sports just aren't as significant—they don't generate a lot of revenue, they don't get national TV, so they don't have the money within the systems . . . Look at the Comets [professional women's basketball team in Houston]: they're subsidized by the Rockets [professional men's basketball team in Houston]. The WNBA is attached to the NBA so they've got stuff but since the Pinks isn't attached to the Texans [professional men's football team in Houston], we've got nothing.

Mary's understanding of the status of the Comets is, in fact, a bit faulty. In the larger study, we discovered that the care provided by the Comets was middle class at best. For example, the Comets did not have a full-time trainer on staff. They relied on contract trainer services. Nevertheless, her general understanding of variations in quality is essentially correct.

Trainers and Facilities

All the players interviewed told us that the team did have good athletic trainers, but that they served on a voluntary basis. The players felt that the overall quality of training and conditioning was enhanced by Coach Williams's contacts as a former professional football player. For example, Coach Williams was recently able to obtain some training time for the women at the PLEX, a sophisticated training complex utilized by the Houston Texans professional football team. Darlene, a defensive back and private sector chemist, emphasized the importance of the coach's personal contacts:

> We have a coach this season who played in the NFL, so he knew about these services and has an existing relationship with the owner of PLEX. If he didn't know somebody, the team still wouldn't have it (professional training facility) . . . he wants his players to be physically and mentally ready.

When the Pinks were able to train at PLEX, there were physical therapists and personal trainers on-site to help athletes build strength in order to reduce risk and incidence of injury. There was even a psychotherapist on staff. Again, the players were now in a position to enjoy services not previously available to them. Since the Pinks did not have the financial resources to hire their own full-time trainer, Danny—the owner of PLEX and a friend of the coach—became a "significant blessing for the team," as Mary said. Yet, even with this recent positive development, Mary noted:

With all the money restrictions, an on-staff trainer is really needed. We are always looking for volunteer trainers, and you don't find them all the time.

The opportunity to train at PLEX was also seen positively with regards to the team's training schedule. In the off-season, players practiced three times a week (Tuesdays, Thursdays and Saturdays). Once the season began, they generally trained twice a week. Occasionally, a third practice is scheduled for some Saturdays and other Saturdays are game days. The players' concern was the relationship of the training schedule with their personal work schedules, since they would train on Saturday only to go to work on Monday with aches and pains. They would then practice again on Tuesday, so, typically, there would very little time for their injuries to heal or for them to seek care. With a facility like PLEX at their disposal, players were now able to go there on Monday or Tuesday at practice and possibly see a health care provider at the facility instead of having to seek treatment outside of the team or instead of ignoring their pain and injuries. Mary added:

> Because PLEX is all-inclusive, you can do everything. A lot of the women were worried about getting membership to a gym, but now they have this facility, and they have trainers at their disposal. Nevertheless, access to PLEX does not extend through the season.

Thus, the semblance of good care afforded the women was not provided during the season when they needed it most.

Paramedics/Emergency Medical Technicians (EMT)

During the games, the league requires the home team to have an EMT in the field. But during practices, the team could not afford to have an EMT present. During practices, if something happens, they have to get in their own cars and drive teammates to the hospital. There have been injuries during practice, but fortunately there have not been any serious injuries requiring immediate hospitalization. A serious incident would require ambulance transport to the local hospital emergency room, but it was not clear who would pay for that.

Health Insurance

The team does not provide health insurance to the players. Most of the players do, however, have health insurance, Mary noted:

> You have to have your own insurance, if something happens you can't tell them that you play football and you hurt yourself during the game.

You tell something else, like you fell down when you were walking in the morning or something.

Another player, Susan, a quarterback and college student, explained her situation:

I'm a college student, I don't have that great of insurance—you just gotta work through it [injuries]. You gotta do what you gotta do, that's life period.

The players who have health insurance are covered either as spouses or dependents, or as employees in their "day jobs." Those players who do not have health insurance depend on Medicaid for coverage. None of this insurance coverage was designed specifically for their "work" as professional football players. For those players who have health insurance through work, a common strategy is to claim that the injury occurred while engaging in exercise or other wellness activity.

Medical Doctors

The team does not have any contract with a medical doctor, but relied on Dr. Francisco, an orthopedic surgeon who sponsors them and comes out to all the games. His services are pro bono at the game. He does, however, invite the women to come to visit him in his office if an injury occurs. Jane noted: 'It's adequate as long as we go out and seek it. . . . But, you still have to pay for it." Jane's point is that Dr. Francisco's services were stopgap and not intended to be comprehensive health and injury care. All follow-up care was scheduled according to regular patient appointments.

In addition to Dr. Francisco, there were several other doctors who acted as team sponsors, and occasionally offered on-site services. Mary approached the issue realistically:

Until this season, players were really relying on "what do I do? Go to your own physician." There's the conflict: being professional but insurance being covered under primary employer—it's a gray area. Players have to go to their doctors.

THE INFORMAL COMMUNITY OF PLAYERS

The players themselves and among themselves comprise an informal community. They take care of each other either in the absence of adequate team care or as a supplement to team care. Let's look at pregnancy. Since this is a women's team and there is no routine clinical care, we asked about the provision of pregnancy tests for the players. Barbara, a linebacker and housewife, told us that they do not have such tests and that, to her knowledge, no such situation (i.e., pregnancy) had occurred:

> We have no idea if someone's out there and pregnant. But in the player contract, it says you can't get pregnant during the season—if you do, notify the team immediately. One player last year, I didn't even know why she stopped, and then I saw her and she was pregnant. They should have a test. Well, we have to pay for physicals ourselves. But women are more responsible. This isn't some kind of flaky thing with an immature teenager out there playing and pregnant. So, the likelihood of that . . . no. Some women won't pull themselves if they're injured, but for pregnancy, they're a lot more responsible. If they're sexually active, they're going to take all the precautions not to get pregnant. That's not an issue. She decided to have a baby, and she quitted, and came back later. We would take care of each other, if I see someone pregnant and trying to play, I would say, "Girl, you better stay off."

The decision to hide or disguise a medical condition is common among both male and female athletes whose employee status on the team is questionable. Among male professional athletes, a visible injury can result in being cut from the team and the loss of significant income.[23] Among female professional football players, a visible physical condition of any kind can result in the loss of a major source of self-esteem and identity. We did not, however, observe any woman playing while pregnant. The point is that the players take serious responsibility for monitoring and controlling each other's health and body status.

For injuries that were visible, the women were very supportive of one another and careful to make the injured player stay away from practice and play until healed. The passion for the game, however, leads players to circumvent that rule. Suzan, a kicker and running back, noted:

> Both my shoulders are tore up right now and, the sad thing is, I don't even have good insurance to have it really looked at right now. I've been blessed and fortunate not to have too many injuries. Alice, the first game we played, she broke her foot and now she has a metal plate in there for life, for us. She's still back playing for us. I watched Vera the other day, she hurt her ankle from skating. And Serena was like, that's nothing, you gotta work through your pain, so I was like, Dang! . . . That's the same kind of mentality I got—work through it. The sad part is that you really can't do anything about it; you just gotta play through it. And if you want it bad enough, that's my mentality, I want it so bad! I'll tape it up, ice it up, take shots to numb it, whatever I have to do to be able to get out there and play.

When we asked whether the trainers or coaches advised her to not play through an injury, Susan's response was:

I don't think they even know. I've never really been like "Hey, can you look at my shoulder?" They might say something crazy like, "Go have your doctor look at it and if you don't get it looked at before the next game, you can't play."

Most of the players believe that women's football is not much different from men's football. They feel that the reason that they may have more injury risk is because of the poor training that they have. Lora, a defensive back and legal assistant who never had an injury explained:

I don't think we're more injury prone (than the men). People say stuff about the breast, but I don't think so. We even have breast plates now. Vicki, she had breast cancer, she came back with a breast plate. So the breast ain't all of that. It's about how you tackle and how you wrap up—if you don't do it right you're going to be injury prone.

Since athletic trainers were not readily available, the three players on the team who were personal trainers would commonly advise other players about what to do with regards to injury. Jane, a receiver and personal trainer, explained how it was helpful for her to be a personal trainer and a football player:

Being a personal trainer helps me a lot. Unlike most of the players in the team, I do exercises all the time. I know how to do things better, that's my job. I think because of that I get less injury [*sic*] than the other players. I never had a major injury. I am in good shape all the time; this is what I do. I sometimes teach other players how to do certain things.

THE SUPPORTIVE COMMUNITY OF WOMEN

With the exception of the emergency care needed for relatively few major injuries incurred, most of the care that was delivered to the Pinks was community-based injury care. Even self-administered care was heavily informed and directed by practical knowledge emanating from the community of women. Players generally used painkillers and ice to immediately manage pain. They took "sick days" off from work or school to stay at home to rest in bed for lingering injuries. Since beginning to practice at PLEX, players have had some access to clinicians for minor injuries, but are only given advice to consult medical doctors for more serious issues.

Since the Pinks are a close-knit and informal group, the team leadership takes special care to monitor players' health—they simply do not have the resources to delegate that responsibility to professionals. Mary, a defensive tackle and team general manager, discussed the "family" nature of health care on the team:

In the locker room, you find that people who've had that injury will support you. We previously had someone who was a chiropractor. She would help. People help each other stretch out. There's always someone who has some kind of pill—Aleve, et cetera. We had someone who was out for a while and she came back but we had to watch out for her. The linemen . . . there's a family right there. She played to my left so it was my responsibility to watch out for her and say when she needed to be taken out. Make sure they eat right, take care of themselves, and remind them when they're at their limit. So it's not so much emotional support but reminding each other that you're part of a whole and if you're not at your best, we're not at our best. So thinking of the line, there can't be a weakest link.

Mary noted that caring also takes place during the game. She is the shortest player on the team, barely reaching five feet, five inches. Line players on her left and right are always looking out for her and asking if she needs help blocking a "chick" who is one hundred pounds heavier than her.

One of the most sociologically interesting if not amazing sites to observe on the sidelines during a game is the number of nurses, nurse practitioners, female physicians and physical therapists there as volunteers. Some are there to recruit clients to their practice, and some are there to be part of the excitement. In conversation with them, however, one learns quickly that the essential reason they are there is to support other women who are courageous enough to play tackle football. Margaret is a neurological physician who claims she lives vicariously through the Pinks:

This is the most exciting sporting event I have ever attended. The girls are tough but sweet—couldn't ask for more. I really do not have an agenda—I just want to help out if needed. . . . I guess my value lies in looking over players who get banged on the helmet, to make sure there are no concussions . . . I have seen two cases this season and neither was in any way serious. If they were, I know we would hold her out of the game.

In a recent season, the team had a player who was a masseuse. The players all agreed that pro bono massages were very helpful, especially after a rough game. The team could not afford to place a masseuse on staff. The players insisted that they help each other whenever they can, whether in health care or good advice. Jane, a quarterback and nurse, suggested differences between men's and women's teams in this regard:

Women are more nurturing by nature, but more women would seek professional help than a male because he might try to just walk it off. These are major injuries so it's not like because they are women they help each other out in many more ways. You can only be more understanding. Because the guys might tell each other to just walk it off, but the girls might ask "are you okay?"

Lora, a linebacker and community college student, described the team's response to a player with a serious health problem:

> If somebody has a problem, we watch each other's back. Last year, someone had breast cancer and we all got together and gave her a little surprise gift: a breast plate. And she was still able to play with her breast plate when the cancer came back. Good things and big things happen.

CONCLUSION

Kaplan has argued that when women defended their roles as athletes it was a mere "supplication of normality, an apology for having dared to step out of the fragile female role and be vigorous."[24] The trouble, she says, is that too many women say, "I can do this *even though* I'm a woman" instead of "This is *what it is* to be a woman." Although it is true that the women in our study commonly compared themselves to men to make a point during interviews, very few of them seemed motivated to play football by feminist ideology, if you will; rather, they like the pleasure of the sport itself or the good feeling it produces. Feminist ideology enters the formula strongly in the way it informs the community of women, which helps supplement the lack of top-quality health and injury care. We found this to be the case for most of the players with whom we spoke. Gloria, a wide receiver and advertising executive, has always had a passion for football.

> When I was young, I had dreams of playing for the Houston Oilers until I realized women were not able to. I played flag football in college and found out from my cousin that there was a professional women's football team in Houston, the Pinks. I decided to look for employment in Houston so I could try out for the Pinks. I'm really happy with my decision . . . It's not about doing what the boys can do, it's fun and we enjoy doing it.

Tracy, the center and a plumber, has always been an athlete:

> In college I played intramural sports. I was a middle distance runner and played soccer. After graduating from college I moved back to Houston and got involved in flag football. I've always been a huge football fan and was really excited when my friend talked to me about a women's pro football team starting. I originally tried out for the Houston team but they wanted a certain type and I'm only half the size of that. But I'm a player that wants the physical contact . . . I just want to hit somebody.

In conclusion, I have reason to believe that the structure and delivery of health care to women professional football players in other leagues and teams is essentially the same as it is for the Pinks. The team owners and management are well-intentioned, but cash-strapped, executives. I propose two follow-up studies to the preliminary one reported here. First, we clearly need a formal inventory of injuries, medical and non-medical responses and the various injury care systems established for all women's football teams. Second, we need to examine the more general, social-psychological features of women football players. Specifically, how do efforts to establish an identity as a football player affect one's risk-taking behavior?

NOTES

1. Funding supported by Grant No. T42CCT610417 from the National Institute for Occupational and Environmental Health (NIOSH)/Centers for Disease Control and Prevention (CDC) to the Southwest Center for Occupational and Environmental Health (SWCOEH), a NIOSH Education and Research Center.
2. Sandstrom, Martin and Fine, *Symbols, Selves, and Social Reality.*
3. Kotarba, "Thoughts on the Body"; "Perceptions."
4. Kotarba, "Social Control Function."
5. Kotarba and Bentley, "Workplace Wellness Participation."
6. Gorrick and Lewis, "Cancer Hazards."
7. Lipetz and Kruse, "Injuries and Special Concerns."
8. Cheung and Steinmann. "Surgical Approaches to the Elbow."
9. Rossi, Lubowitz and Guttmann, "The Skier's Knee.".
10. Lopiano, "Women and Modern Sport."
11. DiClemente, Crosby and Kegler, *Emerging Theories.*
12. Minkler and Wallerstein, *Community-Based Participatory Research.*
13. Lofland, *Analyzing Social Settings.*
14. Collete, "History of Girls' Football."
15. Ibid.
16. Independent Women's Football League, *Official Website.*
17. Ibid.
18. Kantor, "The History of Women's Professional Football."
19. Independent Women's Football League, *Official Website.*
20. DeHaven and Lintner, "Athletic Injuries."
21. Boden, Griffin and Garrett, "Etiology and Prevention."
22. Kotarba, "Professional Athletes' Injuries."
23. Kotarba, *Chronic Pain Experience.*
24. Kaplan, *Women and Sports.*

BIBLIOGRAPHY

American Association of University Women. "History of Women in Sports Timeline." http://www.northnet.org/stlawrenceaauw/timeline.htm (accessed 12 November 2008).

Andrews, James, Gary Harrelson and Kevin Wilk. *Physical Rehabilitation of the Injured Athlete*. Philadelphia: W.B. Sunders Company, 1998.

Beim, Gloria. *The Female Athlete's Body Box*. New York: Contemporary Books, 2003.

Boden, B.P., L.Y. Griffin and W.E. Garrett. "Etiology and Prevention of Noncontact ACL Injury." *Physician and Sportsmedicine* 28 (2000): 53.

Centers for Disease Control and Prevention. "Current Trends Injuries Associated with Horseback Riding—United States, 1987 and 1988." *Morbidity and Mortality Weekly Report* 39, no. 20 (1990): 329 332. http://www.cdc.gov/mmwr/preview/mmwrhtml/00001626.htm (accessed May 6, 2012).

Cervando, Angelita. *Woman's Golf—A History from Aprons to Nine-Irons*. Denver, CO: Hovis Publishing, 1995.

Cheung, E.V. and S.P. Steinmann. "Surgical Approaches to the Elbow." *Journal of the American Academy of Orthopedic Surgery* 17 (May 2009): 325–333.

Clarke, K.S., and W.E. Buckley. "Women's Injuries in Collegiate Sports: A Preliminary Comparative Overview of Three Seasons." *American Journal of Sports Medicine* 8, no. 3 (1980): 187–191.

Coakley, Jay J. *Sport in Society: Issues and Controversies*. 3rd ed. St. Louis, MO: Times Mirror/Mosby College Publishing, 1986.

Cohan, Jillian. "With a Can-Do Attitude, Women Enter the World of Competitive Roller Derby." *Wichita Eagle*, 19 April 2006.

Collete, Mitchi. "A History of Girls' Football." *Toledo Blade*, 5 September 1978.

DeHaven, K.E., and D.M. Lintner. "Athletic Injuries: Comparison by Age, Sport, and Gender." *American Journal of Sports Medicine* 14 (1986): 218–224.

DiClemente, Ralph J., Richard A. Crosby and Michelle C. Kegler, eds. *Emerging Theories in Health Promotion Practice and Research*. San Francisco, CA: Jossey-Bass, 2002.

Drinkwater, Barbara, ed. *Women in Sport: Volume VIII of the Encyclopaedia of Sports Medicine*. Malden, MA: Blackwell Publishing, 2000.

Gill, Diane. "Psychological, Sociological, and Cultural Issues Concerning the Athletic Female." In *The Athletic Female*, edited by Arthur J. Pearl, 19–40. Champaign, IL: Human Kinetics Publishers, 1993.

Gorrick, J.G., and S.L. Lewis. "Cancer Hazards for the Dancer." *Occupational Medicine* 16, no. 4 (2001): 609–618.

Hasday, Judy L. *Extraordinary Women Athletes*. San Francisco, CA: Children's Press, 1957.

Hass, Nancy. "When Women Step Into the Ring." *New York Times*, 1 October 2000, 4C.

Haycock, C.E. *Sports Injuries, Women in Sports*. Lakeland, TN: PSG Publishing Company, 1981.

Independent Women's Football League (IWFL), *Official Website of the Independent Women's Football League*, http://www.iwflsports.com (accessed 13 November 2008).

Kantor, S. "The History of Women's Professional Football." *The Coffin Corner* 22, no. 1 (2000): 1–2.

Kaplan, Janice. *Women and Sports*. New York: Viking Press, 1979.

Kotarba, Joseph A. *The Chronic Pain Experience*. Beverly Hills, CA: Sage, 1983.

———. "Conceptualizing Sports Medicine as Occupational Health Care: Illustrations from Professional Rodeo and Wrestling." *Qualitative Health Research* 11, no. 6 (2001): 766–779.

———. "Perceptions of Death, Belief Systems, and the Process of Coping with Chronic Pain." *Social Science & Medicine* 17, no. 10 (1983): 681–689.

———. "Professional Athletes Injuries: From Existential to Organizational Analysis." In *Sporting Bodies, Damaged Selves: Sociological Studies of Sports-*

Related Injuries, edited by Kevin Young, 99–116. Bridgeport, CT: JAI/ Elsevier, 2004.

———. "The Social Control Function of Holistic Health Care in Bureaucratic Settings: The Case of Space Medicine." *Journal of Health & Social Behavior* 24, no. 3 (1983): 275–288.

———. "Thoughts on the Body: Past, Present and Future." *Symbolic Interaction* 17, no. 2 (1994): 225–229.

Kotarba, Joseph A., and Pamela Bentley. "Workplace Wellness Participation and the Becoming of Self." *Social Science & Medicine* 26, no. 5 (1988): 551–558.

Levy, Allan M., and Mark L. Fuerst. *Sports Injury Handbook.* Toronto: John Wiley and Sons, 1993.

Lipetz, J., and Kruse, R.J. "Injuries and Special Concerns of Female Figure Skaters." *Clinics in Sports Medicine* 19, no. 2 (2000): 369–380.

Lofland, John. *Analyzing Social Settings.* Belmont, CA: Wadsworth, 2006.

Lopiano, D.A. "Women and Modern Sport." *Olympic Review: Women and Sport* 26 (2000): 54–63.

Maguire, Joseph, Grant Jarvie, Louise Mansfield and Joe Bradley. *Sport Worlds: A Sociological Perspective.* Champaign, IL: Human Kinetics Publishers, 2002.

Matheny, Sharon. "Body Image and Sex Stereotyping." *Women and Sport: From Myth to Reality.* Philadelphia, PA: Lea and Febiger, 1978.

McCarthy, Michael. "Battles Yield Winning 'Fighter.'" *USA Today,* 11 April 2005.

Messner, M.A., M.C. Duncan and K. Jensen. "Separating the Men from the Girls: The Gendered Language of Televised Sports." *Gender and Society* 7 (1993): 121–137.

Meyer, Margaret, and Margarite Schwartz. *Team Sports for Girls and Women.* Philadelphia: W.B. Saunders Company, 1965.

Minkler, Meredith, and Nina Wallerstein. *Community-Based Participatory Research for Health.* San Francisco, CA: Jossey-Bass, 2003.

Oglesby, Carol A., ed. *Encyclopedia of Women and Sport in America.* London: Onyx Press, 1998.

Olsen, Odd-Egil, Grethe Myklebust, Lars Engebretsen and Roald Bahr. "Injury Mechanisms for Anterior Cruciate Ligament Injuries." *American Journal of Sports Medicine* 32 (2004): 1002–1013.

Oriard, Michael. *King Football: Sport and Spectacle in the Golden Age of Radio and Newsreels, Movies and Magazines, the Weekly and the Daily Press.* Chapel Hill: University of North Carolina Press, 2001.

———. *Reading Football: How the Popular Press Created an American Spectacle.* Chapel Hill: University of North Carolina Press, 1993.

Paulson, Amanda, and Sara Miller Llana. "In Roller Derby's Revival, Women, Elbow to the Fore." *Christian Science Monitor,* 26 April 2006.

Rossi, M.J., J.H. Lubowitz, and D. Guttmann. "The Skier's Knee." *Arthroscopy* 19, no. 1 (2003): 75–84.

Sandstrom, Kent L., Daniel D. Martin and Gary Alan Fine. *Symbols, Selves, and Social Reality: A Symbolic Interactionist Approach to Social Psychology and Sociology.* Los Angeles, CA: Roxbury, 2003.

Scranton, P.E., J.P. Whitesel and J.W. Powell. "A Review of Selected Noncontact Anterior Cruciate Ligament Injuries in the National Football League." *Foot Ankle International* 18 (1997): 772–776.

Sell, Timothy C., Cheryl M. Ferris, John P. Abt, Yung-Shen Tsai, Joseph B. Myers, Freddie H. Fu and Scott M. Lephart. "The Effect of Direction and Reaction on the Neuromuscular and Biomechanical Characteristics of the Knee during Tasks that Simulate the Noncontact Anterior Cruciate Ligament Injury Mechanism." *American Journal of Sports Medicine* 34 (2006): 43–55.

Shakib, Sohaila, and Michele D. Dunbar. "The Social Construction of Female and Male High School Basketball Participation: Reproducing the Gender Order through a Two-Tiered Sporting Institution." *Sociological Perspective* 45 (2002): 353–378.

Shamoo, Adil E., William H. Baugher and Robert M. Germeroth. *Sports Medicine for Coaches and Athletes: Soccer.* Luxembourg: Harwood Academic, 1995.

Shamus, Eric, and Jennifer Shamus. *Sports Injury: Prevention and Rehabilitation.* New York: McGraw-Hill, 2001.

Shangold, Monica, and Gabe Mirkin, eds. *Women and Exercise: Physiology and Sports Medicine.* Philadelphia: F.A. Davis, 1988.

Shively, R.A., W.A. Grana and D. Ellis. "High School Sports Injuries." *Physician and Sportsmedicine* 9 (1981): 46–50.

Smith, Lissa. *The History of Women in Sports—Nike Is a Goddess.* New York: Atlantic Monthly Press, 1998.

Taylor, Paul M., and Diane K. Taylor. *Conquering Athletic Injuries.* Chicago: Leisure Press, 1998.

Teitz, Carol C. "First Aid, Immediate Care, and Rehabilitation of Knee and Ankle Injuries in Dancers and Athletes." In *The Dancer as Athlete*, edited by Caroline G. Shell, 43–66. Champaign, IL: Human Kinetics Publishers, 1984.

Toth, Cory, Stephen McNiel and Thomas Feasby. "Central Nervous System Injuries in Sport and Recreation." *Sports Medicine* 35, no. 8 (2005): 685–715.

Twin, Stephanie L. *Out of the Bleachers: Writings on Women and Sport.* Old Westbury, NY: Feminist Press, 1979.

Washington, R.E., and D. Karen. "Sport and Society." *Annual Reviews of Sociology* 27 (2001): 187–212.

Witvrouw, Erik, Johan Bellemans, Roeland Lysens, Lieven Danneels and Dirk Cambier. "Risk Factors for the Development of Patellar Tendinitis in an Athletic Population." *American Journal of Sports Medicine, Intrinsic* 29 (2001): 190.

Women's Sports Foundation. *Women's Sports & Fitness Facts & Statistics.* Eastmeadow, NY: Women's Sports Foundation, 2002.

Zacek, Jana, and Joseph A. Kotarba. "Body Image among Women Professional Football Players." Paper presented at the Annual Meetings of the Southwest Sociological Association, Corpus Christi, TX, March 2004.

Zarembo, Alan. "Taking a Real Beating." *Newsweek*, 6 December 1999.

Zelisko J.A., H.B. Noble and M. Porter. "A Comparison of Men's and Women's Professional Basketball Injuries." *American Journal of Sports Medicine* 10 (1982): 297–299.

6 Public Health, Elite Sport and "Risky Behaviors" at the Canada Winter Games

Victoria Paraschak

The Canada Winter Games (CWG) was held in Whitehorse, Yukon, from 23 February to 10 March 2007. This fortieth anniversary of the Canada Games was also the first time that these Games occurred "north of 60," meaning north of the sixtieth parallel in Canada. Sportspeople in the North have had a long-standing interest in hosting the CWG. When the Games were awarded in 2001 to Whitehorse, a community of twenty-three thousand that would require forty-five hundred volunteers over the two weeks of this event, I hoped to be part of and contribute in some small way toward these very memorable Games. A pan-northern (i.e., Yukon, Northwest Territories and Nunavut) hosting approach was adopted for these Games, along with the inclusion of a competition among northern athletes in Inuit and Dene Games, including medals, as a demonstration sporting event. The inclusion of traditional games as an event made the 2007 CWG even more significant in the eyes of those Northerners who had advocated this development for years.[1]

Dr. Paula Pasquali, director of Community Health Programs for the Yukon government, first became involved with the CWG in 2005 as part of liaison efforts between the Department of Health and Social Services, the 2007 CWG Medical Services Committee, the Host Society, the Canada Games Council and her own public health staff. A separate committee was created to coordinate between the Department of Health and Social Services and the Medical Services Committee for the Games. Dr. Pasquali was on the committee to ensure that public health interests were addressed. In notes on these initial meetings, she wrote that the structural approach being taken toward medical services for the Games, which separated and privileged athletes' medical services over others (e.g., volunteers and spectators), "appear[ed] to be at odds with the philosophy of Medicare and the Canada Health Act where access to services is based on need, not who you are."[2]

Reflecting on my sport-centric approach toward viewing sport as a "culture of risk,"[3] I recognized that Dr. Pasquali saw the Games as a different kind of "culture of risk" from a public health perspective. I became curious about the differences in "health risks" between sport and public health. In keeping with my assumptions about social construction and unequal power relations, I wondered how these two different approaches toward risk would take shape and intertwine as preparations for the CWG continued. Dr. Pasquali assisted me in getting permission to explore these two differing perspectives and to see how the Games addressed them both. I took on the role of a participant observer in "health" services for these Games, providing me with insider knowledge about this aspect and a chance to proactively contribute as a volunteer at the same time.

Dr. Pasquali, situated within the Yukon government, was actively attentive to developments tied to public health services for the Games as one part of her job and was able to assign one staff member in environmental health to the CWG. She also oversaw the development of health promotion campaigns tied to the Games. I stayed in Whitehorse for a week in the fall of 2006, and then for two months prior to and two months following the Games. I was thus able to assist during the preparations for the Games, volunteer during the two weeks of the Games and then, afterward, look at organizational documents and interview key individuals who were involved with the Games.

Whitehorse provided a particularly interesting case study, because of the medical limitations regularly faced by citizens due to its remote location. These limitations included only having one hospital in the community, with one medevac airplane on call (i.e., for evacuations linked to more serious injuries or select medical appointments) that would fly patients to cities in southern Canada at a cost of about $20,000 per flight—a health cost that is covered by the Yukon government, but only for Yukoners. The town is serviced by three ambulances and by the number and mix of medical personnel as befits a community of twenty-three thousand people. For the two weeks of the Games, there would be twenty-seven hundred athletes in twenty-two sports from thirteen contingents across Canada.[4] The $18 million budget for the Games included only $100,000 for medical services; the rest would have to be provided by the government of the Yukon, Whitehorse General Hospital, volunteers and donations from various medically based corporations.

In this chapter, I first contrast the social construction of sport performance-based versus public health risks. I then explore how these two types of health risks intertwined (or did not) in the CWG through the bid process, the development of health services (medical versus public health) and the implementation of health services practices during the two weeks of the CWG. Final insights are provided to optimize health services and a health legacy at future elite multisport Games.

THEORETICAL FRAMEWORK

In keeping with Anthony Giddens's duality of structure framework,[5] I assumed that individuals' actions continued to (re-)create the social world around them while concomitantly being shaped by that social world. Individuals chose to act within the boundaries of what they could imagine; those boundaries were made up of formal and informal rules, and the availability of needed financial, human and material resources. I accordingly talked with involved individuals and analyzed organizational files and policies to document the rules and the resources aligned with the management of medical and public health risks for these Games. In keeping with the theory of unequal power relations, I was cognizant of the relative privileging of constructions of "risk" linked to medical versus public health in the ongoing preparations and in the eventual operation of health services linked to the CWG.

In keeping with the strengths perspective,[6] I began by assuming that individuals in any set of conditions already are exhibiting strengths. Thus, I documented the many effective ways that individuals addressed the medical and public health needs tied to the CWG (i.e., the strengths). I then identified ways to further those strengths by using resources available in that environment. This perspective differs from a deficit perspective, which begins by identifying the problems in a situation and then outlines the barriers that are constructing those problems. I have found the strengths perspective to be a more constructive approach for facilitating long-term change with an organization, because it begins by acknowledging the positive steps that have been taken. Recommendations then include the maintenance and support of those positive steps as well as suggested additional actions and/or resources that can further the effectiveness of the approach being taken.

THE SOCIAL CONSTRUCTION OF A "HEALTH RISK"

If a hazard is "a set of circumstances which may cause harmful [health] consequences," then risk is "the likelihood of its doing so."[7] Sport has been identified as a "culture of risk" since 1992, when Howard Nixon first used the term in reference "to the apparent normalisation of injury in some US university sports."[8] Safai further generalized this concept as "the unquestioned tolerance of pain and injury in sport."[9] Porro clarified that it may be more accurate to refer to "high risk practices in sport" rather than "high risk sports."[10] Those high-risk practices in sport are often linked to an increasing expectation of and emphasis on performance. The medicalization of sport (e.g., sport medicine, sport therapy) has contributed toward enhancing sport performances as well as addressing negative health outcomes. Waddington argues that a relationship between sport and medicine has become so normalized "that athletes [now] require routine medical supervision . . . simply because they are athletes."[11]

Safai, looking at the negotiated relationships between sport medicine clinicians and student-athletes, complicated the concept of a "culture of risk" by also identifying a "culture of precaution" and the "promotion of 'sensible risks' by clinicians to injured athletes."[12] Nancy Theberge likewise challenged a default "culture of risk" in sport, arguing:

> Health professionals working in sport negotiate the tensions between their professional obligation to safeguard athletes' health and well-being and the emphasis in sport on performance, manifest both in the toll exacted on athletic bodies by intense training and in pressures to return injured athletes to activity.[13]

Elite athletic performances at the Games—and the associated precautions taken by the Host Society to look after the medical needs of the participants—have thus largely been socially constructed within this sport-specific "culture of risk."

Many potential public health risks can be linked to a multisport event such as the Canada Games. At the 2007 CWG, there were about thirty-five hundred participants (athletes, coaches, managers); four hundred major officials; 120–150 mission staff for the thirteen contingents; six to eight hundred VIPS and corporate sponsors; and 350 media and broadcast staff.[14] Bringing all these individuals together, often in tight quarters from all across Canada during a time of the year when respiratory ailments are high and viruses are particularly active, created an optimal environment for the spreading of communicable diseases. Add in the consumption of 210,000 meals,[15] temporary food venues and water and sewage considerations for large numbers of people, the high probability of exposed bodily fluids including blood in select sporting competitions, and a heightened attentiveness toward potential environmental health risks to participants, volunteers, Games employees, spectators and the local community seems appropriate.

These public health risks were further complicated by a reputational risk faced by the Canada Games Council, the Host Society, their employees and the community if they were unable to effectively plan for and/or address potential health risks. The importance of these Games was captured by Piers McDonald, president of the 2007 CWG and former premier of the Yukon, who said: "This is the largest event ever held North of 60 meaning all eyes will be on us. This event will consume the nation!"[16]

Although both sport performance-based and public health risks were clearly present within the CWG, the socially constructed identification and addressing of health-linked "risky behaviors" were based on a variety of, at times, competing factors. Their selection was a social process shaped in part by what is "culturally identified as important."[17] For example, the Canada Games Council identified that a key success factor for hosting the Games was that they were "athlete-centred."[18] Looking after the "care and comfort of the athletes" was the principle by which the Medical Services Division operated. It was not surprising, then, that procedures to address acute medical risks to participants would be well developed, while procedures geared toward ensuring public healthiness would be less fully understood and/or embraced. Public health "risky practices" (e.g., eating, drinking, going to the washroom, washing your hands), normalized by some as "just a part of daily life," may accordingly not emerge as important within the sporting milieu.

Questions about the relationship between public health risks and sport have, however, arisen recently in Canada, in relation to concerns over the H1N1 virus. In fall 2009, the initial distribution of limited H1N1 vaccines was targeted toward vulnerable populations considered "at risk" of dying from the virus, including young children, pregnant women and individuals with underlying health issues. Concerns were raised in the media when they learned that athletes from the Toronto Raptors and professional hockey teams including the Calgary Flames, the Abbotsford Heat, the Toronto Maple Leafs and the Moncton Wildcats had received this vaccine even though they did not fit the profile of the targeted "at risk" populations. One statement justifying the vaccination of athletes explained how team administrators viewed the "riskiness" of their involvement in sport combined with this virus:

> While all professional athletes are considered high risk to exposure and transmission of the flu due to excessive contact with other players, heavy travel requirements and public exposure, only certain players and staff have received the H1N1 vaccine.[19]

This interpretation was refuted by Canada's chief public health officer, who said:

> There's a difference between being at high risk of getting the flu, and of it causing serious illness or death. We have focused the priorities of who is to be immunized first based on who is at greatest risk of severe disease and dying, not on who is more likely to be exposed . . . Otherwise, school-aged kids would have been the first priority.[20]

Clearly there are important issues to be examined concerning the intersection of the "cultures of risk" in sport and in public health.

CONSTRUCTING AND INTERTWINING "HEALTH RISK" PRACTICES AT THE 2007 CWG

The 2007 CWG was a valuable case study for exploring two different yet intertwined sociocultural sites and their practices concerning "risky health behaviors":[21] elite sport and public health. These constructions began with the Bid Document, submitted by Whitehorse to the Canada Games Committee in 2000, and ended seven years later, as the Whitehorse CWG Host

Society brought their two-week multigame festival to its conclusion on 10 March 2007. An examination of key developments along the way, with special attention given to the construction of rules and provision of resources, helped to document the ways these two aspects of the Games were socially constructed, and the ways they did (or did not) intertwine as they together addressed the "risky health behaviors" of the CWG.

Bid Document

The Sport Committee of the Canada Games Council was responsible for all technical aspects of the Games, including the "care, comfort and safety of athletes," which includes medical services.[22] The council tied this responsibility to their top-ten list of critical success factors for hosting a Canada Games and, in particular, the fourth factor identified: "athlete-centred (care, comfort, competition)."[23] Accordingly, in its outline of bid procedures specific to medical services, the list of services to be provided by the Medical Services Committee during the Games focused on athlete care, including "dentists, doctors, nurses, chiropractors, physiotherapists, athletic therapists and trained first-aid personnel . . . [providing] preventative care . . . and rehabilitation . . . in addition to acute care for illness or injury."[24] A clinic near the residence, infirmary, a medical room for each sport venue, doping control locations and ambulance service/air evacuation for high-risk sport must all be provided. Guidelines for credentials of the chief medical officer (CMO) and chief therapist were given. Guidelines for the care of sponsored professionals who will come from out of town/territory were also outlined.[25] The site evaluation included a tour of the polyclinic and a review of local hospital services and available local medical personnel and their sport experience.[26] In contrast to this, no information was required in the bid document that identified how various public health risks would be addressed. The Canada Games Council bid procedures and requirements thus facilitated the likelihood that athlete medical services would be the top health priority in the bid document and, subsequently, in the approach taken by the Host Society in creating a "healthy Games."

As part of their bid process for awarding the Canada Games to a community, three key criteria were assessed: community capacity (including medical and emergency services), facilities and legacies. However, in looking over the Whitehorse bid document, which clearly fits with the Canada Games Council's principle of geographic equity, there was scant discussion of the medical and emergency services available for athletes. The venue requirements for providing a "safe" environment for athletes, volunteers and spectators in keeping with current public health regulations were likewise absent. Finally, in looking over the potential legacies that are to be outlined for the Games as part of the bid process, health services was absent whereas others, including economic, social and infrastructure legacies, remained a criteria for winning the bid.

These patterns suggested a narrow focus on medical services when addressing "health risks" in the overall bid process. Although the medical needs of athletes are important, the medical needs of others involved in the Games such as coaches, organizers, volunteers, spectators, media and VIPs are less important, and public health concerns are relatively unimportant at the bid stage as compared to sport-specific aspects of the Games. This assessment was further reinforced in comments provided by the volunteer in charge of organizing medical services for the Yukon Games. She had initially hoped to receive a template from the Canada Games Council for organizing medical services and was dismayed to find that no such information was available. This absence of information contrasted with the organizational transfer of knowledge available for other aspects of the Games such as rules governing sporting competitions. Fortunately, the expertise of the community of Whitehorse had been demonstrated by organizing multiple Arctic Winter Games in the past. It was therefore a reasonable assumption on the part of the Canada Games Council that since Whitehorse organizers had previously provided for the medical needs of athletes and spectators, they were capable of doing so for the 2007 Canada Games.

Meeting the formal criteria and documenting adequate resources in the Whitehorse bid document was largely tied to outlining medical services rather than health care capacity more broadly. Required baseline services were outlined. The polyclinic (to be described in greater detail shortly) would be housed in the nursing department at Yukon College, providing a good opportunity for students to get experience through a student practicum tied to the Games. Local health care providers included fifty physicians, three hundred registered nurses, fifty-five licensed practical nurses, nineteen physiotherapists, ten massage therapists, thirteen pharmacists, four chiropractors and many ski patrol and St. John Ambulance volunteers who could all help out with the health care volunteer segment.[27] Sport venues would all have medical coverage during warm-up and competition times based on level of risk for each sport as outlined by the Canada Games Council.[28] Whitehorse General Hospital's features were outlined for Emergency Services and Ambulatory Care. The Yukon Ambulance Service was discussed in terms of current staff, the number of vehicles (three) and the air ambulance service.[29] A variety of skills development sessions would be provided for health care–related professions over the years leading up to the Games, which would increase the number and skill level of health care volunteers—a legacy that would remain in the community afterward. The budget for the Medical Services Division was $100,000, out of a total Games budget of approximately $20 million. This division would be organizationally located under the Athlete Services Division, led by a volunteer "Assistant Vice President (AVP), Medical Services" from the hospital, a medical services coordinator starting in January 2006, and a medical services project assistant starting in September 2006 (both finishing in March 2007).[30] The medical services coordinator should have the expertise in sports medicine, whereas the local AVP Medical Services would contribute expertise about the local health system including public health—these perspectives are complementary and both are needed.

The Canada Games Bid Assessment Summary noted that out of one thousand points total, the care and comfort section was 25 percent or 250 points.[31] Of those points, clinic and infirmary counted for thirty-five points, and other medical services (e.g., first aid for spectators, venue medical rooms, doping control) counted for twenty points—a total of fifty-five points out of one thousand.[32] No aspect of the bid assessment addressed public health issues. As well, the organizational structure provided for the Host Society did not have a division, a committee, or an individual attached to public health who could ensure that Yukon public health legislation and programs were reviewed and applied or modified as appropriate for the two weeks of the Games.

Development of Health Services

Medical Services

The organizational chart for the Host Society[33] located the Medical Services Committee as part of the Athlete Services Division. This committee had one dedicated full-time staff member, who came from Ontario with a background in medical services, beginning in November 2005;[34] an assistant was hired a few months prior to the Games to provide further support. The volunteer AVP in charge of overseeing this committee was Val Pike, whose full-time job was community liaison at Whitehorse General Hospital. She was thus well positioned to effectively coordinate shared services between the polyclinic and the hospital during the two weeks of the Games. She was familiar with Yukon health legislation and programs, and familiar to Whitehorse medical and public health professionals, which enabled her to facilitate the involvement of local professionals in the Games.

Volunteers who had a nursing background and worked at the hospital headed up the various sections of the Medical Services Committee, including medical personnel, medical venues, medical support services and doping control. Spectator services, which included first aid for spectators at the various venues, was initially located within the venues division, although it did eventually move to the Medical Services Committee prior to the start of the Games. The Medical Services Committee was thus centralized effectively for carrying out its duties and resourced with medical professionals who could access medical supplies and services efficiently.

The CMO was the individual overseeing medical treatment of participants at the Games. According to the Host Society medical policies, "participant" was defined as: athlete, coach, manager, artist (National Artist Program), mission staff, and official. All requests for medical information were to be directed to the CMO, and only the CMO or his/her delegate could release medical information.[35] This definition of participant did not include the 120 individuals involved in the Pan North Initiatives,[36] including the thirty athletes and coaches competing in Arctic Sports and Dene Games events during the Games. Volunteers and spectators were required to use the first aid volunteers at venues and, if needed, the regular medical services for the city of Whitehorse, rather than the polyclinic services and/or the medical teams (and their expertise) at the various venues. This was a departure from the Canadian healthcare system, whereby initial triage determines who is most in need of treatment; instead, policies determined categories of people who could access treatment at the site regardless of injuries.

Participants were to be provided "with the right care at the right time by the right professionals."[37] Primary and emergency medical services included: "physicians, nurses, chiropractors, physiotherapists, athletic therapists, massage therapists, pharmacists, paramedics, emergent and non-emergent transportation, lifeguards and ski patrol."[38] Medical referrals for nonsite specialists, available on call, included "dentists, optometrists, counseling, medical specialists and surgeons."[39] The statement that medical service personnel would "provide a safe and healthy medical environment for all participants"[40] aligned with the proactive involvement of public health professionals who could contribute toward that healthy environment. Yet no mention was made in the medical policies about the roles of the Yukon medical health officer, communicable disease officers (CDOs), environmental health officers (EHOs) or health promotion coordinators—all of who would play a role in managing broader public health "risks."

A risk level—high, moderate and low—initially determined by the Canada Games Council was assigned to each sport.[41] Volunteer medical professionals were then allocated to venues based on the assigned risk level for each sport. High-risk sports had a physician, nurse (optional), therapist and EMS on site. Moderate-risk sports had a physician, therapist and an EMS on call. Low-risk sports had a therapist and an EMS on call. This format, passed down to the Medical Services unit from the Canada Games Council, would have worked equally well for categorizing public health risks. Areas of high, moderate and low risk for public health concerns could have been identified, with protocols created in keeping with those ratings.

The polyclinic was the main medical service centre for the Games.[42] Only accredited participants could use this service, and initial care involved a triage process for assessment: "A physician's assessment and *referral* is required for *all* medical services."[43] All medical volunteers had to complete a record of the treatment provided after each participant's visit. In addition, a form had to be completed for any participant with any of the following symptoms identified: "vomiting, abdominal cramps, diarrhea, bloody diarrhea, stiff neck with fever, severe cough, confusion."[44] This process generated the information needed to identify if there was an infectious disease among the participants that could have a broader impact on others at the

CWG or in the broader community, since athletes, coaches and mission staff, for example, are out and about in the community on a regular basis.

The general health and well-being of participants was to take priority in determining their continuation in the competition. Absolute indications for removing a participant from competition included but were not restricted to, transient mental status, impairment, visual impairment, contagious skin conditions, infectious disease, cardiopulmonary instability and suspected spinal column injury. Relative indications for removal from competition were at the discretion of the venue or polyclinic physician (or therapist in charge in the case of some venues where a physician was not present). These relative indications included, but were not limited to, musculoskeletal injuries in which there was significant risk of further injury to the athlete, suspected fractures and suspected visceral injury.[45] Concussion guidelines were available at each venue and had to be followed. It was at the discretion of the on-site physician or therapist (when a physician was not on-site) to determine if the participant was fit to return to competition. A "Reinstated to Competition" form had to be completed for participants returning to competition after an injury. This was to be completed by the venue or Polyclinic physician and approved by the CMO.[46]

Athlete withdrawal from competition was thus well laid out. For example, removing a participant from competition would be done due to "contagious skin conditions [and] infectious disease"[47]—both of which fit with a public health focus. The policy also stated: "A participant suffering from an illness or injury that could harm another participant will be immediately withdrawn from competition."[48] Infectious flulike symptoms or viruses would fit within this policy statement, which could be determined by careful tracking of symptoms. These data were inputted into the medical database, but access to the records by a CDO on a daily basis would have further strengthened that process, since this individual would take charge of the situation if an outbreak occurred. Furthermore, an athlete's return was deemed appropriate "if the venue or Polyclinic physician believes there [was] no longer a risk for further injury."[49] This guideline did not appear to cover athletes who have had infectious conditions that could impact on the health of other participants and nonparticipants; extending the guideline to cover that possibility would have been beneficial, and would have required the involvement of the Yukon chief medical health officer, who was responsible for the health of nonathletes at the CWG.

Doping control[50] was determined in accordance with the policies and procedures set out by the Canadian Centre for Ethics in Sport (CCES), in keeping with the Canadian Anti-Doping Program. The policy approach taken for doping control would also be suitable for public health legislation, which could likewise set the direction for how things must be run at the Games. Personnel at the doping control stations were accredited,[51] and this approach could have been taken for CDOs and EHOs, so that they could have access into Games sites as needed. All controlled drugs had to be handled according to federal legislation for secure storage and account-ability.[52] This recognition of federal policies shaping the approach taken for medical services aligned with what was needed for addressing provincial/territorial public health legislation and standards as well.

Health services in Canada are based on a philosophy whereby access to services is based on need rather than who you are. This philosophy under-pins the triage approach toward decision making in health care, whereby the resources go to those most in need. However, this philosophy did not underpin the structuring of medical services for the 2007 CWG. Within the Host Society organization, the Athlete Services Committee was responsible for overseeing the medical needs of the athletes, such as access to physi-cians, physiotherapists, pharmacists and massage therapists. Meanwhile, the provision of medical services for spectators and volunteers was initially assigned to the Venues Committee, utilizing St. John First Aid providers and the Whitehorse 911 emergency aid system when necessary. First aid services were available to all nonparticipants, defined as "spectator, volun-teer, media representative, VIP."[53] First aid volunteers were present at all competitions and at noncompetition sites. They were to respond at their level of training and then call 911 in case of a medical emergency, thus drawing upon the Whitehorse health care system rather than the temporary medical health system set up for "participants" at the CWG.

This two-tiered structuring of medical services was operational-ized through policies such as the availability of ambulances. Whereas a ground ambulance was present at all "high-risk" venues for specific use by injured athletes, others who might get injured, such as volunteers, specta-tors, media and VIPS, would have to phone for ambulance services. As well, a second airplane—or air ambulance—for use by Canada Games athletes was added to the one plane usually available to evacuate Yukon-ers with serious injuries or life-threatening conditions. It was not clear, initially, how these resources would be regulated—what would happen if athletes needed both planes or if a serious accident in the Yukon meant that residents needed both planes? Who would make such decisions?

Eventually, the protocol was clarified. Once any individual (athlete or nonathlete) became a responsibility of Whitehorse General Hospital, the triage approach toward health care took over. The two-tiered philosophy privileging athletes thus dominated within the Games' medical system, but once athletes were taken to the hospital, the Canada-wide health care approach was reinstated. The two-tiered approach was facilitated by the CWG Medical Services Committee's intention that they create a tempo-rary, parallel medical system so that there would be "no athletes in the hospital."[54] Whitehorse General Hospital's approach to staffing the hos-pital during the two weeks of the Games aligned with this; they assumed that emergency patients to the hospital would be no greater in number than they see at high tourist season each year.[55] A two-tier approach was also evident in the health insurance costs required for out of territory visitors; while athletes were automatically insured for uninsured health costs (e.g., the $20,000 cost to use an air ambulance for more serious injuries not treated in the Yukon), other visitors would need private health insurance to cover costs.

Providing differential medical treatment depending on whom is involved aligned with Kotarba's description of sports medicine as multitiered occupational health care, where "elite" health care is "delivered to the most highly valued workers in an organization,"[56] who are seen as special and difficult to replace. He contrasted this approach with the "managed" health care made available for a price to athletes in minor league systems and the "privileged" health care that may be extended for select athletes who are seen to be even less important, such as the professional wrestlers and rodeo athletes he interviewed. His research supported the contention that multitiered medical care for athletes is a part of sporting culture. There is also evidence of this multitiered health care in the policies aligned with various multisport Games in Canada. While athletes cannot bring their own health care specialists and thus had to draw from a common pool of health professionals for their needs while at the Canada Games, athletes are allowed to bring their own medical support staff when competing at more elite multisport games such as the Olympic Games.

Evidence from the Whitehorse Games suggested that many primary caregivers wanted to volunteer at the Games.[57] However, a few complications arose related to their requests for leave. First, medical staff members were also needed at Whitehorse General Hospital for the duration of the Games. While the staff was subject to operational requirements when asking for leave, physicians, who are not employees of the hospital, were not subject to operational requirements. This required that plans be developed to ensure that physicians staff the emergency room at the hospital adequately throughout the duration of the Games.

Granting leave to volunteers for the Games was also more challenging for the Department of Health and Social Services than many other departments within the Yukon government, because these employees were considered to provide essential services in the Yukon, and thus were not as likely to be released for volunteer duties as "nonessential" government workers—even though their skills would, no doubt, have made an important contribution to the Games.

In light of these restrictions on local health care workers, another potential source for Canada Games health care providers were volunteers from outside the Yukon, referred to as "sponsored professionals." Since the regulations regarding who can practice various medical professions fell within provincial/territorial jurisdiction, there was a need to look at temporary licensing and fees for these potential volunteers, along with the processing time and nature of the application process. For example, the Yukon Registered Nurses Association decided not to waive registration fees for out of territory nurses who wanted to volunteer at the Games; these nurse volunteers were required to pay a $150 fee.[58] Thus, while the need for competent health care professionals was clear, it was also evident that gathering an adequate staff of health care professionals as volunteers would potentially require changes to regulations in the Yukon and the identification of essential health care requirements for Yukoners in general during the Games and the influx of professionals from outside the Yukon.

Public Health Services

Issues that fell under the purview of public health were spread throughout the CWG Host Society organizational chart. The Athlete Services Division also had committees for residence services and food services. Residence services, for example, contacted the EHO for the Yukon government in January 2006 to determine if sheets would be necessary for the mattresses, since sleeping bags were being provided for all athletes. They did end up purchasing and using sheets, as was recommended by the EHO to prevent bugs, bacteria and the like from transferring between athletes and mattresses.[59] Food services staff also spoke to and met with the EHO on different occasions in early 2006 "to discuss plans for food service and safety during the CWG."[60]

The Volunteers Division, which looked after the recruitment, accreditation and training of volunteers, also could have played a role in minimizing public health risks. The Yukon medical health officer only learned partway through the Games that he was, in fact, the overseer of all "nonparticipants" at the Games, which included volunteers. He is reported to have said that if he had known about this responsibility ahead of time, he might have made it a prerequisite that all Games volunteers have a flu shot; this would serve as a preventative step in avoiding a flu outbreak.[61] Additionally, no official CWG protocol was developed for either the removal of volunteers from their role in the Games due to ill health or for their return to work. During the Games, a number of key volunteers in medical services became sick and had to stay home for a period of time. The same thing happened with at least a few volunteers in food services. Such a protocol would be essential for minimizing the potential spread of communicable diseases such as the flu or a norovirus by volunteers to other people at the Games, including athletes and spectators. This division would be a logical place for such protocols to be developed and enforced.

The Pan North Division had responsibility for traditional games located within it. The location of traditional games here rather than in the sport division, where all other sports were located including the demonstration sport of snowboarding, facilitated the likelihood that traditional games athletes would be identified as "nonparticipants" who did not qualify for medical services accorded other athletes and their support personnel. Reading through the medical services policies, traditional games athletes were never labeled as "participants," even though there was a risk analysis done on the "sport" of traditional games, to identify which types of medical professionals needed to attend the competition. Medical files were, however, forwarded to the polyclinic for the traditional games athletes, as was done for the sport "participants." These athletes thus became a hybrid in terms of their fit within medical protocols at the Games. The Pan North Division also had their own food services committee, and thus needed to develop "safe" food preparation practices in keeping with public health guidelines.

The other three divisions that had responsibilities tied to public health included the Community Relations Division, the Venues Division and the Sponsorship Division. The Community Relations Division had responsibility over the North Stay/Accommodations Committee. Due to the need for more accommodations, a Home Stay program was created. This program, providing room and board to the public, in effect created temporary bed-and-breakfast services, which fell under the Public Health and Safety Act and Environmental Health Services. Drinking water obtained from private wells for personal use is not subject to regulation; however, water served to the public through a Home Stay program, at a minimum, needs to meet best practices or guidelines for safety reasons.[62]

The Venues Division had to address all requirements for each CWG venue. That included items like sewage system capacity. For example, sewage disposal at Grey Mountain, the biathlon venue, was straightforward, requiring portable toilets because there were no plumbed facilities. However, at Mount Sima, the ski/snowboarding site, the in-ground sewage disposal system did not have the capacity to handle all the expected visitors—thus portable toilets would be necessary but not popular since indoor facilities would also be available.[63] Spectator Services at each venue would need to address temporary food provision in keeping with public health standards. The Environmental Services Committee, which intended to "green" the Games wherever possible, recommended providing each athlete with a water bottle they could then fill up at water fountains, thus saving on the environmental costs of bottled water. However, public health officials pointed out that to avoid communicable diseases, water bottles should not be filled at water fountains due to potential risk, but could be filled at taps, requiring proper signage at water fountains.[64] In the end, Shoppers Drug Mart (a national pharmacy chain) donated enough bottles of water to provide athletes and volunteers with a source of water throughout the two weeks of the Games.

The Sponsorship Division looked after VIP hospitality, which included providing VIPs with various kinds of food throughout the Games such as local wild meats. However, in the Yukon, the use of local wild meat or smoked fish for sale to the public is considered a high-risk product, because they are not inspected or regulated in the Yukon. This, then, became another risk to the public that needed to be mitigated by public health officials.[65]

Several additional positive, proactive steps were taken to ensure that any "public health risks" would be contained. An Emergency Procedures

Handbook was produced, and an all-day Emergency Procedures Operation was held on 14 February 2007 to test out the many community organizations that would become involved in case of a crisis. The scenario chosen for this mock event was a norovirus crisis, which gave emergency staff practice in addressing ways they would deal with athletes and others should a health crisis such as this occur. Protocols were also created for identifying and addressing a public health outbreak; it would be handled by the Communicable Disease and the EHOs and overseen by Yukon's medical health officer. The EHO liaison for the CWG worked with several committees to establish procedures to deal with many potential environmental health concerns, and an EHO officer remained on call, twenty-four hours a day, for the length of the CWG, which was not the normal practice. Finally there were health promotion campaigns created in light of this national, multisport event for young adult, elite athletes to capitalize on effective ways to address public health issues for this cohort.

The CWG were seen as an opportunity in the Yukon to proactively contribute to community health through the development and dissemination of health promotion messaging. For the 2007 CWG, the Manager of Health Promotion oversaw four CWG-linked projects: helmet safety, customized condoms, the piloting of a *Freestylin' Sexual Health* magazine and a YouTube competition on athlete-generated positive messages for health promotion.

The helmet safety campaign, titled "Same Game, Same Gear" with its motto "Play Safe, Play Hard, Wear Protective Gear," was meant to encourage individuals to put on their helmets for safety when playing winter sports. Four posters were created for bus stops and buses that were used throughout the Games. Young, elite Yukon athletes in four sports—downhill skiing, snowboarding, women's hockey and snowmobiling—were photographed in action with a recreational athlete beside them, and all were having fun while wearing a helmet.

The Medical Services Committee was required to provide eighteen hundred condoms per week for use by athletes. The Community Health Division agreed to create customized condoms special to these Games, selecting the motto "Play Hard. Play Safe." This customized approach has been used in the Yukon in the past for a variety of special events, such as Christmas holidays and high school graduations. Six versions of condoms were created, each with a different slogan: Wanna Take it to the Mat?; Wanna Score?; Wanna Get Your Shred On?; Wanna Parry & Thrust?; A vos marques, pret, deballez!; and Wanna Score Big in the Pairs Event? The ministers responsible for sport and recreation from across the country met just prior to the Games, and the Yukon minister provided each representative with his or her own complete set. Condoms were also placed for distribution in big jars in many of the places where athletes would congregate for the duration of the Games.

The CWG were also used as an event where new ideas in health promotion could be tried. A *Freestylin' Sexual Health* magazine was created, using a format aligned with current magazines popular with the age-group of athletes attending the Games, and they were placed in locations where an athlete might sit and read it during the Games. Finally, a YouTube competition was announced in the magazine—it encouraged athletes to use their phones and shoot a video with a positive health message for other youth. Prizes were offered as part of this competition.

The Host Society identified interdependencies between the various divisions in its structure. Clearly, the Medical Services Committee had a large number of interdependencies, but so did public health issues, although there was no administrative home for this responsibility in the CWG Host Society Organizational Structure. Occasionally, previous CWGs have had a stand-alone health services division, rather than placing medical services as a committee within the Athlete Services Division. For example, the community of Bathurst-Campbellton, which hosted the 2003 CWG, had a Health and Medical Services Division.[66] This organizational structure became a recommendation in the 2007 Final Report from the AVP Medical Services; she felt that such a structure would better ensure that issues related to public health would be coordinated more effectively with those currently falling under the Medical Services Committee.[67] It appeared that although medical services were well defined for "participants," they were less well defined for non participants. As well, the public health issues were spread across several divisions in a manner that did not ensure that they would be effectively addressed, because no one person or committee was accountable for that responsibility. However, proactive efforts on the part of several government of Yukon employees helped to ensure that "public health risks" would be minimized, addressed appropriately, contained if necessary and capitalized upon through positive health promotion messaging.

INTERTWINING/COMPETING
PRACTICES DURING THE GAMES

The intertwining of medical services and public health concerns became more evident during the two weeks of the Games. The Medical Services Committee had worked hard to effectively prepare for medical needs at the CWG. Sponsored professionals were brought in, provided with transportation and accommodation and invited to special "social" information sessions at night. The CMO gave daily morning reports on athlete injuries to mission staff from the thirteen contingents, and was the individual through whom all information on the athletes' health was channeled. Acute medical injuries were effectively addressed. Policies were followed for concussions, for removal of athletes and for their return to competition. Data inputted into the medical computer program on each participant's treatment faced some challenges when volunteers unclear on medical terms could not input them correctly; physicians helped out by inputting their own information to address the problem. As well, athletes with chronic diseases such as cystic fibrosis, who needed access to the polyclinic on a daily basis, had initial challenges because their unique needs had not been incorporated into existing policies, but arrangements were quickly made by polyclinic staff to accommodate them.

Effective practices had also been proactively created to address areas of concern in public health. Hand-sanitizing stations had been placed strategically for athletes where they ate meals. When respiratory problems increased among athletes in the first week, additional units were brought into the residences, and athletes were encouraged actively to use them by their mission staff. The helmet safety campaign was widely available to the public as well as CWG participants, and their use of Yukon athletes fostered pride in local athletes. The customized condoms were a hit with the athletes, who traded them much as pins get traded at other Games. The *Freestylin' Sexual Health* magazine was made available for easy access by the athletes. The YouTube competition was held, but generated minimal involvement from the athletes.

Public health concerns did, in the end, arise among athletes and needed to be addressed. In an update on winter viruses to all Yukon health care providers, the Medical health officer and CDO noted that since mid-January, there had "been 27 laboratory-confirmed reports of Influenza A . . . five were in visiting athletes participating in the Canada Winter Games and two were in Yukon athletes. All were in residence in the Athletes village at the time of onset of illness . . . Norovirus, a 'laboratory-confirmed winter gastrointestinal illness . . . ' has also been confirmed as the causative agent of acute gastrointestinal illness among some Canada Winter Games participants."[68]

This was one situation where the intertwining of medical and public health services could have been improved. As the incidence of athletes with the flu increased in week one, the AVP Medical Services continued to stress in daily updates to the mission staff that hand washing was a critical practice in reducing the spread of influenza. The Yukon government's CDO was not contacted until later in week two, when she was informed that there was an increased incidence of a norovirus-like symptom among athletes; at this point she was brought in to oversee the situation. If she had been given daily access to the medical database, similar to the CMO, then she could have been monitoring the situation throughout the Games on behalf of the Medical Services Committee. In addition, she was not accredited and thus had difficulty getting access into the polyclinic to do her job. The same situation—a lack of accreditation—was faced by the EHOs, which made their job of overseeing CWG locations where public health issues needed to be monitored very difficult. In addition, access to parking was always a challenge for the short time they needed to be at venues to do their inspections, and yet they could not obtain parking passes from the Host Society.

One requirement that the Host Society agreed to was that the polyclinic would be closed down before the end of closing ceremonies, so that it could be returned to the college in time for their use. The polyclinic closure at this time became problematic with a number of athletes ill and vomiting at the end of the Games. Athletes were temporarily housed in the largest venue available—the Canada Games Centre—until their flights home, with a skeleton crew of medical staff to watch over them. Sick athletes were then sent home on planes, bringing that virus back home with them.

The turnaround that happened at the end of the first week, when athletes from week one head home and accommodations for incoming athletes are prepared, was another point where public health issues became relevant. These accommodations, and in particular the beds that had been used and would be used again, needed to be fully sanitized in a very short period of time. After the Games ended, sleeping bags left (and perhaps used) by athletes were sold to the public. Athlete beds were then packed up and shipped to Yellowknife for the Arctic Winter Games that would happen in a year. Having protocols in place for each of these cases that were informed by public health practices would help to ensure that public health problems were minimized for athletes and also for the public.

Volunteers worked long hours in the medical services area, often around sick participants. This combination of factors no doubt contributed toward the periods of time where various key volunteers in this area had to remain home due to sickness. The importance of a medical policy governing both the removal of volunteers from their position and approving their return to work became evident. This was also the point at which the CMO clarified that the Yukon's medical health officer was in charge of all "nonparticipants"—a responsibility that should have been identified in CWG medical policies, explaining that the medical health officer would be the person endorsing medical protocols for nonparticipants. Inviting all medical volunteers and government staff who were actively supporting the healthiness of participants and nonparticipants to evening socials (e.g., CDO, environmental medical officer, nonmedical professionals who were volunteers), instead of just sponsored professionals and select local medical professionals, would also seem to have been appropriate in light of their key roles in the CWG.

Finally, despite the popularity of the customized condoms among athletes, and the proactive public health campaign using the *Freestylin' Sexual Health* magazine, officials from the CWG refused to publish an article about these campaigns in their official daily newspaper or to place it on their website. This happened even though all of the ministers responsible for sport and recreation across Canada requested a full set of the condoms to take home, and the local newspaper included an article about these campaigns. For reasons that were never explained, the public and "official" linkage of sexual health with CWG athletes was not one the CWG officials were willing to endorse—they thus required that the condoms be made available, but were limited in their ability to promote the use of the condoms to athletes.

RECOMMENDATIONS FOR ADDRESSING "HEALTH RISKS" AT THE CWG

Numerous strengths were evident in the ways that medical and public health concerns were managed at the 2007 CWG. Policies were created and followed so that acute health care for participants and nonparticipants was clearly—and differently—resourced. Risk management by the Host Society, along with the creation and running of a mock emergency, prepared emergency services for addressing potential risks. The interdependencies for the Medical Services Committee were effectively identified. However, the lack of a similar focus in the Host Society for public health issues suggested that recommendations for improvement in that area, along with a few recommendations specific to medical services, were appropriate.

In terms of improving medical services for participants, it would seem that the creation of a medical policy that recognized and created a protocol for athletes with chronic problems requiring special use of the polyclinic would have been appropriate. As well, the treatment of Traditional Games athletes as "nonparticipants," even though they had roles like other athletes, while nonathlete coaches, officials and mission staff had access to "participant" medical services, clearly needed to be addressed. Traditional Games athletes, because of their placement in the Pan North Division, were provided with different and less-full medical services than all other athletes who fell under the responsibility of the sport division, including athletes from the demonstration sport of snowboarding.

Another recommendation to improve the management of health services in future Games would be the creation of a separate Health Services Division, including both public health and medical services, with a chair of public health who would be accountable for ensuring that public health protocols were followed. The CMO/medical health officer roles need to be clarified at the start, and the medical health officer needs to be actively involved in the creation of medical policies for nonparticipants just as the CMO oversees policies for participants. There needs to be proactive identification of local (i.e., provincial/territorial) public health legislation, programs, risks and practices during or just after the bid process, so that sport-based medical practices can be modified as needed, and public health practices also modified on a temporary basis as needed. Medical officials who work in sport need to partner with local public health professionals to ensure that "healthiness" for participants and nonparticipants is achieved throughout the Games. The generation of risk categories for non-sport-related activities and settings that have the potential to create public health risks (e.g., accommodation, eating arrangements), comparable to the risk categories for CWG sports, would be a logical step. Then public health protocols could be assigned to the various categories accordingly, ensuring that a reasonable approach to public health requirements is achieved, given the temporary nature of the CWG. As these professionals work in partnership, it would be reasonable that the CDO be given access to daily medical records so that potential problems can be identified and addressed immediately. Accreditation and parking privileges would make sense for CDOs and for EHOs, so that they could effectively monitor potential public health concerns. This partnership would also contribute to the proactive creation of a health services legacy, broadly conceived to include both medical and public health services.

CONCLUDING INSIGHTS

This case study provided important practical insights for how future Canada Games could approach "health services," in particular for smaller, more remote hosting cities, which now include not only Whitehorse, but also Yellowknife and Iqaluit. These smaller communities, along with other underresourced Games such as the North American Indigenous Games and the Canadian Transplant Games, would benefit by carefully combining medical and public health services from the start of their organizational efforts, to ensure that optimal "healthiness" is achieved.

Exploring the intertwining of "cultures of risk" at the 2007 CWG also provided some insight for academic explorations of the "culture of risk" in sport. Multitiering of health services based on "risk" and "participant" definitely occurred in the CWG, aligning with Kotarba's findings that elite sport health care is provided to the most valued workers (or elite athletes) in an organization.[69] In keeping with Safai's insights on a "culture of precaution" alongside a "culture of risk,"[70] it seemed that the Medical Services Committee was committed to addressing public health concerns once they arose, but they had difficulty welcoming in public health professionals as equal partners in that process. It does seem that a "culture of precaution" could be enhanced if such a partnership was facilitated.

Privileging athletes' medical health had the effect of reinforcing a high tolerance for *individual* risk, with medical services available on the ready, which allowed athletes to push the envelope of what is possible and to perform as close to the danger zone as possible without going over to optimize performance. If athletes' access to medical services was not prioritized, the threshold for risk tolerance might be lower.

The combination of privileging athletes and high tolerance for individual risk supported a myopic view of health and the health system—it focused on the health, well-being and fitness of the individual, primarily in relation to acute injuries and conditions. Even where an athlete is downed because of infectious disease, it was still about how the infection was impacting the performance of the individual—not about the additional impact that the illness could have on others.

The irony is that although there is a high tolerance for individual risk, there is something between neglect and the minimizing of risk to others situated in a social network of concentric circles around the individual athlete—his/her roommates and fellow athletes, coaches and support staff, mission staff and games officials, volunteers and spectators, the community at large. By downplaying or ignoring good public health practices (including prevention, surveillance, early identification, etc.), Games organizers were actually assuming a very large risk to the Games as a whole. While the risk to individual athletes may have been great resulting in his/her inability to compete, the risk of ignoring public health was that a significant portion if not the whole Games may have been shut down. Although the probability of that was low, its impact, if the Games had to be interrupted for even a day or two due to widespread illness, would have been immense.

In conclusion, a comprehensive approach toward "public healthiness," incorporating the public, volunteers and the athletes, would complement already well-developed protocols for "individual athlete healthiness" at future CWG. Careful attention to public health regulations, programs and services would help to ensure the care, comfort and safety of all participants to the Games, while hopefully producing a health services legacy that would benefit the host community well after the Canada Games were done.

NOTES

1. For example, feedback from the NWT delegates on a draft of the Sport Canada Policy on Aboriginal Peoples' Participation in Sport noted the following: "For Aboriginal athletes to be part of the mainstream system a level playing field is needed. The inclusion of Aboriginal events at the Canada Games would be an excellent opportunity to expose other provinces to these events. At the Arctic Winter Games both Aboriginal and non-Aboriginal athletes compete in traditional games" (Sport Canada, "Aboriginal Peoples' Participation," 21).
2. Dr. Pasquali Pasquali, "Personal Notes on CWG Involvement," personal files, 27 March 2006.
3. For example, Donnelly, "Sport and Risk Culture."
4. Canada Winter Games Organizing Committee, "Whitehorse 2007 Jeux du Canada Games Host Society Power Point Presentation on the Games," personal files, 2006.
5. Giddens, *Constitution of Society.*
6. For example, Saleebey, "Introduction."
7. Fox, "Postmodern Reflections," 12.
8. Donnelly, "Sport and Risk Culture," 32–33.
9. Safai, "Healing the Body," 128.
10. Cited in Donnelly, "Sport and Risk Culture, " 33.
11. Waddington, "Development of Sports Medicine," 179.

12. Safai, "Healing the Body," 127.
13. Theberge, "Sport Medicine," 177.
14. Canada Winter Games Organizing Committee, "Whitehorse 2007."
15. Ibid.
16. Ibid.
17. Lupton, "Risk as Moral Danger," 428.
18. Canada Games Council, *2007 Canada Winter Games.*
19. Wingrove, Mehler Paperny and Walton, "Hockey Players Jump," para. 7.
20. Ibid., para. 8, 9.
21. Lupton, *Imperative of Health.*
22. Canada Games Council, *2007 Canada Winter Games*, 10.
23. Ibid., 11.
24. Ibid., 32.
25. Ibid., 32–33.
26. Ibid., 63–64.
27. Whitehorse Bid Committee, *Whitehorse Bid*, 13.
28. Ibid.
29. Ibid., 14.
30. Ibid., 44.
31. Canada Games Council, *Canada Games Bid Assessment Summary*, personal files, 2000.
32. Ibid.
33. Canada Winter Games Host Society, *Organizational Chart*, personal files, April 2006.
34. Canada Winter Games Host Society, "Project Charters Binder," *Medical Services Committee Project Charter*, personal files, 4 November 2005.
35. Canada Winter Games Host Society, *Medical Policy*, Policy 1.0.
36. Pan North Division, "Information Handout from the Canada Winter Games Organizing Committee," personal files, 2006.
37. Canada Winter Games Host Society, *Medical Policy*, Policy 5.0.
38. Ibid.
39. Ibid.
40. Ibid.
41. Ibid., Policy 13.0.
42. Ibid., Policy 8.0.
43. Ibid. (emphasis in original).
44. Ibid., Policy 14.0.
45. Ibid., Policy 9.0.
46. Ibid., Policy 10.0.
47. Ibid., Policy 9.0.
48. Ibid.
49. Ibid.
50. Ibid., Policy 3.0.
51. Ibid.
52. Ibid., Policy 4.0.
53. Ibid., Policy 15.0.
54. Personal interview with H. Morgan, medical services coordinator, November 2006.
55. Personal interview with V. Pike, AVP Medical Services. January 2007.
56. Kotarba, "Conceptualizing Sports Medicine," 767.
57. Dr. Pasquali Pasquali, "Personal Notes on CWG Involvement," personal files, 27 March 2006.
58. Ibid. The government of the Yukon eventually paid this fee for the nurse volunteers.

59. E. Bergsma, "2007 Canada Winter Games Activity Log for Eric Bergsma," personal files, 26 October 2006.
60. Ibid.
61. Dr. Pasquali Pasquali, "Update during Canada Winter Games," personal files, March 2007.
62. Dr. Pasquali Pasquali, "Personal Notes on CWG Involvement," personal files, 27 March 2006.
63. Ibid.
64. Ibid.
65. Ibid.
66. Bernadette Theriault, "Health and Medical Services Final Report Presentation, Bathurst Campbellton Host Society," personal files, 2003.
67. Medical Services Committee, *Whitehorse 2007*.
68. E-mail memorandum to all Yukon Health Care Providers from B. Larke (MHO) and C. Hemsley (CDO), personal files, 14 March 2007.
69. Kotarba, "Conceptualizing Sports Medicine."
70. Safai, "Healing the Body."

BIBLIOGRAPHY

Canada Games Council. *2007 Canada Winter Games Bid Procedure and Requirements*. Ottawa: Canada Games Council, 2000.
Canada Winter Games Host Society. *Whitehorse 2007 Jeux du Canada Games Host Society Medical Policy*. Whitehorse: Canada Winter Games Host Society, 2007.
Donnelly, Peter. "Sport and Risk Culture." In *Sporting Bodies, Damaged Selves: Sociological Studies of Sports-Related Injury*, edited by Kevin Young, 29–57. London: Elsevier, 2004.
Fox, Nick. "Postmodern Reflections on 'Risk,' 'Hazards' and Life Choices." In *Risk and Sociocultural Theory: New Directions and Perspectives*, edited by Deborah Lupton, 12–33. Cambridge: Cambridge University Press, 1999.
Giddens, Anthony. *The Constitution of Society: Outline of the Theory of Structuration*. Berkeley: University of California Press, 1984.
Kotarba, Joseph. "Conceptualizing Sports Medicine as Occupational Health Care: Illustrations from Professional Rodeo and Wrestling." *Qualitative Health Research* 11, no. 6 (2001): 766–779.
Lupton, Deborah. *The Imperative of Health: Public Health and the Regulated Body*. Thousand Oaks, CA: Sage, 1995.
———. "Risk as Moral Danger: The Social and Political Functions of Risk Discourse in Public Health." *International Journal of Health Services* 23, no. 3 (1993): 425–435.
Medical Services Committee. *Whitehorse 2007 Jeux du Canada Games Medical Services Final Report*. Whitehorse: Canada Winter Games Host Society, 2007.
Safai, Parissa. "Healing the Body in the 'Culture of Risk': Examining the Negotiation of Treatment between Sport Medicine Clinicians and Injured Athletes in Canadian Intercollegiate Sport." *Sociology of Sport Journal* 20, no. 2 (2003): 127–146.
Saleebey, D. "Introduction: Power in the People." In *The Strengths Perspective in Social Work Practice*, 5th ed., edited by D. Saleebey, 1–23. Boston: Pearson Education, 2009.
Sport Canada. *Sport Canada's Policy on Aboriginal Peoples' Participation in Sport: Draft #8*. Ottawa: Sport Canada, 2003.

Theberge, Nancy. "'It's Not about Health, It's about Performance': Sport Medicine, Health, and the Culture of Risk in Canadian Sport." In *Physical Culture, Power, and the Body*, edited by Jennifer Hargreaves and Patricia Vertinsky, 176–194. New York: Routledge, 2007.

Waddington, Ivan. "Development of Sports Medicine." *Sociology of Sport Journal* 13, no. 2 (1996): 176–196.

Whitehorse Bid Committee. *Whitehorse Bid for the 2007 Canada Winter Games*. Whitehorse: City of Whitehorse, 2000.

Wingrove, Josh, Anna Mehler Paperny and Dawn Walton. "Hockey Players Jump the Flu Queue—and Land on Thin Ice." *Globe and Mail*, 4 November 2009. http://www.theglobeandmail.com/life/health/h1n1–swine-flu/hockey-players-jump-the-flu-queue-and-land-on-thin-ice/article1351587/ (accessed 14 June 2010).

7 The Benefits and Challenges of Complementary and Alternative Medicines for Health Care in Sport

Elizabeth C.J. Pike

Athletes' usage of complementary and alternative medicines (CAM) is a common but relatively underresearched aspect of sport medicine. A recent survey of injured participants in the sport of rowing found that 59 percent of females and 10 percent of males had used CAM in the recovery from sport-related injuries.[1] The reasons identified for such high usage included dissatisfaction with more orthodox medical practices, a preference for what were perceived to be natural and holistic health care modalities, a sense of greater control over the medical encounter and a more pleasurable experience of treatment particularly for women. This is consistent with broader surveys of usage that indicate that, in the Western world, between 20 percent and 49 percent of the population report visiting CAM practitioners each year.[2] Usage is particularly high in Germany and France, where CAM modalities are mostly practiced by trained medical doctors.[3] In the US, approximately $40 million per annum is spent on CAM, with twice as many consultations made with such nonorthodox practitioners as with mainstream family doctors.[4] In the UK, where the research for this chapter is based, it is estimated that 10.6 percent of the population have used the most established forms of CAM (acupuncture, chiropractic, homeopathy, hypnotherapy, medical herbalism, osteopathy), amounting to twenty-two million visits in a year.[5]

Despite the apparent popularity of such medical practices, there is no clear definition of CAM and the concept itself has even been discarded as "a dubious piece of phraseological rebranding."[6] At the heart of this debate is the *A* of CAM and what is offered by way of alternativeness to orthodox allopathic medicines. In the UK, this stems from the UK Medical Registration Act (1858), which defined the system of allopathic medicine practiced by doctors as "orthodox," and in so doing provided these practitioners with the exclusive right to the term *medical practitioner*. It was not until 1960 that the Professions Supplementary to Medicine Act regularized some paramedical professions, including physiotherapy and chiropody. This labeling process created a state-approved hierarchy of medical professionals within which doctors were allotted a dominant position.[7] Any therapies outside of those regulated were then variously classified as "complementary," "alternative" or "nonorthodox." This terminology indicates the varied perceptions of such treatments: for example, the term *complementary therapy* suggests that there is some collaboration with orthodox medicine,[8] while classification as "alternative" indicates a conflict with allopathic treatments, and indeed "alternative" primarily refers to those modalities reliant on principles that are indifferent to scientific principles of conventional medicine.[9] The label of "nonorthodox" is a marker not of the knowledge base of the treatment per se, but of whether the approach has formal state recognition and support from the medical profession.[10] In other words, the label is a clear indicator of the "differentials in power and prestige evident in post-industrial medical systems."[11]

In the UK, statutory regulation has so far only been awarded to those professions, such as osteopathy and chiropractic, that are similar to the "paramedical" professions mentioned earlier in their use of joint mobilization and manipulation techniques to treat neuromuscular conditions, including the kinds of injuries many athletes experience. These approaches often combine their techniques with nutritional advice and sometimes pharmacological approaches, and so the CAM are most closely aligned to the orthodox biomedical model of practice.[12] Other CAM modalities that have had greater difficulty in achieving state recognition include various forms of herbal medicine (such as traditional Chinese medicine [TCM] and Ayurvedic herbal medicine) and acupuncture, which involves inserting needles into specific anatomical points to redirect the body's energy flow. I will discuss the reasons for these difficulties in a later section. In this chapter, I will use the definition of CAM as those modalities that do not fit into the state-approved definition of medical orthodoxy, and yet claim to be curative or preventative; have a systemized body of knowledge about illness and health; and involve technical intervention by an expert practitioner.[13]

When juxtaposing the ways in which the struggle for definition and recognition of CAM is contrasted with their popularity among their many users, the complexity of these approaches and their likely acceptability in sport medicine practice becomes clear. In this chapter, I examine the relationship between CAM and the athletic community. I outline the demographics of the CAM using community and what athletic users perceived to be the benefits of CAM. The chapter further examines the divisions between CAM and "orthodox" medicine that center upon philosophical differences toward the use/primacy of evidence based approaches to medicine, and thus act as a constraint on the more widespread use of CAM within sport and sport medicine.

Data were collected from athletes who had sought a variety of medical treatments for sport-related illnesses and injuries, along with information gathered from coaches and other members of their sporting network. The data from the athletes was collected via a questionnaire survey of two hundred male and female rowers during one regatta season in the UK. The questionnaire identified the broad issues pertaining to injury risk and subsequent medical treatment in this sporting subculture. The questionnaire data were analyzed through descriptive statistics. There followed a two-year period of participant observation and semi-structured interviews with twelve female rowers and four of their male coaches in two women's rowing clubs in the South of England. The qualitative data from the sporting subculture were analyzed through theoretical and thematic coding.[14] It should be noted that all names used are pseudonyms. Finally, an in-depth semi-structured interview was conducted with the executive director (ED) of a UK-based, international nongovernment organization (INGO) that draws on the expertise of practitioners from orthodox and alternative medicines and seeks to shape the regulatory and scientific framework to incorporate natural health, by challenging EBM and the established approach to healthcare.

A SOCIALLY EXCLUSIVE MEDICAL ENCOUNTER

The political struggle for state recognition of CAM has had a very real consequence for potential users. With many lacking state recognition, CAM are denied direct funding, which means they remain primarily a private form of treatment in the UK. Additionally, the absence of a cohesive professional power base, or role in state policy, makes it difficult for CAM to be able to look beyond the level of individual clients.[15] As a result, such practices arguably have little to offer those with low economic capital who are priced out of alternative treatments. Lupton goes as far as to suggest that alternative therapies "may be regarded as all the more insidious because they overtly offer an alternative to the prevailing model of health care while covertly legitimizing social inequality."[16] Unsurprisingly, therefore, evidence identifies that the people most likely to use nonorthodox practitioners are the middle classes.[17]

Although the distribution of demand is primarily a matter of price, with most CAM offered through private rather than state-funded health care, it is suggested that people with high cultural capital and low economic capital (for example, teachers and others in the public sector) are also likely to follow ascetic consumption patterns.[18] This includes a more critical consumption of health care and a preference for "natural" approaches that contributes to a propensity to use nonorthodox therapies.[19] In the case study of the rowers, it was notable that the women involved in this study who used nonorthodox health care supported this trend, being either university-educated professional workers (73 percent of questionnaire respondents) or full-time students (25 percent). Several did identify the problems they encountered funding their CAM treatment but, as Pauline explained, since the only advice she had received from her doctor was to rest for six months, she said of the minimum £20 for a CAM session, "I think what is that compared to not being able to do exercise?"

In addition to the "classed" nature of the CAM encounter, it is also evident that this is a gendered experience. The athletes identified that one of the main reasons that they explored CAM as treatment for their sport-related injuries and ill health was a perceived inadequacy of traditional medicine. A key challenge for the female athletes was the fact that their rowing clubs did not have any contacts with medical practices, physiotherapists or other specialists. For example, 40 percent of the questionnaire respondents stated that they received no treatment for their injuries, and 50 percent did not receive any meaningful rehabilitation program.[20] This is far from unique, and female athletes often identify that it is not only the frequency of injury, but also the relative absence of medical care, which is a reality of their sport. For example, in her work with women's ice hockey players, Theberge identified that, in contrast to male teams that had therapists working with players as a matter of course, the women's team had no therapist attached to it.[21] This is indicative of what Duquin called "the silence of the injured":[22] that women are less socially visible and as a result are doubly-dominated, traditionally suffering the most from male domination in both sport and the medical experience (see also Kotarba's contribution in this collection).

It has been argued that, in addition to the practical reasons for choosing alternative treatments, CAM appeal to women through the "femininity" of treatments such as massage and aromatherapy that use fragrant oils,[23] and the holistic approaches to health balancing body, mind and spirit, "which appear to offer women a measure of control and power over their lives."[24] Many of the rowers talked of self-prescribed techniques of self-massage, exercise, strappings and pain relief medication, much of which had been informed by visits to CAM practitioners (see also Atkinson's contribution to this collection). This is indicative of "democratic professionalism," an approach to professional services that aims to empower service users and members of different professional groups, and is argued to be more "woman-friendly" as it is based on egalitarian relationships between the medical professionals and their informed clients.[25] Democratic professionalism is in contrast to the more aggressive, mechanistic and arguably more "masculine" treatment of the body in orthodox medical care that focuses on the repair and elimination of symptoms rather than overall well-being.[26] It should be acknowledged that there is a counterargument that CAM modalities are actually disciplining, because their "holistic" approach makes all areas of a person's life available for the surveillance of the CAM practitioner and encourages disciplinary techniques of self-monitoring and self-control.[27] In effect, while ostensibly offering "control" to the client, it has been argued that the reality is an emphasis on individual responsibility for health, which rewards the "right" behavior in a way that is also evident in orthodox medicine. In turn, this continues to obscure the impact of collective problems including the pressures to engage in injurious behavior in the first place, and the limited access to appropriate health care for those who lack the economic or cultural capital to avail themselves of such modalities.[28] However, it was the sense of control in the medical encounter that was attractive to many women in this study.

ACTIVE MEDICINE

Key features of patient dissatisfaction with orthodox medical practice are related to a perception that doctors lack interest or empathy with their needs, and are overreliant on drug prescription to eliminate symptoms, rather than spending time to give more efficacious treatment.[29] During the interviews with the rowers, Valerie commented that her hospital doctor made a diagnosis even though "he could not have been there for more than twenty seconds. He didn't even look at me or anything"; a questionnaire respondent argued that "doctors just say 'rest and take Ibuprofen.'"[30] Similar concerns were expressed with other forms of treatment that conformed to the orthodox model. For example, physiotherapy practice is incorporated into orthodoxy as a subordinate profession allied to medicine;[31] this was rejected by Clare, who argued that physiotherapists "treat the symptoms but not necessarily fix the structure that is underneath it."[32]

In contrast, CAM are seen to be more empowering, particularly because they require the active involvement of the client in the collaborative nature of the treatment process.[33] Indeed the language of "client" rather than "patient" is a move away from passivity, or what Frank refers to as "a moral order that subordinates him [*sic*] as an individual" to the "active" physician.[34] This seems important because several of the women enjoyed their status as, what Goffman would call, a person of action. For example, Helen talked of her dissatisfaction with her doctor's diagnosis for her neck injury, which led to a period of rest during which she "started feeling very unfit." She turned to a chiropractor and enjoyed the prescribed activity of "a lot of stretching" and, at the time of the interview, intended to see a "sports physio quite soon to see what kind of training I can do," as part of the process of returning to full activity.[35] Treatment that enables the active engagement of the client also presents them with the opportunity to retain management of their own lives during their recovery from injury. This is particularly significant for athletes, as the rehabilitation process is otherwise often an isolating and disempowering experience.[36] Physical activity is central to the lives of athletes, they have a heightened awareness of their corporeal abilities and requirements and they rely on their bodies to maintain their lifestyles. Any corporeal failure through injury or illness, along with the related treatments, often means that they are unable to engage with their usual networks of physically active individuals, which in turn compromises their daily routines and even their self-identity. In contrast, "active patients involved in their own treatment feel less vulnerable because they are taking control."[37]

ORTHODOX VERSUS ALTERNATIVE: THE CULTURE OF MISTRUST

The evidence suggests that there is not a clear-cut choice between either using orthodox medicine or using CAM. In reality, it appears that those who use CAM do not absolutely reject orthodox practices, are often high users of biomedicine and so are generally high consumers of medicine.[38] Certainly the majority of the rowers in the case study had used a combination of orthodox medicines and CAM. Sharma refers to people who "shop around" as "eclectic users,"[39] who display a consumerist attitude to health care that is indicative of the direct competition between practitioners in a market-led health care system.[40]

Despite this overlap in usage, a British parliamentary report outlines how there remains suspicion and distrust between orthodox and nonorthodox practitioners that has created an environment whereby clients do not tell the former that they are using the latter, and make their own decisions about appropriate treatment.[41] This is in part because patients fear ridicule or disapproval from orthodox practitioners, and also recognize that orthodox medicine has authority and they may need to continue to benefit from the services it offers.[42] For example, Valerie, one of the rowers in the case study, did tell her doctor that she was having alternative treatments for an injury, and subsequently described her General Practitioner (GP) as "a narrow-minded doctor" who had said of her osteopath that "he just wanted money."[43]

It appears to be the case that critics of nonorthodox therapies, including many medical personnel, believe that they lack scientific proof and are a return to magic and superstition.[44] Therefore, while a British survey found that approximately 93 percent of GPs and 70 percent of hospital doctors claim to have suggested referral for alternative medicine, many perceived themselves to be under pressure to refer and are not necessarily convinced of its value.[45] It is also worthy of note that while the General Medical Council allows GPs to refer patients for nonorthodox care, the patient remains the responsibility of the GP, even though the National Health Service (NHS) is unlikely to pay for the treatment. In this way, the orthodox practitioner maintains some "control" over the nonorthodox therapy,[46] which might undermine the possibility of satisfactory treatment because this may limit the ability of the nonorthodox practitioner to offer a truly alternative treatment and the sense of empowerment that might be experienced by the client.[47] The troubled relationship between orthodox practice and CAM is developed in the next section.

THE CONSEQUENCES OF "PROFESSIONALIZATION" FOR CAM

The consumer demand for CAM has contributed to moves toward "professionalization" of these practices. Some, such as chiropractic and osteopathy, have developed their own regulatory councils and refuse to support a pro-posal for a new Complementary and Alternative Medicines Council that would embrace all CAM. Other bodies, such as physiotherapy, register through specialist sections of the Health Professions Council.[48] In the UK government's White Paper, *Trust, Assurance and Safety*,[49] other CAM were refused the right to develop their own statutory councils. Instead, in 2008, the Complementary and Natural Healthcare Council (CNHC) was established to support approved complementary health care practitioners to register with them and so join the process of achieving self-regulation. The consequences of this are that all CAM now have to conform to more orthodox practices if they wish to achieve recognition. For example, one of the currently approved practices is Sports and Remedial Therapies. As with other CNHC-approved CAM, the treatment is primarily grounded in physiological and biomechanical techniques, aiming to prevent, recognize and treat sports-related injuries and to maintain and improve fitness. The main focus of this approach is to work on neuromuscular and circulatory systems, using posture and gait analyses and treatments that incorporate mechanical and electrical approaches, all of which embrace a biomedical approach to diagnosis and rehabilitation.[50]

Therefore, it is possible that the increased plurality of medical practices challenges the hegemony of the biomedical model as it has to legitimate itself in contrast to alternative practices.[51] In reality, however, for those CAM modalities wishing to become professionally recognized, pressures have been placed upon them to produce evidence of their effectiveness, in ways congruent with current scientific knowledge.[52] Such pressures have led to changes both in the knowledge claims and practices of some forms of CAM, which many regard as reinforcing, rather than challenging, the hege-mony of biomedicine[53] and "selling out" on the principles of the practices.[54] These include all or some of the following (depending on the specific ther-apy): a standardized curriculum leading to accreditation of the modality; a modification of knowledge claims from "alternative" to "complementary" to orthodoxy; aligning the knowledge base of the modality to the positivist scientific paradigm; and engaging in the registration of qualified practitio-ners as a statement of expertise and specialism with the effect that practice is restricted to a small highly qualified group.[55] This follows the neoliberal model of "expert professionalism," which gives primacy to specialized and marketable scientific knowledge.[56] It is possible that what Goffman calls the "the social consequences of professionalization"[57] may undermine the benefits of CAM for clients and the challenge that CAM present to the limitations of orthodox medicine. It is even possible that CAM may become absorbed into the system against which they are defined as complementary and/or alternative.[58]

At the heart of this debate is the concept of evidence-based medicine (EBM; see also Nancy Theberge's contribution to this collection). For exam-ple, at the time of writing, the UK Department of Health had not awarded entry into the Health Professions Council or CNHC nor given state regulation to acupuncture, herbal medicine and TCM primarily because the evidence base for these treatments was not considered to be sufficiently robust. Without such an evidence base, it is unlikely that public funding from the NHS will be made available. Interestingly, although these healing methods are fully accepted in many countries, and are considered to be thousands of years old,[59] in the UK and other Western nations they are regarded as "less established, aspirant professions."[60] The Department of Health recognizes the importance of acknowledging the long tradition of these alternative approaches, but still calls for "increasingly detailed data that grows into a convincing portfolio of evidence that balances rigour (internal validity) and relevance (external validity)."[61] Most crucially, the required evidence includes randomized controlled trials (RCT), alongside case studies and qualitative data. And, of course, all of this is to be conducted by professions that are denied state funding to undertake such research.

In contrast to the experience of these forms of CAM, which are having to find funding in order to undertake the required research to prove their value, in the interview with ED, he argued that the majority of health care funding is actually channeled into orthodox "modalities which have general acceptance," but, crucially "when you really look at the evidence base there really isn't much of one, especially when results from the clinical environment and external, published data are evaluated together." This is an example of what Latour calls scientific legitimation:[62] that once something is established as a scientific fact (that the biomedical model for health care is the most effective and safe), it is accepted as truth, becomes legitimated and no longer needs referencing or scrutiny.[63]

Several recent studies have taken a Foucauldian perspective to critique EBM, drawing on Foucault's examination of the ways in which people's lives can be managed by the state and other authorities through the presentation of "truths" and expertise that operate in panoptic surveillance.[64] Normalization is created through definitions of risks, which leads to the introduction of systems constraining behavior and lifestyle choices, while simultaneously privileging some individuals over others.[65] In this case, the perceived "risks" are the questions over the safety of nonstatutory regulated professions, the constraints are the consequences of limited funding, the privileged are the orthodox medical practitioners, whereas CAM are "othered." Holmes et al. have argued that this is a system of microfascisms, which "is outrageously exclusionary and dangerously normative with regards to scientific knowledge."[66] This is particularly significant for those athletes who find CAM to be a more effective, holistic treatment for their sport-related injuries than orthodox health care, as illustrated by many of those interviewed during this research. Furthermore, there is a hidden politics within the presentation of such "evidence": that the so-called experts often have vested interests in promoting a product for consumption. As ED argues, "corporations' and government views have been distorted by a number of different presences, many of them driven largely by financial interests." It is worthy of note that any CAM modality wishing to register with the CNHC and work toward achieving the status of a regulated profession has to pay registration fees to this body.

Criticisms are also leveled at the role of RCT in EBM. The initial basis of EBM was to develop an approach to medicine based firmly on evidence, with the evidence provided from two main areas: published scientific research and the clinical environment.[67] However, as ED explains, in contemporary science EBM is interpreted rather differently, and, to the frustration of the instigators of the EBM concept, "it generally ignores the experiential, clinical side of it . . . looking less at observational data and more at randomized trials." The problem that ED has discovered with the increasing reliance on RCTs is that there is a "big discrepancy between what people are experiencing at a clinical level and what studies based on RCT are saying." In other words, in the experimental RCT situation, the very nature of the controlled situation means that the experience for the client is completely different to the real-world situation: the relationship between client and practitioner, the mental and even spiritual experience, are all removed in the RCT. Following Goldacre, CAM is more than just the actual treatment, "it's about the whole cultural experience of a treatment, your expectations beforehand, the consultation process you go through while receiving the treatment, and much more."[68] For many athletes this is largely related to how actively they might be involved in their treatment and, for some, the gendered nature of the process, as demonstrated in an earlier section of this chapter. Indeed, one criticism the rowers in the case study made against their orthodox practitioners was the apparent disinterestedness and failure to dedicate sufficient time to their treatment. This is a more general criticism of orthodox medicine. As Goldacre explains, "a GP can't do much in a six-minute appointment,"[69] yet athletes contrasted such experiences with the style of engagement exhibited by CAM practitioners. The challenge for the RCT is that it fails to replicate the often lengthy and holistic interaction of client and practitioner, and so invalidates what really happens in the clinical environment. When the RCT finds a lack of evidence supporting the effectiveness of the approach, there is a failure to recognize that it may be the scientific method, rather than the practice, that is problematic. And where there is significant evidence of positive experiences, as in the case of thousands of years of TCMs or Ayurveda, and even the stories of the rowers consulted in this research, this evidence is often dismissed as "anecdotal." ED argues that the RCT attempts to measure and quantify *efficacy* in an experimental situation and that in so doing, it often fails to provide useful data on *effectiveness* in the real world. He goes on to state that the policy makers and those responsible for state registration are overly preoccupied with EBM based on RCTs "without appreciating the huge limitations of RCTs," and so state registration becomes based on efficacy rather than effectiveness. Notably, the Department of Health report is most concerned that CAM produce "codified detailed accounts of the long-term *efficacy and safety*."[70] The paucity of RCT evidence or, where such data are available, the often conflicting results obtained continue to delay state registration of CAM modalities in many European countries, including the UK, with negative implications for their many users, including athletes requiring CAM treatment for sport-related injuries and illness.

CONCLUDING THOUGHTS

The evidence from the case study of athletes, and more general surveys of usage, demonstrates that CAM are experienced as effective health care treatments for injured athletes and the wider population. While the use of CAM by athletes is symptomatic of broader social trends, it also appears to be the case that athletes are particularly inclined to use CAM as they fulfill a specific need of this population for an active and holistic treatment that is consistent with the athletic identity. However, the ongoing reliance on a positivist scientific paradigm that privileges EBM grounded in RCT serves to reinforce the hegemony of allopathic medicine. This appears to be to the detriment of a more inclusive health care system and to the clients themselves, who desire their services but are constrained by the economic and regulatory structures that often force consumers into the "care" of the orthodox practitioner. It is clear that the professionalization of health care is valuable when it results in safe, effective practice. However, the evidence presented in this chapter suggests that there is increased need for the development of a democratic professional model for CAM modalities, such that the voices of all professional groups and service users, including athletes, are heard and inform future practice.

NOTES

1. Pike, "Doctors Just Say."
2. Cant and Sharma, "Alternative Health Practices."
3. Ernst, "Role of Complementary and Alternative Medicine."
4. Rees and Weil, "Integrated Medicine."
5. Thomas, Nicoll and Coleman, "Use and Expenditure."
6. Goldacre, *Bad Science*, 28.
7. Sharma, *Complementary Medicine Today*.
8. Ibid.
9. Saks, "From Quackery to Complementary Medicine."
10. Ibid.
11. Hardey, *Social Context of Health*, 12.
12. Rees and Weil, "Integrated Medicine."
13. Pike, "Doctors Just Say"; Sharma, *Complementary Medicine Today*.
14. Flick, *Introduction to Qualitative Research*. For further details of the research findings from the rowing study, see Pike, "Doctors Just Say"; "Risk, Pain and Injury."

15. Hardey, *Social Context of Health*.
16. Lupton, *Medicine as Culture*, 128.
17. Crawford, "Healthism"; Sharma, *Complementary Medicine Today*.
18. Lupton, "Your Life"; Urry, *Tourist Gaze*.
19. Savage et al., *Property, Bureaucracy and Culture*.
20. Pike, "Doctors Just Say."
21. Theberge, *Higher Goals*.
22. Duquin, "Body Snatchers."
23. Hardey, *Social Context of Health*.
24. Wilkinson and Kitzinger, *Women and Health*, 129.
25. Sandall et al., "Social Service Professional."
26. House of Lords, *Sixth Report*; Lupton, *Imperative of Health*; Taylor, "Alternative Medicine."
27. Braathen, "Communicating the Individual Body"; Crawford, "Healthism"; Lowenberg and Davis, "Beyond Medicalisation-Demedicalisation."
28. Coward, *Whole Truth*; Lupton, *Medicine as Culture*.
29. House of Lords, *Sixth Report*.
30. Pike, "Doctors Just Say," 207.
31. Larkin, *Occupational Monopoly*.
32. Pike, "Doctors Just Say," 208.
33. Cant and Sharma, "Alternative Health Practices"; Hardey, *Social Context of Health*; Lupton, *Medicine as Culture*.
34. Frank, *Wounded Storyteller*, 93.
35. Pike, "Doctors Just Say," 211.
36. Wilkinson and Kitzinger, *Women and Health*.
37. Charmaz, "Experiencing Chronic Illness," 288.
38. Cant and Sharma, "Alternative Health Practices."
39. Sharma, *Complementary Medicine Today*, 50
40. Hardey, *Social Context of Health*.
41. House of Lords, *Sixth Report*.
42. Sharma, *Complementary Medicine Today*.
43. Pike, "Doctors Just Say," 212.
44. Cant and Sharma, "Alternative Health Practices."
45. Perkin, Pearcy and Fraser, "Comparison."
46. Hardey, *Social Context of Health*.
47. Sharma, *Complementary Medicine Today*.
48. Kuhlmann, Allsop and Saks, "Professional Governance."
49. Department of Health, *Trust, Assurance and Safety*.
50. See www.cnhc.org.uk. Accessed 1st August 2011.
51. Kuhlmann, Allsop and Saks, "Professional Governance."
52. British Medical Association, *Alternative Therapies*; Cant, "From Charismatic Teaching"; House of Lords, *Sixth Report*.
53. McClean, "Doctoring the Spirit."
54. Cant, "From Charismatic Teaching."
55. Ibid.; Cant and Sharma, "State and Complementary Medicine"; Pike, "Doctors Just Say."
56. Sandall et al., "Social Service Professional."
57. Goffman, *Asylums*, 296.
58. Schneirov and Geczik, "Alternative Health."
59. Galambos, "Origins of Chinese Medicine."
60. Department of Health, *Report to Ministers*.
61. Ibid., 32.
62. Latour, *Science in Action*.
63. Jackson and Scambler, "Perceptions of Evidence-Based Medicine."

64. Foucault, *Power/Knowledge.*
65. Holmes et al., "Deconstructing the Evidence-Based Discourse"; Markula and Pringle, *Foucault, Sport and Exercise*; Murray et al., "No Exit?"; Neilson, "Anti-Ageing Cultures"; Pickard, "Governing Old Age"; Piggin, Jackson and Lewis, "Telling the Truth."
66. Holmes et al., "Deconstructing the Evidence-Based Discourse," 181.
67. Sackett et al., "Evidence Based Medicine."
68. Goldacre, *Bad Science*, 37.
69. Ibid., 76
70. Department of Health, *Trust, Assurance and Safety*, 31 (emphasis in original).

BIBLIOGRAPHY

Braathen, E. "Communicating the Individual Body and the Body Politic: The Discourse on Disease Prevention and Health Promotion in Alternative Therapies." In *Complementary and Alternative Medicines: Knowledge in Practice*, edited by S. Cant and U. Sharma, 151–162. London: Free Association Books, 1996.
British Medical Association. *Alternative Therapies. Report of the Board of Science and Education.* London: British Medical Association, 1986.
Cant, S. "From Charismatic Teaching to Professional Training: The Legitimation of Knowledge and the Creation of Trust in Homeopathy and Chiropractic." In *Complementary and Alternative Medicines: Knowledge in Practice*, edited by S. Cant and U. Sharma, 44–65. London: Free Association Books, 1996.
Cant, S., and U. Sharma. "Alternative Health Practices and Systems." In *The Handbook of Social Studies in Health and Medicine*, edited by G. Albrecht, R. Fitzpatrick and S. Scrimshaw, 426–40. London: Sage, 2000.
Cant, S., and U. Sharma. "The State and Complementary Medicine: A Changing Relationship?" In *The Sociology of Health and Illness Reader*, edited by S. Nettleton and U. Gustafsson, 334–344. Cambridge: Polity, 2002.
Charmaz, K. "Experiencing Chronic Illness." In *The Handbook of Social Studies in Health and Medicine*, edited by G. Albrecht, R. Fitzpatrick and S. Scrimshaw, 277–92. London: Sage, 2000.
Coward, R. *The Whole Truth: The Myth of Alternative Health.* London: Faber and Faber, 1989.
Crawford, R. "Healthism and the Medicalization of Everyday Life." *International Journal of Health Services* 19 (1980): 365–388.
Department of Health. *Report to Ministers from The Department of Health Steering Group on the Statutory Regulation of Practitioners of Acupuncture, Herbal Medicine, Traditional Chinese Medicine and Other Traditional Medicine Systems Practised in the UK.* London: Stationery Office, 2008.
———. *Trust, Assurance and Safety—The Regulation of Health Professionals in the 21st Century.* London: Stationery Office, 2007.
Duquin, M. "The Body Snatchers and Dr. Frankenstein Revisited: Social Construction and Deconstruction of Bodies and Sport." *Journal of Sport & Social Issues* 18 (1994): 268–281
Ernst, E. "The Role of Complementary and Alternative Medicine." *British Medical Journal* 321 (2000): 1133–1135.
Flick, U. *An Introduction to Qualitative Research.* London: Sage, 1998.
Frank, A. *The Wounded Storyteller: Body, Illness and Ethics.* London: University of Chicago Press, 1995.
Foucault, M. *Power/Knowledge: Selected Interviews and Other Writings 1972–1977.* London: Harvester, 1980.

Galambos, I. *The Origins of Chinese Medicine—The Early Development of Medical Literature in China.* 2000. http://www.logoi.com/notes/chinese_medicine. html, accessed 1ˢᵗ August 2011.

Goffman, E. *Asylums: Essays on the Social Situation of Mental Patients and Other Inmates.* London: Penguin Books, 1961.

———. *Interaction Ritual.* New York: Doubleday Anchor, 1967.

Goldacre, B. *Bad Science.* London: Harper Perennial, 2009.

Hardey, M. *The Social Context of Health.* Buckingham: Open University Press, 1998.

Holmes, D., S. Murray, A. Perron and G. Rail. "Deconstructing the Evidence-Based Discourse in Health Sciences: Truth, Power and Fascism." *International Journal of Evidence Based Healthcare* 4 (2006): 180–186.

House of Lords, Science and Technology Committee. *Sixth Report: Complementary and Alternative Medicine.* London: United Kingdom Parliament, 2000.

Jackson, S., and G. Scambler. "Perceptions of Evidence-Based Medicine: Traditional Acupuncturists in the UK and Resistance to Biomedical Modes of Evaluation." *Sociology of Health & Illness* 29 (2007): 412–429.

Kuhlmann, E., J. Allsop and M. Saks. "Professional Governance and Public Control: A Comparison of Healthcare in the United Kingdom and Germany." *Current Sociology* 57 (2010): 511–528.

Larkin, G. *Occupational Monopoly and Modern Medicine.* London: Tavistock, 1983.

Latour, B. *Science in Action: How to Follow Scientists and Engineers through Society.* Cambridge, MA: Harvard University Press, 1987.

Lowenberg, J., and F. Davis. "Beyond Medicalisation-Demedicalisation: The Case of Holistic Health." *Sociology of Health & Illness* 16 (1994): 579–599.

Lupton, D. *The Imperative of Health: Public Health and the Regulated Body.* London: Sage, 1997.

———. *Medicine as Culture: Illness, Disease and the Body in Western Societies.* London: Sage, 1998.

———. "Your Life in Their Hands: Trust in the Medical Encounter." In *Health and the Sociology of Emotions*, edited by V. James and J. Gabe, 157–172. Oxford: Blackwell, 1996.

Markula, P., and R. Pringle. *Foucault, Sport and Exercise: Power, Knowledge and Transforming the Self.* London: Routledge, 2006.

McClean, S. "Doctoring the Spirit." *Health: An Interdisciplinary Journal for the Social Study of Health, Illness and Medicine* 7 (2003): 483–500.

Murray, S., D. Holmes, A. Perron and G. Rail. "No Exit? Intellectual Integrity under the Regime of 'Evidence' and 'Best Practices.'" *Journal of Evaluation in Clinical Practice* 13 (2006): 512–516.

Neilson, B. "Anti-Ageing Cultures, Biopolitics and Globalisation." *Cultural Studies Review* 12 (2006): 149–164.

Perkin, M., R. Pearcy and J. Fraser. "A Comparison of the Attitudes Shown by General Practitioners, Hospital Doctors and Medical Students towards Alternative Medicine." *Journal of the Royal Society of Medicine* 87 (1994): 523–525.

Pickard, S. "Governing Old Age: The 'Case Managed' Older Person." *Sociology* 43 (2009): 67–84.

Piggin, J., S. Jackson and M. Lewis. "Telling the Truth in Public Policy: An Analysis of New Zealand Sport Policy Discourse." *Sociology of Sport Journal* 26 (2009): 462–482.

Pike, E. "Doctors Just Say 'Rest and Take Ibuprofen': A Critical Examination of the Role of 'Non-Orthodox' Health Care in Women's Sport." *International Review for the Sociology of Sport* 40 (2005): 201–219.

————. "Risk, Pain and Injury: 'A Natural Thing in Rowing'?" In *Sporting Bodies, Damaged Selves: Sociological Studies of Sports-Related Injury*, edited by K. Young, 151–162. Oxford: Elsevier, 2004.

Rees, L., and A. Weil. "Integrated Medicine." *British Medical Journal* 322 (2001): 119–120.

Sackett, D., W. Rosenberg, J. Muir Gray, R. Haynes and W. Richardson. "Evidence Based Medicine: What It Is and What It Isn't." *British Medical Journal* 312 (1996): 71–72.

Saks, M. "From Quackery to Complementary Medicine: The Shifting Boundaries between Orthodox and Unorthodox Medical Knowledge." In *Complementary and Alternative Medicines: Knowledge in Practice*, edited by S. Cant and U. Sharma, 27–43. London: Free Association Books, 1996.

————. *Professions and the Public Interest*. London: Routledge, 1995.

Sandall, J., C. Benoit, S. Wrede, S. Murray, E. van Teijlingen and R. Westfall. "Social Service Professional or Market Expert: Maternity Care Relations under Neoliberal Reform." *Current Sociology* 57 (2009): 529–554.

Savage, M., J. Barlow, P. Dickens and T. Fielding. *Property, Bureaucracy and Culture: Middle Class Formation in Contemporary Britain*. London: Routledge, 1992.

Schneirov, M., and J. Geczik. "Alternative Health and the Challenges of Institutionalization." *Health: An Interdisciplinary Journal for the Social Study of Health, Illness and Medicine* 6 (2002): 201–220.

Sharma, U. *Complementary Medicine Today: Practitioners and Patients*. London: Routledge, 1992.

Taylor, R. "Alternative Medicine and the Medical Encounter in Britain and the United States." In *Alternative Medicines: Popular and Policy Perspectives*, edited by J. Salmon, 191–228. London: Tavistock Publications, 1984.

Theberge, N. *Higher Goals: Women's Ice Hockey and the Politics of Gender*. New York: State University of New York Press, 2000.

Thomas K., J. Nicoll and P. Coleman. "Use and Expenditure on Complementary Medicine in England: A Population Based Survey." *Complementary Therapies in Medicine* 9 (2001): 2–11.

Urry, J. *The Tourist Gaze: Leisure and Travel in Contemporary Societies*. London: Sage, 1990.

Wilkinson, S., and C. Kitzinger. *Women and Health: Feminist Perspectives*. London: Taylor Francis, 1994.

8 Challenges to the Implementation of a Rationalized Model of Sports Medicine
An Analysis in the Canadian Context

Nancy Theberge

Analyses of the emergence of modern sport have emphasized the significance of the historical process of rationalization. Particular attention has been drawn to the application of scientific knowledge about the sources and determinants of human performance to the study of sporting performance. In his account of the evolution of sports science over the course of the twentieth century, Hoberman has shown how scientific interest in the "biological wonders of the human body," initially divorced from any concern with practical applications, was transformed into "today's attempts by teams of athletes, trainers, doctors and scientists to produce record-breaking performances."[1] Additional elements of the historical analysis of rationalization are provided by Waddington in his examination of the development of sports medicine as an instance of the application of scientific knowledge to improving human performance. Waddington locates the acceleration of this process in the post–World War II era, marked by rising nationalism, leading countries to place emphasis on performance in international competition as a way to enhance visibility and prestige, and increased commercialism, leading to greater material rewards from sporting performance.[2]

The social bases of the rationalization process have been extensively examined in Beamish and Ritchie's analysis of contemporary high-performance sport.[3] They argue that advances in scientific understanding of human capacity have yielded a new paradigm of performance.

> The new paradigm of sport science is dominated by an instrumental, technological rationality where the results of experimental research from around the globe concerning performance enhancement are placed directly at the finger tips of applied sport scientists, coaches, and athletes as they explore and experiment with training techniques, and methods to enhance athletic performance. Athletes, professionals in sport medicine, and coaches now find themselves at the centre of a well-funded, high stakes drive to push human performance to its outer limits.[4]

The "well-funded, high stakes drive" has been institutionalized in national sport systems, marked by investments in administrative and technical support aimed at the production of medal winning performances in international sport. Green and Houlihan have examined the implementation of this model in a comparative analysis of elite sport processes and policy change in the United Kingdom, Australia and Canada.[5] Their analysis of the Canadian case is particularly relevant to the present discussion. The last half century has been marked by the emergence in Canada of a "centrally planned and bureaucratic elite sport development model" that includes, among other features, "a relatively sophisticated cluster of sports science, sports medicine and physical therapy services for elite athletes."[6] In their analysis of policy and process, Green and Houlihan conclude that in Canada (and similar to the other countries studied, the UK and Australia), despite the growth of sports science programs and the establishment of medical committees in national sport organizations, "sports have been fairly slow to explore the potential of sport science in relation to competitors." This is contrasted with greater engagement of scientific research related to equipment and apparel, and Green and Houlihan suggest that the explanation for the difference lies in the commercial profits to be made from product development rather than research into training, nutrition and athlete preparation for competition.[7]

References to the rationalization of sport often conflate the terms *sports medicine/sports science*, whereas a full understanding of the application of this paradigm recognizes that the manner and degree to which research in medicine and sports science is incorporated into clinical practice is an empirical question. This point is acknowledged by Safai in her discussion of the historical development of sports medicine in Canada, where she indicates that although the interest to apply medical science has become incorporated into the ideology and organization of sport in Canada, "the degree to which high performance athletes experience or perceive the medicalization of sport is unknown."[8] To this it may be added that there has been little investigation of the process whereby this occurs.

In an effort to advance our understanding of the social organization of sports medicine as a historically specific form of rationalization, this chapter examines the administration and delivery of sports medicine services to high-performance athletes in Canada. Drawing on interviews with administrators, coaches, health care providers and athletes, this chapter explores accounts of what an effective model for the delivery of sports medicine entails and some of the challenges attendant to the implementation of this model. The discussion focuses on challenges in two contexts. The first is internal to sport and entails aligning the interests and actions of different stakeholders around a vision of an effective sports medicine system. The second challenge lies at the intersection of sport and the system of sports medicine professions and involves negotiation over which professions, and professional services, will be supported within the support structure for high-performance athletes. This issue is examined in a discussion of the place of massage therapy within this structure.

DATA COLLECTION AND ANALYSIS

The analysis reported here is taken from a larger study of the social organization of sports medicine in Canadian high-performance sport. As in other contexts, in Canada the term *sports medicine* is used to refer to a multidisciplinary field that includes medicine and allied health professions. Historically, the primary allied professions in Canada were physiotherapy and athletic therapy, the designation in Canada for the profession known in the US (and formerly in Canada) as athletic training. The roots of athletic therapy, and its continuing base, lie in university athletic programs and on professional sports teams in the US and Canada, where athletic therapists (or trainers) historically were the primary providers of site coverage of athletic events, including immediate care of athletic injuries.[9] In more recent years both chiropractic and massage therapy have gained greater prominence in the system of sport medicine in Canada. The provision of health care to athletes occurs in a variety of settings, including at major competitions such as the Olympics, when teams are away at training camps, and in private clinical settings. One of the main contexts and a focus for much of the discussion presented here is a network of eight Canadian Sport Centres, or CSCs, which are located in major urban centers across the country. The CSCs provide support for high-performance athletes and coaches in a variety of areas, including sports science and sports medicine. The CSCs also assist in funding some health care services, for care not covered by public health insurance programs (this point is discussed in more detail below, in a consideration of funding provide to athletes for massage therapy).

Data were obtained by means of interviews with four groups of participants: administrators responsible for the organization or delivery of sports medicine services for national team athletes in different contexts; coaches who are affiliated with national team programs; athletes who are affiliated with national team programs; and health care providers who work with national-level athletes. The sample includes five administrators, five coaches, thirty-six athletes and thirty-four health care providers, including ten physicians, eight athletic therapists, ten physiotherapists and eight chiropractors. Among the administrators and coaches, the majority of study participants are men whereas the sample of athletes and practitioners is more evenly balanced between men and women. The sports that the athletes compete in, and other members of the sample work with, include men's and women's as well as team and individual. In the interests of preserving study participants' anonymity, their gender and the sports they are affiliated with are not identified. Additionally, because in the case of the non-physician professions, identification of a provider's profession might compromise anonymity, this information also is not indicated and physiotherapists, athletic therapists and chiropractors are referred to as "care providers."[10]

Participants were recruited to the research in several ways. The recruitment process began with inquiries to administrators at CSCs, who provided referrals to other administrators as well as practitioners, coaches and athletes who might be interested in participating in the study. In the case of practitioners, additional respondents were identified from lists of health care providers at recent Olympic Games posted on the website of the Canadian Olympic Committee. Another means was a snowball technique whereby participants were asked to suggest the names of others in the subgroups of interest who might be interviewed for this research.

The interviews covered a range of topics related to the delivery of health care to athletes and professional practice in different contexts, such as the Olympics and when teams are away at training camps.[11] The present analysis draws in particular upon interview discussions of the following topics. Administrators and practitioners were asked about the state of sports medicine in Canada and/or in the specific contexts in which they work and challenges and opportunities related to their assessment of current conditions. These groups were also engaged in extensive discussions about their work routines, as a way to elicit observations on the organization and delivery of health care to elite athletes. Participants in all the groups were asked about the place of different professions in the system of sports medicine professions; in the case of administrators and practitioners, this question was asked in a general fashion, whereas coaches were asked about the professions represented on the medical teams in their sports and athletes were asked to discuss the providers they worked with (i.e., the profession and not the individual) and the conditions that led them to work with different practitioners. The interviews were semi-structured and of a conversational nature, allowing for wide-ranging discussions. The interviews were conducted in 2004 and 2005.

The interviews were audiotape-recorded, transcribed and entered into a qualitative data management software tool (QSR NVIVO, 2002). A preliminary coding scheme was devised and then revised on the basis of reading of the transcripts. Sections of interviews based on the codes were extracted and then examined to develop the analysis.

"UPGRADING THE LEVEL OF PROGRAMMING" OF SPORTS MEDICINE

Discussions of the state of sports medicine, whether posed broadly or with regard to specific programs, yielded extensive commentary on a common theme: the need for coordination of the activities of sports medicine practitioners. A portrait of the challenges attendant to implementing a coordinated program is offered in the following account, which draws on the observations of three participants: an administrator at a national sport center responsible for the provision of sports medicine for high-performance athletes, the head coach and a care provider in a sport affiliated with the center where this administrator works. This account begins with the following statement by the administrator concerning his/her efforts to "upgrade" sports medicine programs. The statement that follows was preceded by the administrator's indication that, in the past, the organization of sports medicine was generally understood as "coordinating the services." S/he explained: "That means line up this physio with that athlete or this surgeon with that athlete who's blown his knee out or whatever." The administrator then elaborated on his/her efforts to improve the organization of sports medicine services:

> What I'm trying to do is upgrade the level of programming that our coaches and athletes are involved in. So one of the areas is that it's all well and good to have a team [of providers from different professions]. But if none of those people are talking with each other, if that program isn't coordinated, it's not effective. . . . We're not trying to set up a performance enhancement team of individuals around the team. We want it to operate as a team. Which means that they actually meet, they discuss individual athletes. They have specific—they come with a coordinated plan to deal with each individual athlete, as opposed to trying to separate all these services out.

A parallel view of the process was provided by the head coach of a team that is affiliated with the center where this administrator works; comments in the interviews indicate these two participants have worked together on the development of sports medicine programs in the coach's sport.[12] In discussing his/her vision for sports medicine support for this team, the coach indicated s/he was trying to set up a "system" and that a key issue in this process is timely access to expert practitioners with whom this coach and athletes have ongoing relationships:

> [What] I've tried to implement here has been setting up the system, the structure with our sports med/sport science professionals, our expert sports med/sport science committee, so we have a network where the athlete will be able to get into an orthopedic surgeon, get in to see the chiropractor, physio, so they won't be denied access and the timing of that access as well as the quality of practitioner. We have the best people that we can get. So we have a system in place so that I can direct them to experts in each area. . . . I want to have a small group, custom group where I'm going to them all the time. I'm not going to this person here. I'm not going over there; I'm not going over there. You have to develop a relationship.

The coach was asked how well this system is functioning. His/her answer indicates the importance of communication, as emphasized by the administrator quoted earlier:

> Nowhere near the way it should and nowhere near the way I'd like it to. But at least we have something in place that we're moving toward. And we need to enhance our communication skills. You know, and we have these online diaries, which [an assistant coach] set up, links for communication. So that we will try. We're almost there in setting it up. But I would like to see it tried. For example, online medical files, obviously there are some issues of confidentiality but, yeah, I think we can overcome that part of it. But really that would be the best scenario, for example, I send the athlete to the GP, he sends a note, you know, referral to the orthopedic surgeon or it comes back to the therapist or massage or chiropractor and then to the coach. And then also—that's the initial contact. What is equally important is the continued follow-up and assessment and evaluation. So it's happening; it is happening but not as formally as I would like.

The coach was then asked what is needed to improve the operation of the sports medicine team. S/he noted "buy in" to the concept is in place but "hurdles" to its implementation remain, citing the example of finances:

> Well, we need a communication skill. We need to get on the same page. Like, for example, some of the practitioners don't use the e-mail as much. Some prefer to call me and then try to get a hold of somebody. . . . Now I think everybody's bought into the concept to enhance our communication, but we have some hurdles yet to develop a good system. And part of that is the dollars, to actually make that work.

A care provider who works with the same sport offered an account that again stressed the importance of a coordinated effort that brings together the sports medicine team, coaches and athletes. The care provider noted that the coach supports the concept but challenges to implementing a "system that will work" remain:

> It's not well integrated in [name of sport]; no. . . . With [name of coach], s/he believes in the concept and since I came on board I've been pushing for it because I think it's something that we should do and the [administration at the national training center], they also believe in the whole concept and we've been kind of trying to work out a system that will work. But it comes back again to funding; it comes back to time involved and getting the system going. I think in [name of sport], I think some of the people believe in it. They understand the concept. I don't think everybody has. I think maybe some people think it doesn't

matter. [They think], "You just get out and do your thing." But I'm of the belief that, I see with the clients that I think it makes a difference.

The comments from the coach and practitioner quoted in the preceding both indicate the need for greater financial support to implement effective sports medicine teams. This point offered one of the notable comparisons with the views of the administrator, who argued that an emphasis on the lack of financial support for improving the organization of sports medicine is misplaced. This participant offered the following account:

> My feeling is that the reason that Canada does badly internationally, or we do below par or we perform below our levels of expectation, is because our athletes aren't well prepared. It's not because they're not talented athletes. It's not because they're not committed, and it's not because the government doesn't put enough money into it. The fact is right now if the government shovels in truckloads of money into our program, we will have a more expensive lousy program. That's what the result is. Without proper programming and planning, we will not be successful. Our athletes are getting shortchanged on the programming and planning part of their preparation. And there is, this is just a matter of getting down to the details of developing a good program.

Although the preceding comment was made before the 2010 Winter Olympic Games in Vancouver, British Columbia, the interview occurred after the announcement of the awarding of the Games to Canada and a subsequent infusion of monies into athlete support. The administrator was asked about the likely impact of the staging of a domestic Olympic Games on high-performance sport in Canada. His/her response provided another occasion to stress the higher priority of an "effective" system:

> I think the focus has provided new money. But I've never been, I'm not as concerned about the money. The value of the money for me is that it's a hammer. So that what it means is that we'd like you to do this professionally and, if you're not prepared to do it, then your funding is going to be affected.

I then said, "But having hammers can be very useful," to which the participant responded:

> Yeah, I think so. But as far as the money itself, I mean, as I said before, I don't think injecting a whole bunch of money into a system without the system being clearly articulated and effective is just making it a more expensive crappy system, and I don't want to do that. But having it in my pocket makes me more effective.

The accounts provided earlier from individuals affiliated with the same sport indicate common agreement on the need for a coordinated system for the delivery of sports medicine services. Participants also agree that whereas not everyone affiliated with this sport is "on board," key individuals—notably coaches, sports medicine practitioners and officials at the national training center—are in support of the effort to improve the administration of services. There are some notable contrasts in the accounts offered by the three study participants. Perhaps most obvious is the different views of the importance of finances to improving the coordination of programs, where the administrator discounts the view expressed by the others that lack of finances is a main reason for the failure to implement a more effective program. Rather, s/he emphasizes the importance of "proper programming and planning."

Another contrast has to do with different understandings of what coordination entails. For the coach, *coordination* refers to ready access to a network of expert practitioners and enhanced communication among the members of that network, coaches and athletes. Although this certainly figures in the administrator's conception of a coordinated program, this participant advances a more demanding view that coordination involves an "upgraded" level of programming that is clearly articulated and realized through practices such as regular meetings and detailed plans for individual athletes. These accounts suggest that one of the challenges the administrator faces is revising the understanding of how the sports medicine team shall work and what its effort would entail. Whereas the view that more finances are needed provides a readily identifiable barrier to improved programming, transforming the understanding of the content of an effective sports medicine program and the planning process that underlies the activities of sports medicine professionals is a more complex matter and, arguably, a greater challenge to attaining the vision of a well-coordinated and effective program.

THE OTHER SIDE OF AN EFFECTIVE SYSTEM: POORLY COORDINATED SPORTS MEDICINE SUPPORT

The accounts provided in the preceding presented a vision for the effective coordination of sports medicine services and depictions by a coach and a care provider of some progress toward achieving this vision in one sport. The gap between this vision and the state of programming of sports medicine in Canadian sport was highlighted in accounts of other sports where the provision of sports medicine services is marked by an absence of communication and coordination. In making the case for a system that is "clearly articulated and effective," the administrator quoted earlier provided an example that illustrated the problems that arise when services are available but not coordinated. The example concerned an athlete who competed in an Olympic Games and then sustained an injury that plagued her for years, preventing her from competing in a subsequent Olympics. The sport in which she competes is well supported, with an extensive sports medicine team and coaching staff. The participant said during the course of this athlete's injury and rehabilitation: "None of those people had spoken (to each other)." S/he went on to provide details of the athlete's situation, which involved recurrence of the injury:

> The reason that she was breaking down was because she was weak. She maybe had an injury, you know, in the beginning. That injury was addressed so that it was no longer painful but she was not at a strength level that would help stabilize that [joint], so that every time she [returned to training], as soon as her workload would go up she would reinjure her [joint]. Well, the thing is that she wasn't lazy; she's not undermotivated. The problem with her was that she's weak. Well, why isn't the coach talking with the strength and conditioning consultant who's talking with the physio who's talking with the exercise physiologist? . . . That was totally unnecessary.

Interviews with athletes provided a number of additional examples of poorly coordinated care. An athlete provided the following account of "falling through the cracks" following surgery:

> It was a bit frustrating because we couldn't figure out what was going on with it and I think, in retrospect, I fell through the cracks a little bit after my surgery. I couldn't get to [site of training center] right away to see our physio because I couldn't drive there and the physio [where the athlete lives, a two-hour drive from the training center] wasn't really good enough. So I think it's just [that] at opportune times that I was supposed to be moving on to the next step for my muscles firing and making sure that was all happening the way it should, I didn't see them and it was just kind of one thing grew into a bigger thing into a bigger thing. So then once they figured it out, it still took another few months, you know, the symptoms ended up kind of showing up in January and it still was almost end of March or April until they really said, "Okay, this is what it is." So the severity of the situation really wasn't maybe diagnosed right away and then it just kind of got worse and worse and worse.

Another athlete provided a similar account of a rehabilitation process that suffered from lack of coordination. The issues identified by this participant include professional tensions and lack of communication between providers. The following excerpt began with the athlete's indication that a "big gap" in managing her rehabilitation is communication between providers and with her coach:

What I see as the big gap there is the communication between all of them. . . . As far as the physician I see and the physio . . . they're not linked together and they're not in one place and some of them don't enjoy each other's conversations [*chuckles*] so they don't support each other. . . . And I don't really know the whole story or what the issue is, but I definitely know that there's not the support of each other. . . . And then the other big link there is to the coach. And that's something that's really tough because my coach has other athletes and it's pretty tough to manage, to have that discussion. . . . [The physio and coach] don't have any problems with each other or anything like that. It's just that there's never been that link before. They know each other but there's never been a phone call [between them]. It's always the athlete coming back to the coach and saying, "This is what's going on."

The preceding accounts of athletes who experienced poorly coordinated sports medicine services indicate a variety of problems. In the example recounted by the administrator, the issue is the lack of communication and coordinated effort among providers. In the other cases, both athletes indicate that one problem is distance between themselves and expert providers. In the first case, this evolved into the athlete "falling through the cracks" and a delay in identification and then resolution of problems with rehabilitation. In the following example, in addition to distance from providers, the athlete identifies lack of communication between providers, due in some cases to interprofessional tensions, as well as demands on the coach's time, which limited attention to the athlete's condition. These accounts make clear that the delivery of expert medical care to athletes is heavily conditioned by social and organizational factors, and that, in some sports, the gap between the promise of medical science and the reality of medical support in athletes' lives is often considerable.

RATIONALIZING THE PROVISION OF SERVICES: "WALKING SOFTLY" AND WORKING TOWARD AN EVIDENCE-BASED MODEL

One element of the project to rationalize the organization of sports medicine is the coordination of clinical care within a team of providers; another aspect involves the determination of what that support entails. One of the main issues is determination of which professions will be included within the medical support made available to athletes. Discussions of the composition of the sports medicine team occur within the context of the evolution of the system of sports medicine professions in Canada and associated debates about the contributions of different professions to the performance-focused agenda of high-performance sport. An account of the historical evolution of sports medicine in Canada is contained in Safai's analysis of the Sports

Medicine and Science Council of Canada (SMSCC).[13] The SMSCC was established in 1978 (originally as the Sports Medicine Council of Canada, or SMCC) as the governing body of sports medicine in Canada. Although the council subsequently fell victim to political battles in Canadian sport and jurisdictional conflicts in sports medicine that led to its eventual dissolution in the early 1990s, in the interim, the council achieved considerable success in solidifying the presence of sports medicine within the organization of Canadian sport. The most notable indicator of this was improvements in the provision of sports medicine services for Canadian athletes at international games such as the Olympics to a very high standard. Another outcome of the advancements under the auspices of the SMSCC was the accelerated development of the clinical practice of sports medicine within medicine and the allied professions.[14]

When the SMSCC was established, its membership was comprised of physicians, physiotherapists and athletic therapists, as well as sport scientists. In subsequent decades other professions, specifically chiropractic and massage therapy, sought inclusion and the legitimation this would provide for their efforts to be recognized as health care providers to Canadian athletes. Expansion of the professions included in the council was resisted by the established members, who put forward two main arguments. The first was that including these professions would duplicate services already available and thus was redundant. The second argument questioned the scientific basis of the professions. Inability to resolve debates over the expansion of professions in the SMSCC contributed significantly to the demise of the council some twenty years after its establishment.[15]

Notwithstanding their unsuccessful efforts to gain membership in the SMSCC, both chiropractic and massage have made important inroads into the system of sports medicine professions in the last two decades. One measure of their acceptance is their regular inclusion in the medical missions for major sporting events such as the Olympic Games. And yet, although both these professions are now established within the system of sports medicine professions, as the following discussion of massage therapy will show, concerns about efficacy and scientific legitimacy continue to figure prominently in deliberations about the place of this profession in the programming of health care for athletes.[16] The discussion also will show that in decisions about the provision of services, this concern is balanced against a client-based model of health care that accords significance to athletes' preferences and understandings of their needs.[17]

The importance of respecting athletes' preferences figured prominently in discussions of the support structure in sports medicine. One administrator said:

> For years we've always had this debate. Do we tell the athletes what they need? Or do the athletes just tell us what they need and we react? And it's sort of a mix of both because I think there's a lot of cases where

they don't know what they need and we need to be providing some leadership. Not to say, "You do this or else" but to say, "You know what? Given what you're telling us, here's some pretty good choices as to what you could do."

Another administrator made a similar point while adding that his/her intention is, over time, to move to a position of grounding decisions about the provision of services in an evidence-based model. The following excerpt is taken from an interview conducted at a time when the administrator was in the early stages of formulating a plan to rationalize the provision of sports medicine services:

> At this point, my approach is (to) walk softly and try to get some small things in place and not push too hard. I'm quite willing for them to work with [for example] a naturopath right now. I'm not saying that we're going to be doing that for the next four years but, right now, the worst thing I could do is say, "You know what? We're not going that way. We need to use a sports medicine physician and here's the line." I'm not going to do that.

The participant was then asked how his/her approach would evolve in the move to a more efficiently organized sports medicine program. S/he answered:

> I guess we would base our decision on what we perceive (is) the value that's been added to the teams and whether the advice and the expertise that these groups are getting seems valid in our opinion.

Following the above comment, the participant was asked: "So is it fair to say you'd be moving towards an evidence-based decision?" S/he answered: "Yes. Yes. It's very fair to say that." This administrator's references to the value-added and evidence-based foundation of professional practice as determinants of their inclusion in the support structure provided to athletes references concerns about redundancy and validity, couched in contemporary terminology.

RATIONALIZING SERVICES: THE CASE OF MASSAGE

The observations of study participants from all four groups provided testimony to the established presence of massage therapy within sports medicine. Many athletes reported regular use of massage therapy and/or a wish to access massage more frequently, and participants from the other groups typically included massage in their enumeration of professions within sport. Whereas there was common recognition that massage now has an

established place in sports medicine, discussions of this profession also generated divergent ideas about the contributions of massage, indicating that
earlier debates about redundancy and validity continue. Debate about the
contributions of massage provides a case study of administrators' efforts to
rationalize the provision of services in a context where it is recognized that
athletes' wishes should be taken into account.

The administrator quoted earlier on moving to an evidence-based model
of health care elaborated on the challenges attendant to this effort with a
specific reference to massage. His/her comments were prefaced by an observation on the increasing presence of allied health professions, including
massage in sports medicine:

> There's a traditional medical approach [in sports medicine] which would
> be, you would have a sports medicine physician that is in charge of your
> sports medicine program and then there'd be other allied health profes-
> sionals. So physiotherapists, for example. . . . And then you'd get into
> other sort of allied health people like massage therapists. Which, if you
> ask an athlete about, are absolutely essential and nonnegotiable people
> to help them. . . . Now if you ask *me* about massage therapists I'll say,
> "Well, there's no good evidence that it actually enhances recovery and
> regeneration," but you talk to the athletes, they'll say, "Yes it does."

In light of these different understandings and given budget limitations, the
participant was asked how s/he formulated policies governing access to massage therapy. Consistent with another administrator's statement quoted earlier about not dictating to athletes on the utilization of specific forms of care,
s/he indicated that, notwithstanding personal skepticism about the efficacy
of massage, it is included among the services that are provided to athletes:

> At this point, we don't try to be micromanagers of that kind of thing.
> And in fact we try to be very positive about the role of massage. I'm not
> saying it doesn't work. I don't think I have enough knowledge to make
> the decision that it doesn't work. I'm still a skeptic. But I wouldn't
> impose those views on coaches or athletes.

The participant then went on to say that policies in regard to massage, as well
as on other services not covered by provincial health care insurance plans,
attempt to bring some order to utilization patterns by requiring athletes to
take some responsibility for partial payment. Health insurance in Canada is
administrated on a provincial basis and most provincial health care plans do
not cover massage therapy. Additional funding for health care is provided
to national team athletes through privately purchased insurance and funds
made available through the CSCs. The CSC where this administrator works
provides limited funds to athletes for services including massage therapy.
After providing some detail of payment plans, s/he said:

In terms of athlete responsibility, we have a policy in place where in fact we won't subsidize the whole thing. What that does is it makes them think about when and how they want to use massage. It makes them show up for their appointments [*small chuckle*] and be accountable. If we pay for the whole thing then, yeah, they might show up, they might not. They'll just use it indiscriminately. . . . So we want to make it, we want to make them accountable and responsible and make them think about what they're actually engaging these professional services for.

The reference to athletes' use of massage "indiscriminately" figured in a number of accounts. Another administrator said:

It's not surprising that athletes say they would love a massage. If you asked any general person on the street, "Would you rather, you know, go to the dentist or go to the massage therapist?" "Oh, I'd rather go to the massage therapist." "How often would you like to go?" "Wow, I'd like to go every week if I could." Everybody would say that because it's nicer to go, right? So that doesn't surprise me.

These accounts are backed up by providers who indicate they must rationalize the time they devote to massage, as demand exceeds the time available. One provider provided the following account of his/her experience when on tour with a national team:

I actually end up doing a lot of massage on tour. . . . If we had a massage therapist on tour, there would be a lot bigger lineups for treatment [*small chuckle*]. I don't—I basically save massage treatments for the more senior players who have been banged up more or somebody with, you know, a serious problem. A lot of the younger players, they like the massage and they feel like they need it, but I don't have the time to give it to them on tour.

Comments from study participants that question the efficacy of massage also were supported by the observations of practitioners, who offered a range of views on this issue. A physician offered the following assessment that speaks to both efficacy and the funding context:

When you're really training hard and your sport has a heavy emphasis on endurance so that you're constantly in for muscle fatigue and pain, I think massage therapy can be helpful. But in terms of it being scientifically proven, they don't have a lot of science on it. So from an administrator's point of view, when they're looking at what to spend money on, I can understand why they have trouble with massage therapy. . . . I think the acute stage of any injury, yes, there are some things you can do to try to hasten improvement through that acute stage, but what really counts is what do you do for your rehab after that acute stage is over. And . . . is what you're being given sport-specific enough? Does it have enough core stability in it? That sort of thing. I'm not as certain that massage—I'm not against massage therapy. I just think [that] when you're priorizing [*sic*] what a person needs, massage may not be the first thing.

A position on massage put forward by some respondents is that the concern with scientific evidence of the effect of massage on performance is misplaced. One provider, speaking of the understanding that athletes may seek massage because "it feels good" said: "If an athlete's feeling good, they're probably going to perform better." In support of this point, a physician said: "Making them feel good might make them perform better, too. So that's the whole unknown."

ATHLETES' UTILIZATION OF MASSAGE: MULTIPLE REASONS AND ATTRIBUTIONS OF BENEFITS

Administrators' questions about the place of massage in athletes' health care is given some basis by the observations of athletes about the utilization of massage. Several points made in these discussions are of note. First, the view of administrators expressed earlier that athletes frequently want greater access to massage is confirmed in the athlete interviews. Many athletes indicated that they would like more regular access to massage therapy and that the main reason they did not access massage as often as they like is due to funding limitations. As already noted, national team athletes typically receive some, but limited, funds for massage therapy.

Another point evident from athlete interviews is the varied ways in which the treatment is understood to be beneficial. Following is a representative selection of statements by athletes on the benefits they derive from massage. Following each statement, a parenthetical summary has been inserted of the specific benefits indicated in the interview excerpt. The variety of outcomes cited, including recovery, rehabilitation, prevention, relaxation and improved performance, is notable:

> When we're training so much and your muscles just get so tight and massage therapists just kind of loosen everything up. A lot of releases and stuff like that. They help take out a lot of knots in muscles and stuff and I find that really helps me . . . in terms of my range of motion. (Recovery from training)

> It helps for me for recovery. I was hit by a car two years ago. So I broke my collarbone. So starting back (training) I was getting a lot of muscle tension and so just to prevent injury and just to help kind of allow me to

train. So now it's more for maintenance and again, more for injury prevention. Just to make sure that things aren't getting too tight and just to
keep things balanced. (Recovery from training; injury prevention)

More from a relaxation point of view, a recovery point of view and also
more of an injury prevention situation as well. . . . Basically, it completely relaxes me, it stretches me out and that relaxation allows me to
rehab. Like all the aches and pains associated with practicing four, five
times a week are now not as much of a factor because I go into the next
practice a lot more fresh. (Relaxation; recovery; injury prevention)

I personally like massage therapists [*laughs*]. Really relaxing. . . . It's
nice to have. I don't think it really—I think it helps. You know, my performance would be a lot better if I'm healthy and I'm feeling, my body's
feeling good. (Relaxation; improved performance from "feeling good")

I find that with massage you can get into, your muscles and things
like that are always compensating or changing, depending on training
or injury or how you're using your body and a massage therapist can
really tell the compensations and help, well for me she helps work with
me to relax or to try and de-stress I guess [*chuckles*] the muscles and
make them not so tight. (Relaxation; correction of muscle imbalance
problems)

I take massage to recover, to flush like all the work that we've been
doing. So I take the massage as a recovery for my body like from work-
outs. (Recovery from training)

I'm a big massage fan. When I'm getting a massage, my body feels just
so good, right? ("Feels good")

[At a tournament] after every match I'd get massage and I was able
to [compete] through, and I don't think I would've been able to do
that considering the amount of stress that my body went through that
weekend, without the massage 'cause as soon as I was done the masseuse was there to flush my system and I was ready and I was up. . . . I
don't know how that is physiologically, but I felt—as long as I kept on
[competing in my sport] and he kept massaging me leading up to that,
I didn't even use ice throughout the competition until the last couple of
matches. (Recovery during competition)

Although the preceding accounts provide ample testimony to athletes' beliefs
about the importance of massage in their lives, the accounts also may be
seen to offer support for the skepticism voiced by administrators. Returning to the observations of the administrator who indicated an intention to

move to an evidence-based model, where access to services is endorsed on the basis of their contribution to performance, a number of concerns are suggested by athletes' accounts. The very variety of benefits cited by athletes may prompt skepticism about whether massage can make a meaningful contribution to performance in all the ways identified earlier. Even if the answer is "no," or "unlikely," it is appropriate to ask: which effects do impact performance? An additional question raised by some study participants, which speaks to the issue of "value added," is: might the benefits of massage be obtained in some other ways?

The issue of alternative sources of some of the benefits of massage was discussed by a physician. This observation occurred in the context of a discussion of the expanding array of services that has emerged under the client-centered model of sports medicine. This participant suggested that this model has contributed to a decline in athletes' responsibility for their well-being. S/he provided the following account that referenced athletes' reliance on massage:

> At some point, there's this whole business of . . . where these guys cannot compete unless they have everything. . . . Without their massage, they won't be able to go the other [i.e., next] day. You kind of have to temper it a little bit. Like one of the coaches [in sport where the physician works], he was standing there watching everybody waiting for their massage and he was, you know, "Whatever happened to the cool down?" You know? And frankly, it's probably more valuable than a massage. And because they're not doing, because they're getting the massage, they don't even do the cool down because the masseur will flush everything out. So you've gotta, you have to put everything in balance.

It should be emphasized that interrogating the place of massage in athletes' lives is not an endorsement for withdrawing massage from the treatments made available to athletes or excluding massage therapists from professions included in sports medicine teams. Moreover, a number of participants endorsed the view that athletes' beliefs that massage has identifiable outcomes, with regard to recovery, rehabilitation or even relaxation, constitute a valid basis for including it in the menu of services provided to them. Notwithstanding some concern that the availability of massage may prompt athletes to forgo forms of self-care, such as a "cool down," the larger consideration is weighing the contributions of massage in a context where resources are limited and it is recognized that athletes' preferences are important considerations in deciding on the provisions of services. One way in which reservations about effects are tied to an effort to ration resources is requiring athletes to pay some part of the costs of massage treatment in order to hold them accountable for an efficient utilization of the resource.

DISCUSSION AND CONCLUSION: THE LIMITS TO A RATIONALIZED MODEL OF SPORTS MEDICINE

Historical accounts of the development of modern sport have documented the emergence of a paradigm of sporting performance grounded in an instrumental and technical rationality. One of the main contexts for the application of scientific knowledge is the delivery of sports medicine support for athletes. The present analysis has contributed to our understanding of the incorporation of sports medicine into the support structure for athletes by examining the observations of administrators, coaches, sports medicine professionals and athletes concerning the content of effective sports medicine programs and some of the challenges attendant to their development and implementation.

Discussions of the content of sports medicine programs highlighted the need for coordination of care. This point was explored through the observations of administrators on their planning objectives and illustrated in the accounts of participants from other groups of inadequate care deriving at least in part from poor coordination between not only health care providers, but between providers, athletes and coaches. One of the notable features of these accounts is the variety of circumstances that were cited as contributing to lack of coordination. In many instances, poor coordination was accompanied by, or an outcome of, poor communication. Comments also spoke to variations in the support among key personnel, both coaches and health professionals, for efforts to achieve a coordinated program. Additional problems cited in the accounts of athletes concern accessing health care providers, in some cases due to geographical distances, professional or interpersonal tensions between practitioners and limitations on coaches' time. The last is significant because of the centrality of coaches to all aspects of athletes' training programs.

One of the most telling aspects of the discussion of challenges to implementing a well-coordinated program is evident in the narrative of conditions in one sport drawing upon the observations of an administrator, coach and care provider. Whereas the coach and provider indicated that difficulties in coordinating sports medicine services were due in part to limited financial resources, the administrator argued that a focus on funding as a key to program development was misplaced. Rather, s/he felt that emphasis must be placed on "the details of developing a good program" and following through on this with proper planning and coordinated activity among the key members of the athlete's support structure, notably coaches, trainers and sports medicine personnel. In this observation, the administrator suggests that deficiencies in the delivery of sports medicine are grounded in the social organization of the surrounding support structure. These observations suggest that there is a considerable gap between the instrumental paradigm of sport science that has seen such advances in the generation of knowledge of performance and its application to the social organization of sport.

The second form of challenge to the implementation of a rationalized model of the delivery of sports medicine examined here occurs at the intersection of the social organization of high-performance sport and the system of sports medicine professions. This topic is examined in a discussion of the place of massage therapy in the support structure for athletes. In recent decades, massage therapy has become established within the system of sports medicine professions. This has occurred despite ongoing debate about its benefits. Doubts about the efficacy of massage are countered by the recognition that athletes wish to have access to this treatment, supported by the understanding that "if an athlete's feeling good, they're probably going to perform better." In their efforts to implement a rationalized or evidence-based model of health care in high-performance sport, administrators must weigh concerns about the efficacy and value-added contributions of specific forms of health care against athletes' preferences and beliefs about treatments. The client-centered nature of sports medicine along with the established position of massage within the system of sports medicine professions combine to create a specific challenge for administrators' efforts to implement an evidence-based model of sports medicine. It may also be said that this effort points to the limits of the model of technical rationality that derive from the human dimension of sport performance.

In conclusion, the analysis presented here suggests that whereas the dominant paradigm of performance in sport has indeed placed scientific and medical knowledge about performance at "the fingertips" of applied sports scientists,[18] including sports medicine clinicians, the implementation of this model is conditioned, and often constrained, by features of the social context in which sports medicine and science is applied. The discussion in this chapter has highlighted how the social organization of sport and its intersection with the system of sports medicine figure powerfully in the translation of scientific knowledge into clinical applications. Although the quest to maximize performance remains the defining feature of the ideology of modern sport, its realization remains dependent on the social formations embodied in the worlds of sport and sports medicine.

NOTES

1. Hoberman, *Mortal Engines*, ix.
2. Waddington, "Development of Sports Medicine."
3. Beamish and Ritchie, *Fastest, Highest, Strongest.*
4. Ibid., 64–65.
5. Green and Houlihan, *Elite Sports Development.*
6. Ibid., 50. See also Macintosh and Whitson, *Game Planners*; Safai, "Critical Analysis."
7. Green and Houlihan, *Elite Sports Development*, 177.
8. Safai, "Critical Analysis," 335.

9. Walk, "Athletic Trainers."
10. Among the nonphysician health care providers (i.e., physiotherapists, athletic therapists and chiropractors) interviewed for this research are individuals who have close and long-standing relations with specific sports. It is for this reason that identifying an individual by his/her profession may risk compromising the anonymity of the interviews.
11. Theberge, "Professional Identifies."
12. So as to preserve the anonymity of the study participants, when a given participant referred to another participant during an interview, the fact that the person mentioned was also a participant in the study was not divulged.
13. Safai, "Demise."
14. Ibid.
15. Ibid.
16. An examination of the integration of chiropractic into the system of sports medicine is provided in Theberge, "Integration of Chiropractors."
17. Theberge, "Integration of Chiropractors"; "We Have All the Bases Covered."
18. Beamish and Ritchie, *Fastest, Highest, Strongest*, 64.

BIBLIOGRAPHY

Beamish, Rob, and Ian Ritchie. *Fastest, Highest, Strongest: A Critique of High-Performance Sport.* New York: Routledge, 2006.
Green, Mick, and Barrie Houlihan. *Elite Sport Development: Policy Learning and Political Priorities.* Abingdon: Routledge, 2005.
Hoberman, John. *Mortal Engines: The Science of Performance and the Dehumanization of Sport.* New York: Free Press, 1992.
Macintosh, Donald, and David Whitson. *The Game Planners: Transforming Canada's Sport System.* Montreal: McGill-Queen's University Press, 1990.
Safai, Parissa. "A Critical Analysis of the Development of Sports Medicine in Canada, 1955–1980." *International Review for the Sociology of Sport* 42, no. 3 (2007): 321–341.
———. "The Demise of the Sports Medicine and Science Council of Canada." *Sport History Review* 36 (2005): 91–114.
Theberge, Nancy. "The Integration of Chiropractors into Health Care Teams: A Case Study from Sports Medicine." *Sociology of Health & Illness* 30, no. 1 (2008): 19–34.
———. "Professional Identifies and the Practice of Sports Medicine in Canada: A Comparative Analysis of Two Sporting Contexts." In *Sport and Social Identities*, edited by John Harris and Andrew Parker, 49–69. London: Palgrave MacMillan, 2009.
———. "We Have all the Bases Covered; Constructions of Professional Boundaries in Sports Medicine." *International Review for the Sociology* 44, nos. 2–3 (2009): 265–281.
Waddington, Ivan. "The Development of Sports Medicine." *Sociology of Sport Journal* 13, no. 2 (1996): 176–196.
Walk, Stephan. "Athletic Trainers: Between Care and Social Control." In *Sporting Bodies, Damaged Selves: Sociological Studies of Sports-Related Injuries*, edited by Kevin Young, 251–268. Oxford: Elsevier, 2004.

Part III

Sports Medicine Practices

9 Docile Bodies or Reflexive Users?
On the Individualization of Medical Risk in Sports

Lone Friis Thing

I went out for a run one day. And then my knee just started to hurt so badly that I couldn't, I couldn't run back. So I called the doctor who had done the arthroscopy to hear what it could be that would hurt that way all of a sudden. Then he said that it could be cartilage formations on the kneecap or behind the kneecap somewhere. He recommended that I signed up for another arthroscopy, so I did that. And then there were cartilage formations in the knee, and he removed them, and then I was okay with that knee. I remember he asked me why I didn't get my cruciate ligament fixed. And then I said I thought it was working quite okay. I guess I was a bit scared to have it fixed. (Bolette, 37)

In medical sociology, the question of whether recent biomedical technologies create docile bodies or produce reflexive users is frequently posed.[1] The potentially oppressive effect and the pathologizing medicalization tendencies of the technology are discussed in relation to the more positive aspects of medical technology.[2] On the one hand, critics highlight the unintentional and negative consequences of new technology[3]; on the other, the potentially liberating aspects of new technological discoveries are emphasized.[4] Williams and Calnan state that the macro-theoretically based medical sociology has established knowledge that shows that the public accept and trust modern medicine.[5] However, people's relationship to medical knowledge is still ambivalent and ambiguous, and the use of the knowledge complex. Thus, new research argues that laypeople are not passive and dependent on modern medicine, but that the picture is much more complex.[6] This can be illustrated through behaviors ranging from people's use of alternative medicine,[7] to bodybuilders' expert use of pharmaceuticals (see also Pike's and Atkinson's contributions to this collection).[8]

The present revolution of information and communications technology has given a much wider audience access to knowledge.[9] Williams and Calnan emphasize that empirical studies are necessary before the medical use of technology can be evaluated and before conclusions can be drawn.[10] The satisfaction surveys used up until now in the health care system are criticized for being superficial.[11] It has also been argued that questions relating to treatment quality are such sensitive issues that they may be difficult for individuals to evaluate. Instead there are calls for in-depth qualitative and ethnographic studies with the capability to more adequately evaluate medical care.[12] The present chapter must be seen in this context as it attempts a detailed exploration of the perspectives of laypeople on treatment technology.

This chapter uses athletes' risk management in relation to injuries to explore these issues.[13] It will be illustrated how body and risk are dealt with in the long journey from the moment of injury in the sports arena to treatment in the health care system of the Danish welfare state. The case illustrates the patient as "docile body" or "reflexive user" through exploration of the experiences of laypeople being treated using biomedical technology. The empirical statements are "injury narratives"[14] showing the illness period in its entirety of being.[15] I analyze the patients' encounter with the health care system. I look at patient narratives about illness and at the choices made by the patients as well as patients' thoughts about surgery and sports medicine. Finally, a number of future scenarios for the debate about the medical use of technology will be explored, in the hope that treatment institutions will take seriously the questions of user democracy and dialogue in the health care system.[16]

METHODOLOGICAL CONSIDERATIONS

The present chapter is based on a larger study of the rehabilitation of Danish women handball players with anterior cruciate ligament (ACL) injuries. ACL injury is the most frequent serious sport injury in Danish women's handball. The injury is serious in the sense that, at best, the player must go through rehabilitation several times a week for six months, and at worst she may not be able to play handball even after several years of rehabilitation. Cruciate ligament reconstruction entails surgically implanting an artificial ligament. The new ligament is taken from the thigh and attached through channels drilled in the femur, often with a variety of medical nails and screws.[17] Research shows that only half of the patients who have had an ACL reconstruction can expect to resume sports that are as hard on the knee as the sports they played before the injury.[18] The ACL injury, thus, potentially signals the end of the injured player's handball career. It may also change her social life in general, as this type of injury may lead to unintended consequences.

The study is based on long-term fieldwork at a private physiotherapy clinic and is based on in-depth qualitative interviews with female sports patients. Interviews were conducted with seventeen handball players from nineteen to thirty-seven years of age (mean value twenty-five years). All were white and middle class.[19] Two of the seventeen patients in the study have not had a reconstruction, but have only received physiotherapy rehabilitation after their injury. Fourteen patients were observed during their post-reconstruction rehabilitation, and just one person has been interviewed prior to reconstruction.

Rehabilitation takes place in a small gym in groups of approximately three patients and one therapist. I was seated in the corner, observing the rehabilitation and taking field notes immediately after the treatment session. An ACL patient who has undergone reconstruction usually participates in rehabilitation for one hour, three times a week, for at least six months. The fieldwork includes several hundred consultations. Whenever possible, I was with every single patient for training. Parallel to the observational study at the clinic, I have carried out in-depth qualitative interviews with the patients, either in their private homes or in my office. Most of the patients were interviewed toward the end of their rehabilitation, that is, after I had been observing their process at the clinic for between six months and a year. I therefore knew the informants well at the time of the interview.

The duration of the interviews was one and a half to two and a half hours. I focus on the embodied, lived experiences of being sports injured with a view to understanding the meaning in the human lifeworld and the phenomenology of the body.[20] The project does not investigate *why* ACL injuries occur. The focus and purpose of the study is to show *how* the sports patient experiences the injury and the encounter with the treatment system. The interviews are inspired by the phenomenological tradition, which means that consciousness of the body has also been prioritized in the interview by seeking concrete and bodily descriptions of narratives rather than explanations of the injury event. Taking the event of the injury as their point of departure, the patients narrate the entire course of their period of injury. The narratives therefore stretch from the injury situation through reception at the emergency ward, to diagnosis and decision for or against ACL reconstruction and the rehabilitation process. It must be noted that almost all the ACL injured persons in the study experienced difficulties being diagnosed. They have thus had a very long period of illness and have, after diagnosis, experienced periods of waiting for reconstruction of approximately one year. The quotes used in this chapter are presented in full. They have been translated into English but not edited, abbreviated or otherwise manipulated. The empirical statements from the women have been compared to the observational studies and constitute the starting point and empirical basis of the chapter.

SPORTING BODIES AND TECHNOLOGY USE

Yes, I had no doubts. I mean, if I was going to play handball again, and that was the goal, right, then I had to have an operation. I don't believe I could play handball at that level without an operation, not at all. My meniscus was totally ruined. I had to have that fixed. I found it quite a natural thing to have my cruciate ligament fixed, 'cause without it I could damage my knee even more. So for me there was no doubt about it. (Johanne, 23)

In contemporary societies, we are surrounded by technological cultural artifacts, but technology is more than toasters that fail, hairdryers that burn out or computers that stop working.[21] The use of technology is not limited to objects of use—the body, too, is an object of technology as technology is invading our bodies, sometimes literally getting under our skin (for a discussion, see Kondo and McNamee's contribution in this collection).[22] Artificial ligaments, nails and screws are modifying athletes' bodies and constitute, in contemporary sports, an essential feature of striving for performance. Monaghan states that experts, and expert systems of knowledge, have a particular place in the "risk society," because they contribute to the production of risk and to its management.[23] In the world of sports, the dependence on knowledge of sports medicine is manifest, for example, in technological ingenuity in the treatment of the sports injured body, but also in knowledge and information of diet and nutrition, training plans and sports psychological counseling/therapy in relation to elite performances.

Sports injuries, and therefore their treatment, are not simply "natural," but "social" in the sense of being socially constructed human products or risks.[24] Sports injuries are phenomena of second modernity and cannot be understood or explained as the result of the so-called "natural" weak body of the woman. I emphasize this because much research in sports medicine, and on ACL injuries in particular, seeks to explain injuries in female sports as the result of the woman's biological body. Reference is made to the hormonal effect of the menstrual cycle on the occurrence of injury, and the position and size of the woman's pelvis in relation to her knees. Research is conducted on women's coordination of movement in relation to takeoff and landing as particularly nonfunctional in relation to ball games.[25] My idea is to remove the focus from the biological body and look, instead, at the social events and the result of the ambiguous development processes of sports. Let me explain this.

Modern sports can be interpreted as a perfect image of the "tradition of progress,"[26] as the essence of sports is a search for, and a transgression of, existing and present limits for human achievement.[27] It can be said that sport is a "border war,"[28] an imaginary manifestation in which imaginary territories are challenged in a bodily and silent way. In that sense, sports injuries are the offspring of sports, although an illegitimate offspring, and injuries can be regarded as the unintended results of the cultural "battle of the body."

Although the nature of sport may always have been to transgress limits, and although athletes have always been involved in doping and injuries,[29] we need to differentiate qualitatively between applied sports technologies and their effect: the uncontrollable results. Early examples of drug (ab)use, such as cyclists using stimulants in the Tour de France, were not the result of highly developed products from the pharmaceutical industry. Rather, (ab)use consisted of individual and isolated attempts to endure the hardships of a physically demanding event. Late modern doping, however, but also modern treatment, is largely *expert dependent* and scientific *knowledge based*. Technologies in the shape of pharmaceutical production and operational techniques are, in Beck's sense, the result of the late modern development, which involves an escalation of the interdependency between sports and medicine beyond the institutional intentions. Processes of sportization are, even in a long-term perspective, neither planned nor intended by discrete groups.[30] In the early years of sports (around 1900), doping and the treatment of injuries were not *systematized, scientified* or *commercialized*.[31] The social and political implications of the cost aspects of sports were neither global nor paramount in their manifestation. Today, the picture has changed. At one end of the continuum, sport-related medical technology in the shape of pharmaceuticals, treatment technology, training plans, etc., are produced. At the other end, the performative body is controlled by knowledge of sport medicine. The use of sports-medical biotechnology is not just a question of survival *or* care; here the technology is also largely the "helping hand" of the logic of achievement. The cultural development in the global world of sports creates a technological awareness leading to the transgression of what has hitherto been regarded as "pure" nature and to the modeling of it on the basis of the force of ideologies. Sport medicine seeks to optimize the functionality for the athlete through pharmaceuticals that, for example, enhance performance, but also *after* the injury in the hope of winning medals for the nation-state and in the hope of a continued sports career. But although sport medicine is part of the public health program aiming to maximize public health with a view to prevention, sports medicine is not limited to curative technology such as diagnostic techniques or rehabilitation procedures in general. Sport medicine is also deeply involved in the production of sports results. Sporting bodies are both media for, and the results of, new biomedical knowledge in the sport world.

Thus the development of sport medicine and knowledge is not "pure" nature, but a culture with the moral intention of optimizing performance, which is expressed on the basis of scientific/medical knowledge. The present technological development of contemporary sport medicine largely enables the athlete to free herself from the limitations imposed by injuries, although the treatment opportunity gives rise to uncertainty and fear, as we saw from Bolette's comment in the beginning of the chapter. Technological development creates the possibility of seeing bodies not as "pure" nature, but rather as a material that can be modeled, formed and repaired even if it takes blood, sweat and tears.[32] Or, as Giddens puts it, the body is decreasingly considered a given, determined by external factors; it is mobilized individually and reflexively.[33] But technologies are not just liberating; they invoke new mechanisms of compulsion.[34] The mechanisms of compulsion can be seen, for instance, in expert dependency. The experts guide the free choice of the athletes, but no choice is without responsibility. Often the expert guidance results in a kaleidoscopic journey between expert statements and testimonials.

The story of Lisbeth, twenty-six, illustrates this kaleidoscopic behavior. Lisbeth's process of injury is different from most other research subjects because she was submitted to the hospital immediately after the injury, with her knee "locked." Her meniscus was operated on two days after the injury, and she was therefore quickly diagnosed with ACL injury. Lisbeth then had the option of being put on a waiting list for an ACL operation, which means that Lisbeth has not invested energy or knowledge in the struggle to get a diagnosis. She was offered an operation six months after the injury, as the doctor found that rehabilitation after the meniscus operation was necessary before the ACL operation. During the interview, Lisbeth had no doubts about reconstruction. She had been active all her life and wanted to continue to play handball and to water-ski. She wanted to have an operation as quickly as possible. She seeks information from various experts. Lisbeth finds the information contradictory and very unclear. The surgeon who is going to operate tells her that she is free to choose a type of operation different to the one they "normally" use at that hospital. But, according to the patient, the doctor makes it clear which types of technology have, in their experience, been most successful. Lisbeth expresses that she finds it difficult to make a choice about medical technology. She makes use of other laypeople's knowledge of ACL operation by talking to a handball friend who has had an operation, and this management strategy is not unique. The women handball players make wide use of each other's experiences in relation to choice of hospital and treatment technology, and they use each other as a social network in relation to the psychosocial problems of being injured (see Kotarba's contribution in this collection). Lisbeth confronts the surgeon at the public hospital with the treatment technology of a private expert. She finds that this process has made her "wiser" as she has become more knowledgeable about ACL injury and the different types of treatment, but she repeats that she was, and is, confused. She was not sure that she made the right decision. Sometimes she feels it would have been easier had the doctor made the decision for her (the docile body). But Lisbeth does not want the old-world authority back. Lisbeth makes a pragmatic choice (is a reflexive user) by choosing the type of operation she *assumes* that the surgeon is best at, and she feels dependent on the expert.

EXPERT DEPENDENCY:
BETWEEN CERTAINTY AND DOUBT

Certainty and doubt are not, in the patients' experience, an "either–or" question. Expert dependency is, as we saw in Lisbeth's story, characterized both by certainty *and* doubt. Patients need expert advice, knowledge and guidance as a background for their own ability to act, and there is a need for open dialogue about the options and possibilities for action, but the individual patient is relatively autonomous and independent when it comes to the final decision about treatment. Uncertainty can be found among laypeople, and they also have a strong interest in searching for information and dealing actively with the illness process. This phenomenon can be observed in relation to all the interviewees, both in terms of their considerations in relation to the choice of having surgery or not and in their search for information to help them deal with the illness process.

> It was just like I knew a bit more about a cruciate ligament operation than the doctor did, and of course I only knew that because all my friends had had operations, you know. So there were many questions I had to ask myself. So I don't think he was very good at making it clear what was actually going to happen and things like that, 'cause he was very busy. (Kate, 21)

Giddens emphasizes laypeople's dependence on expert systems,[35] whereas Beck emphasizes the fact that evident knowledge is not static, but subject to change.[36] Petersen criticizes both Beck's and Gidden's sociological analyses of "risk" in late modern society, arguing that the analyses are problematic in that they are too modernistic in their understanding of the relationship between self, knowledge and society.[37] The strong focus on the individual, rationality and reflexivity, and the belief in the possible validity of science are not, in Petersen's Foucauldian view, realistic. But although Beck and Giddens see risk as an important issue in late modern society, and although they both attribute importance to the concept of risk, Petersen overlooks important differences between the two theorists. Whereas Giddens stresses the necessity of believing in experts and in the scientific production of knowledge, Beck largely outlines the social conditions that create the framework of this doubt and belief for citizens in the Western world. The difference between Beck and Giddens is by no means slight. Beck does not pay tribute to the processes of individualization and their effect, although he does believe in rationality. He explains that objective life conditions force individuals to behave the way they do.[38] Beck problematizes the consequences of the actions of individuals in search of visionary thought. The autonomous and self-reflexive individual has not, in Beckian thought, come out of nothing, but is a consequence of external circumstances, such as the labor market, the global economy, the family, the institutionalization, media and consumerism.[39] The individualized life is, in other words, a condition to which citizens are subjected.

Williams and Calnan conclude that the relationship between medicine and laypeople is largely structured around the reflexively organized dialectics of certainty and doubt.[40] Certainty and doubt are partners; they coexist in the sense that, in the medical context, they are not mutually exclusive. Certainty and doubt must be constructed continually from one case to the next and from one meeting to the next. The nature of knowledge means that the authoritative status of experts is challenged, albeit in different ways depending on the patient's social group, gender, age and ethnic group. Beck points out that the "objects" of scientification become "subjects" because they need to deal actively with the various scientific offers of interpretation (the way that Lisbeth does).[41] Users of knowledge cannot just choose between highly specialized and contradictory validity claims, but also *play them off against each other*. Beck maintains that this results in new opportunities for influence and creativity for the users. Thus, the methodological doubt developed by science has won. Beck puts it this way: "Users liberate themselves more and more *from* science *by means of* science."[42] But the question remains: what are the consequences of this autonomy for the users, and the injured athlete in particular?

"DOCTOR SHOPPING" AS A MANAGEMENT STRATEGY

Evidence suggests that some laypeople seek control over the dialectics of certainty and doubt by engaging in consumer behavior.[43] They go "doctor shopping" in their attempt to understand the situation and in the hope of acquiring new knowledge that will enable them to find their bearings. Quite paradoxically, however, several of the interviews show that the phenomenon of "doctor shopping" is not seen as something positive by the users, although the experts believe that this is so. On the contrary, the shopping mentality is described as psychologically testing and time-consuming and as a necessary sociocultural evil. The patients in this case maintain that, when it comes to sport injuries, this shopping and self-management strategy is an absolute necessity. The patients experience is that no other mechanisms/persons in the system take care of their injuries. They are "forced," so to speak, to take on the role of "the self-expert."[44]

The doubt in relation to expert knowledge is illustrated in the patients' experiences with the Danish hospitals and the patients' experience with the diagnosis of an ACL injury. Emergency room experiences, in particular, are criticized in the patient narratives. Several of the female handball players express the opinion that it is better to avoid the emergency room, as it leads nowhere. Susanne, twenty-two, discusses her first visit to the emergency room shortly after she was injured during a handball match. Susanne's phenomenological injury narrative illustrates a very typical pattern for ACL injuries in Denmark. Susanne was injured in a tackle, and it is clear from her retelling that she was in great pain. She heard a clear "pop" inside her leg and was baffled by the strong pain that disappeared as suddenly as it had come. She felt it "as if a rubber band had snapped":

And then I'm put in a room, and then this lady comes in, I don't know if she was a resident or what, but a woman doctor anyway. I looked quite okay, and my parents were like: "Well, surely it can't be the cruciate ligament" because I looked okay and I was joking a bit about it and being a bit humorous. It didn't actually hurt so much, I was just lying there, you know, and it doesn't really hurt when you're just lying down, not at all. I didn't think that it was something very serious either, or anything. But at the same time I knew, I mean thinking of that popping sound, and many of my friends have tried it, so deep inside I guess I knew that okay, there's something really wrong here. (Susanne, 22)

The emergency room sends her home without a diagnosis. Not long after this experience, Susanne takes control of the situation. She contacts a private sport medicine doctor whom she has heard about from her boyfriend at the time who was also an athlete. She goes "doctor shopping," and decides that she is willing to pay for another consultation. The background for her doubts about the "lack of" diagnosis from the emergency room is primarily based on the stories and experiences of other women with ACL injuries. Several friends tell her that with the way she fell, and with her description of the injury, it "looks like" an ACL injury. The feeling that "something's wrong" stimulates Susanne to act.

Experiences in the emergency room form a part of the phenomenon of doctor shopping, but cannot solely be put down to the lack of knowledge and expertise in Danish emergency rooms. The phenomenon must also be attributed to the complexity of knowledge in the late modern society: the speed of knowledge development. Even the experts disagree about the "latest findings," and even experts discuss the emergence and consequences of knowledge. Medical knowledge is no longer a question of truth or fiction, but a field in which everything is up for discussion, and where the doctor knows that contradictory evidence often exists in relation to the treatment. The result is that patients go doctor shopping in an attempt to gather as much information as possible and in the attempt to understand the illness, its consequences and the treatment options. Schmidt argues that the modern patient is a competent patient, and that this involves the risk of the general practitioner, in his eagerness to respect the autonomy of the patient, no longer daring to be an authority.[45] I believe, however, that this is a misinterpretation of the situation, and I will show why, based on this empirical case.

Today's patients are competent in the sense that laypeople are knowledgeable and active users who are largely capable of making choices and creating possibilities for action.[46] Schmidt argues that the doctor does not *dare* to be an authority, but this analysis misses the point. The kind of authority requested by Schmidt could, in Foucauldian terms, be called the *pastoral power*: the hierarchical hegemony expressed top-down. This authoritative relationship is long gone, and to the best of my knowledge, there is no point in mourning its loss. Schmidt's characterization of the doctor–patient relationship lacks contextualization, which would bring the relationship in touch with the modern world. The relationship between lay-people and experts can no longer be described by means of metaphors of opposition and is no longer hierarchical with the expert as superior to the layperson.[47] Contemporary patients can largely be described as knowledge-able users of science. In my study, this is manifested when Nina, who is a medical student herself, actively discusses the possibility of continuing her handball career with the orthopedic surgeon in the hospital where she is having a reconstruction, and when, after the operation, she chooses to seek more knowledge about sport injuries by choosing to do her medical internship at the very same hospital ward where she had the surgery.

Another example shows that it is not just the highly educated patient groups who are able to search for information and perform risk management in relation to biomedical technology. During her period of illness, Ida, who works as a purchasing agent for a company, surveys the waiting lists of all hospitals in Denmark and compares them to the prices of private hospitals in an attempt to assume control over the course of her own rehabilitation:

> Yes, I looked on the Internet to find out about waiting lists, and also about the doctors, when I asked in the sports club. Then I got some names of some hospitals. So I took the one that had the shortest waiting list. (Ida, 28)

This woman also gathers information about the experts' competence within the area of orthopedic surgery, in order to decide between private and public treatment. The concept of the "lay expert" has been used to describe contemporary patient categories.[48] These examples show that Schmidt's analysis is conservative and retrospective. Future scenarios of dialogue and democratization of the doctor–patient relationship will be more analytically productive as the social context is radically changed. Knowledge development in late modern society has, if you will, caused citizens to actively seek to understand their illness process. A characteristic feature of this case study is the patients' active involvement in the process of their illness, when it comes to diagnosis and the choice for or against surgery, but particularly when it comes to the management of the rehabilitation process itself.

The experienced handball player has knowledge of bodily technology and a practical experience with the body, which should be involved and integrated into the treatment of injury in the Danish emergency room. The women's narratives show exactly that the doctors (still) exhibit "traditional authority." The study shows that fourteen of the seventeen women were discharged without a diagnosis from the Danish hospitals, often with remarks like: "Go home and take some painkillers." Several women were told that their knee was probably "sprained." None of the fourteen women were told that they might be seriously injured and that they should take precautions in relation to a possible ACL injury. For the women, the lack of a diagnosis leads to anger and frustration that is managed through, among other things, "doctor shopping." The patients' reaction or strategy is not to confront the doctor with their uncertainty and doubt. The patients do not explain their dissatisfaction to the doctor; rather, they look for a new doctor:

> When I was injured again with my knee, then I had no doubts whatso-
> ever that I should have an operation. And I told my doctor so. When I
> had just returned from the emergency room, I was both sad and a bit
> angry, because they had just sent me home. I really wanted to have a
> knee operation as soon as possible. (Linea, 20)

It would therefore seem that the doctor–patient dialogue would benefit from involving the patient's own bodily self-experience in diagnosing ACL injury. The patients feel they are being ignored, and perceive their dialogue with doctors as limited. Although the patient may well be a self-expert, and although the patient is not seen as a passive recipient, patients still feel that doctors do not properly acknowledge them, and thus that the care the health system provides is incomplete.[49] The patient is dependent on the expert, although the patient is knowledgeable and considers the health care system a public service.

Analytically, the patients' risk management has a dual character of certainty and doubt. The patients are not only reflexive and autonomous users who know all there is to know. Rather, there is a duality between compliance and reflexive action. The patients in this study are active in relation to their surgery and they make active choices when it comes to which hospital or clinic to contact. They gather information about the doctors and their competence. They check out the reputation of the orthopedic surgeon. Does he/she know how to operate? What surgical technique does he/she use? They ask about the long-term consequences of particular techniques.

But in the face-to-face encounter, the patients in the study are still passive, loyal and compliant. Here, they are not demanding, they do not ask a lot of questions, and the patients do not feel that the doctors have time for them. I both observe this in the clinic and find it in the interviews about the relationship to the doctors at the hospital. Some sports patients prepare for the consultation with the doctor, e.g., by making a *list* of questions to make sure they ask the doctor all their questions, and by drawing on other people's experiences (which tell them that the doctor does not have time and does not listen). In the face-to-face situation the patients do not always know what questions to ask, and they become *intimidated users* when the doctor's information does not correspond to their own understanding of the knee problem.

SUMMARY AND CONCLUSION

In the past, sport injuries have represented danger and the "compulsion of nature" over the individual. The injured body was an event not easily overcome. From a historical and temporal perspective, an ACL injury meant the end of a career in handball less than twenty years ago. Now, due to technology in the form of surgery and specialized clinical rehabilitation, career resumption is possible. The player performs risk assessment and risk management in order to survive as an athlete. The player reflexively considers advantages and disadvantages of surgery and chooses for or against it.

The answer to the question of whether patients are *docile bodies* or *reflexive users* is that they are both. This case shows that, at a distance, the patients are users. The modern techniques of power have, in the Foucauldian sense, produced resourceful knowledge users of the health care system,[50] but the study demonstrates that the authority is still attributed to the role of doctor and expert in the face-to-face situation. The doctor–patient relationship on equal terms is the consequence of the processes of individualization that, in the field of health and illness, are manifested as issues of responsibility assumption: the patient has to be *competent* and assume *responsibility* for her own illness. Patients must be capable of acting and dealing with illness, in spite of methodological doubts about both diagnosis and treatment technology. The weak aspects of individualization are, in this case, the women's uncertainty and the feeling of being left alone with their illness. The women feel a huge responsibility, and for some of them the years of their youth taken by the ACL injury have had serious consequences and implications. Although the women act knowledgeably and reflexively, the experience takes its toll. In other words, sport injuries are hazardous, but not only to physical health. The patients/players share information and support each other in their effort to manage their own illnesses. But their self-management practices are not wholly satisfying—they still claim and wish to have good communication with their doctors. Or, as Fox, Ward and O'Rourke say, "the expert patient" is a double-edge sword.[51] The patients have become knowledgeable in a wide range of approaches but still *feel* on their own.[52]

The open question of user involvement and democracy in the health care system, the question of how to empower the patients and how to communicate the interpretational plurality of knowledge in such a way that enables the patient to manage the methodological doubt and uncertainty entailed in big biographical decisions, remains unanswered. The conclusion is that *freedom of choice* and *doctor shopping* are not the expression of supercilious consumers who egotistically try to take center stage. Influence is necessary exactly because knowledge *is* subject to interpretation. The present revolution of information and communication technology has given a much wider audience access to knowledge, and this knowledge cannot be ignored by the treatment system. The patient must be consulted. This is not a question of letting the patient be her own health care professional, an autonomous self-therapist. And it is not a question of reducing the patient to a "demanding" and maladjusted consumer because she goes "doctor shopping," because she (thinks she) knows better. The patient inhabits a knowledge society, and the diversity of knowledge must be taken seriously. The plurality of knowledge is not, as the governmentalist tradition of Rose has it, just a matter of freedom.[53] The plurality of knowledge requires resources, and we need to create a new framework—new relationships of authority that are based on *negotiation treatment* on equal terms, as called for in national strategies for quality development in the health care system.

There is no doubt that authorities are challenged by the active and knowledgeable layperson. But the knowledgeable layperson is not flawless, and doubts are lurking just around the corner. With Beck, we might outline a future scenario that combines macro-sociological-level political debates about health policy with micro-sociological aspects such as the relationship between layperson and expert.

NOTES

1. Williams and Calnan, *Modern Medicine*, 263; Wilson, "Policy Analysis"; Rose, "Biopolitics."
2. Williams, Birke and Bendelow, *Debating Biology.*
3. Beck-Germsheim, "Health and Responsibility."
4. Denny, "New Reproductive Technologies."
5. Williams and Calnan, *Modern Medicine*, 3.
6. Shaw and Baker. "Expert Patient"; Fox, Ward and O'Rourke, "Expert Patient."
7. Baarts and Pedersen, "Derivative Benefits."
8. Monaghan, *Bodybuilding, Drugs and Risk.* See also Atkinson in this collection.
9. Beck, *Risiko Samfundet.*
10. Williams and Calnan, *Modern Medicine*, 263.
11. Williams and Calnan, "Convergence and Divergence."
12. Malterud, "Qualitative Research."
13. See also Thing, "Risk Bodies"; "Scars on the Body"; "Voices."
14. Bury, "Chronic Illness"; Frank, *Wounded Storyteller.*
15. Kleinman, *Illness Narratives.*
16. Beck, *Risiko Samfundet; Reinvention of Politics.*
17. Jørgensen, "Rekonstruktion af forreste korsbånd."
18. Poulsen et al.,"Rekonstruktion."
19. The patients were selected as they turned up in the treatment situation, as sports injured personalities. Over a period of a year and a half, only two patients at the clinic did not want to participate in the study. My aim was to have a comparatively heterogeneous group consisting of both elite and nonelite players, of patients at different stages of rehabilitation, of different ages and educational backgrounds. The clinic selected for the study is one of the most active and leading clinics in the country for sports injuries. The physiotherapists are regarded as knowledgeable specialists in this area.
20. Denzin, *On Understanding Emotion*; Valle and Halling, *Existential-Phenomenological Perspectives.*

21. Elam, "Når maskiner eksploderer"
22. Featherstone, *Body Modification*.
23. Monaghan, *Bodybuilding, Drugs and Risk*, xi.
24. Beck, *Risiko Samfundet*.
25. Aagaard, "Korsbåndsskader og Faren ved Keratin."
26. Beck, *Risiko Samfundet*.
27. Møller and Povlsen, *Sportens forførende skønhed*.
28. Haraway, *Simians, Cyborgs, and Women*.
29. Pedersen, "Doping."
30. Maguire, *Global Sport*, 69.
31. Henderson and Petersen, *Consuming Health*.
32. The Human Genome Project has also affected sport. In the US, research is done on the human genome in the hope of being able to form/create the *ideal* elite athlete.
33. Giddens, *Modernitet og selvidentitet*, 252.
34. Beck, *Risiko Samfundet*.
35. Giddens, *Modernitet og selvidentitet*.
36. Beck, *Risiko Samfundet*.
37. Petersen, "Risk," 190.
38. Beck, *Risiko Samfundet*, 207.
39. Consequently, I do not think that seeing risk management as a (self-)management strategy (Castel, "From Dangerousness to Risk") is very far from Beckian thought. Although Beck operates with a more ontological concept of risk in his analyses of issues such as the environment, pollution and global economy, I do not think his thoughts go against the governmentality tradition. This can also be seen when Lupton ("Your Life") debates the risk society at the level of the body. The thought of management rationality emphasizes the individual as an entrepreneur who has the freedom and autonomy to create his or her own world because the social conditions constantly try to make citizens independent, autonomous individuals.
40. Williams and Calnan, *Modern Medicine*.
41. Beck, *Risiko Samfundet*, 257.
42. Ibid., 287.
43. Lupton, "Your Life," 164; Henwood et al., "Ignorance Is Bliss."
44. Rose and Novas "Genetisk risiko"; Rose, *Politics of Life Itself*.
45. Schmidt, "Sundhedspædagogikken."
46. Rose and Novas, "Genetisk risiko."
47. Maranta et al., "Reality of Experts."
48. Rose, "Biopolitics."
49. Gadamer, *Enigma of Health*.
50. Wilson, "Policy Analysis."
51. Fox, Ward and O'Rourke, "Expert Patient."
52. Lupton, *Emotional Self*.
53. Rose, "Biopolitics."

BIBLIOGRAPHY

Aagaard, Per. "Korsbåndsskader og Faren ved Keratin (Cruciate Ligament Injuries and the Danger of Creatine)." *Puls* 12, no. 2 (2001): 23–25.
Baarts, C., and I.K. Pedersen. "Derivative Benefits: Exploring the Body through Complementary and Alternative Medicine." *Sociology of Health & Illness* 31, no. 5 (2009): 719–733.

Beck, Ulrich. *The Reinvention of Politics. Rethinking Modernity in the Global Social Order.* Cambridge: Polity Press, 2005.

——. *Risiko Samfundet. På vej mod en ny Modernitet* (Risk Society. Toward a New Modernity). Copenhagen: Hans Reitzels Forlag, 1997.

Beck-Germsheim, E. "Health and Responsibility: From Social Change to Technological Change and Vice Versa." In *The Risk Society and Beyond. Critical Issues for Social Theory,* edited by B. Adam, U. Beck and J. Van Loon, 122–135. London: Sage Publications, 2000.

Bury, Michael. "Chronic Illness as Biographical Disruption." *Sociology of Health & Illness* 4, no. 2 (1982): 167–182.

Castel, Robert. "From Dangerousness to Risk." In *The Foucault Effect. Studies in Governmentality. With Two Lectures by and an Interview with Michel Foucault,* edited by G. Burchell, C. Gordon and P. Miller, 281–299. Chicago: University of Chicago Press, 1991.

Denny, Elaine. "New Reproductive Technologies: The Views of Women Undergoing Treatment." In *Modern Medicine. Lay Perspectives and Experiences,* edited by S. J. Williams and M. Calnan, 207–227. London: UCL Press, 1996.

Denzin, Norman. K. *On Understanding Emotion.* San Francisco, CA: Jossey-Bass Publishers, 1984.

Elam, Mark. "Når maskiner eksploderer, hjul falder af og brødristere går amok! Om objektivistiske versus konstruktivistiske repræsentationer af teknologisk viden og praksis (When Machines Explode, Wheels Fall Off and Toasters Go Berserk. About Objectivistic versus Constructivistic Representations of Technological Knowledge and Practice)." In *Socialkonstruktivisme. Bidrag til en kritisk diskussion* (Social Constructivism. A critical Contribution to a Discussion), edited by M. Järvinen and M. Bertilsson, 68–87. Copenhagen: Hans Reitzels Forlag, 1998.

Featherstone, Mike. *Body Modification.* London: Sage Publication, 2000.

Fox, N.J., K.J. Ward and A.J. O'Rourke. "The 'Expert Patient': Empowerment or Medical Dominance? The Case of Weight Loss, Pharmaceutical Drugs and the Internet." *Social Science & Medicine* 60 (2005): 1299–1309.

Frank, Arthur W. *The Wounded Storyteller. Body, Illness, and Ethics.* Chicago: University of Chicago Press, 1995.

Gadamer, Hans-Georg. *The Enigma of Health. The Art of Healing in a Scientific Age.* Stanford, CA: Stanford University Press, 1996.

Giddens, Anthony. *Modernitet og selvidentitet. Selvet og samfundet under senmoderniteten* (Modernity and Self-Identity. Self and Society in Late Modern Age). Copenhagen: Hans Reitzels Forlag, 1996.

Haraway, Donna J. *Simians, Cyborgs, and Women. The Reinvention of Nature.* London: Free Association Books, 1991.

Henderson, S., and A. Petersen. *Consuming Health. The Commodification of Health Care.* London: Routledge, 2002.

Henwood, F., S. Wyatt, A. Hart and J. Smith. "'Ignorance Is Bliss Sometimes': Constraints on the Emergence of the 'Informed Patient' in the Changing Landscapes of Health Information." *Sociology of Health & Illness* 25, no.6 (2003): 589–607.

Jørgensen, Uffe. "Rekonstruktion af forreste korsbånd—operativ teknik, postoperativ behandling, årsager til funktionssvigt og kvalitetskontrol (Reconstruction of the Anterior Cruciate Ligament—Operative Technique, Postoperative Care, Causes of Dysfunction and Qualitative Control)." *Dansk Sportsmedicin* 3, no. 4 (1999): 6–10.

Kleinman, Arthur. *The Illness Narratives. Suffering, Healing & the Human Condition.* New York: Basic Books, 1988.

Lupton, Deborah. *The Emotional Self.* London: Sage Publications, 1998.

————. "'Your Life in Their Hands': Trust in the Medical Encounter." In *Health and the Sociology of Emotions*, edited by V. James and J. Gabe, 157–172. Cambridge: Blackwell Publishers/Editorial Board, 1996.

Maguire, Joseph. *Global Sport*. Cambridge: Polity Press, 1999.

Malterud, Kirsti. "Qualitative Research: Standards, Challenges, and Guidelines." *Lancet* 358 (August 2001): 483–488.

Maranta, A., M. Guggenheim, P. Gisler and C. Pohl. "The Reality of Experts and the Imagined Lay Person." *Acta Sociologica* 46, no. 2 (2003): 150–165.

Møller, V., and J. Povlsen. *Sportens forførende skønhed. En antologi om sport og æstetik* (The Seductive Beauty of Sport. An Anthology of Sport and Aesthetics). Odense: Syddansk Universitetsforlag, 2002.

Monaghan, Lee F. *Bodybuilding, Drugs and Risk*. New York: Routledge, 2001.

Pedersen, Inge Kryger. "Doping and the Perfect Body Expert: Social and Cultural Indicators of Performance-Enhancing Drug Use in Danish Gyms." *Sport in Society* 13, no 3 (April 2010): 503–516.

Petersen, Alan. "Risk, Governance and the New Public Health." In *Foucault, Health and Medicine*, edited by A. Petersen and R. Bunton, 189–206. London: Routledge, 1997.

Poulsen, M., J. Fabrin, J.P. Carstensen, L. Ulnits and G.S. Lausten. "Rekonstruktion af forreste korsbånd med bone-patellar tendon-bone graft eller fascia lata-graft (Reconstruction of Anterior Cruciate Ligament Using Bone-Patellar Tendon-Bone Graft or Fascia Lata Graft)." *Ugeskrift for læger* 165, no. 7 (2003): 682–685.

Rose, Nikolas. "Biopolitics in the Twenty First Century—Notes For a Research Agenda." *Distinktion. Scandinavian Journal of Social Theory* 3(2001): 25–44.

————. *The Politics of Life Itself. Biomedicine, Power, and Subjectivity in the Twenty-First Century*. Princeton, NJ: Princeton University Press, 2007.

Rose, N., and C. Novas. "Genetisk risiko og fødslen af det somatiske individ (Genetic Risk and the Birth of the Somatic Individual)." *Slagmark* 35 (2002): 99–130.

Schmidt, Lars-Henrik. "Sundhedspædagogikken og jagten på et livsindhold (The Health Pedagogy and the Quest for a Life Content)." *Månedsskr. Prakt. Lægegerning* 79, no. 9 (September 2001): 1127–1136.

Shaw, J., and M. Baker. "'Expert Patient'—Dream or Nightmare? The Concept of a Well Informed Patient Is Welcome, but a New Name is Needed." *British Medical Journal* 328 (2004): 723–724.

Thing, Lone F. "Risk Bodies. Rehabilitation of sports patients in the physiotherapy clinic." *Nursing Inquiry* 12, no.3 (2005): 184–191.

————. "Scars on the Body: The Risk Management and Self-Mastery of Injured Female Handball Players in Denmark." In *Sporting Bodies, Damaged Selves: Sociological Studies of Sport-Related Injury*, edited by K. Young, 195–210. New York: Elsevier Press, 2005.

————. "'Voices of the Broken Body.' The Resumption of Non-Professional Female Players' Sports Careers after Anterior Cruciate Ligament Injury. The Female Player's Dilemma: Is She Willing to Run the Risk?" *Scandinavian Journal of Medicine and Science in Sports* 16, no. 5 (2006): 364–375.

Valle, R., and S. Halling. *Existential-Phenomenological Perspectives in Psychology. Exploring the Breadth of Human Experience*. London: Plenum Press, 1989.

Williams, S.J., L. Birke and G.A. Bendelow. *Debating Biology. Sociological Reflections on Health, Medicine and Society*. London: Routledge, 2003.

Williams, S.J., and M. Calnan. "Convergence and Divergence: Assessing Criteria of Consumer Satisfaction across General Practice, Dental and Hospital Care settings." *Social Science & Medicine* 33, no. 6 (1991): 707–716.

———, eds. *Modern Medicine. Lay Perspectives and Experiences.* London: UCL Press, 1996.

Wilson, P.M. "A Policy Analysis of the Expert Patient in the United Kingdom: Self-Care as an Expression of Pastoral Power?" *Health and Social Care in the Community* 9, no. 3 (2001): 134–142.

10 Sports Medicine, Client Control and the Limits of Professional Autonomy

Ivan Waddington

In several publications since the early 1990s, Howard L. Nixon II has made a major contribution to our understanding of the sociology of risk, pain and injury in sport.[1] Central to Nixon's work is his concept of "sportsnets," by which he refers to the webs of interaction between members of social networks in sport-related settings. Nixon argues that the structural characteristics of sportsnets—which he described as a "conspiratorial alliance" of coaches, administrators and sports physicians—expose athletes to "biased social support" that can influence and impose messages that foster the acceptance by athletes of risk, pain and injury and insulate them from, and inhibit them from seeking, medical care from outside the sport system. Walk has suggested that one implication of Nixon's work is that "medicine is practiced differently, more competently, and/or more ethically in nonsports contexts."[2] Young had earlier raised similar questions when he suggested that sports workplaces are the sites not just of medical mastery, but also of "extraordinary medical neglect."[3] These comments represent the starting point for this chapter, the central object of which is to consider whether there are aspects of the practice of sports medicine that might be considered as something less than what Walk calls "proper medical care." More specifically, the chapter sets out to examine whether the network of relationships in which sports medicine practitioners are involved limits their professional autonomy and constrains them to make medical compromises that their colleagues in other branches of medicine are less constrained to make.

The chapter begins by outlining some of the major role conflicts facing team physicians and associated sports medicine personnel. This is followed by an examination of codes of medical ethics and the laws relating to medical practice that provide guidance in relation to managing these conflicts. I then compare the documented behavior of team physicians and related medical personnel with the ethical guidelines. Finally, I seek to account for any discrepancies between the ethical guidelines and how team physicians actually behave by drawing on a combination of Nixon's research and Eliot Freidson's work on medical practice and client control.[4]

CONFLICTS IN THE ROLE OF THE TEAM DOCTOR

The role of the club doctor is often likened to that of the "family doctor," where the relationship with the patient is normally underpinned by three fundamental assumptions:

1. The doctor's skill is used exclusively on behalf of the patient.
2. The doctor is not acting on behalf of anybody else whose interests may conflict with those of the patient.
3. The doctor may be trusted with private or intimate information, which he/she will treat confidentially.

However, this comparison is somewhat misleading for these assumptions may not apply in the same way in the work situation of elite sport. Of particular significance in this regard is that the team doctor "provides medical services to athletes that are arranged for, or paid for, at least in part, by an institution or entity other than the patient."[5] Such an arrangement raises a series of potential problems for, as the British Medical Association (BMA) noted in its handbook of medical ethics:

> Doctors who are employed by sports teams and by sports clubs may find themselves subject to the tension of conflicting loyalties. On the one hand they are agents of the team or club with the contractual obligations of an employee, and, on the other, as doctors, they are advocates for the individual athletes or players who are their patients.[6]

Clearly the club, which employs the doctor, has a legitimate interest in the management of players' injuries. But, as Roy and Irvin note, where medical staff members are employed by the team management, "this may lead to an explicit expectation on the part of the management or coaching staff of loyalty to them . . . [which] may not always be in the best interests of the athlete."[7] For example, there is, as numerous studies have documented, often a clear expectation that, wherever possible, players will continue to play through pain and injury;[8] as Young, White and McTeer have noted, "Overt and covert pressures are brought to bear on injured players to coerce them to return to action,"[9] and within this situation club medical staff may be subject to strong pressure to agree—possibly against their better medical judgment—to players returning to play before they have fully recovered from injury.

Additional problems relate to medical confidentiality. Crane, a former football club doctor, has written that the rules of confidentiality governing relationships between the club doctor and players are *not* those that apply in general practice, but rather those that apply to the relationship "between an occupational physician and an employee of a company." In this respect, he noted that the physician "may be employed by the company primarily to serve its interest. *There may arise, therefore, a conflict of loyalties.*"10 A similar point has been made by Graf-Baumann. Writing as a member of the Sports Medical Committee of the Fédération Internationale de Football Association (FIFA), he noted: "Pressure from officials, the media or even sponsors can lead to a conflict of interests," and he described confidentiality issues as "a particularly sensitive problem in football and in all prominent sports."[11]

These appear to be the two key concerns of sports physicians. In a study of sixteen sports physicians working with elite teams and athletes in New Zealand, the issue of greatest concern was that of maintaining patient confidentiality and privacy in the face of demands from coaches and management. The second major issue concerned "difficulties between the medical requirements of the patient and the pressure [from the player, coach or other team members] to return the individual to the field."[12]

SPORTS MEDICINE, MEDICAL ETHICS AND THE LAW

Notwithstanding the potential conflict of loyalties outlined in the preceding, the ethical guidelines—and the law—relating to the obligations of sports physicians are quite clear. For example, the BMA provides the following unambiguous advice on confidentiality in the physician–athlete relationship:

> Ethically, sports doctors need to be aware that their chief loyalty is to their patients, and that, contractual issues notwithstanding, the duty of medical confidentiality remains unchanged . . . Unless expressly indicated in the terms of the player's or athlete's contract, confidential information can be released only with the expressed consent of the patient, and breaches of confidentiality can be justified only when there is a risk of serious self harm or harm to a third party.[13]

The BMA statement simply reaffirms what has long been the general understanding, of both patients and medical practitioners, in relation to such issues: that when a patient provides information to his/her doctor that information will, save in exceptional circumstances (for example, where information is required by due legal process), be treated confidentially. As the General Medical Council (GMC), the statutory body regulating the medical profession in the UK, succinctly puts it: "Patients have a right to expect that [doctors] will not disclose any personal information . . . unless they give permission."[14] Significantly, guidance on ethics for occupational physicians (cf. Crane) was one of the first issues addressed when the Faculty of Occupational Medicine was founded in 1978. The faculty reiterated the long-established position that the consent of the patient is required—again save in exceptional and defined circumstances—before access to clinical information is granted to others.[15]

The BMA also notes that individuals may experience pressure to continue playing after sustaining injury, even when there is a risk of exacerbating injuries and/or longer-term damage. In this context, it notes that "the doctor's chief obligation must be to the long term health and wellbeing of individual players."[16] More recently, Devitt and McCarthy have noted that the primary obligation of the team doctor is "to uphold the welfare of the player notwithstanding results or the success of the team."[17] In the US, the Team Physician Consensus Statement similarly emphasizes that the "principal responsibility of the team physician is to provide for the well-being of individual athletes."[18]

The physician's primary responsibility to the player-as-patient is also a clearly established legal principle. Thus Mitten has pointed out that, in law, the team physician's "paramount responsibility should be to protect the competitive athlete's health."[19] Mitten notes that in the sporting context there "may be an undesirable custom of not disclosing or minimizing certain medical risks to encourage an athlete to play," but he points out that the team physician "should fully disclose to an athlete the material medical risks of playing with an injury . . . and the potential health consequences of a given medication or treatment . . . in plain and simple language."[20] This was upheld in the case of *Krueger v. San Francisco Forty Niners*, in which a California court held that a professional football team's conscious failure to inform a player that he risked a permanent knee injury by continuing to play was fraudulent concealment. As Junge has noted, one implication of the Krueger case is that a "sports player is entitled to rely on the physician's advice without concern that the physician is placing the team's interest above patient care."[21]

Team physicians' ethical obligations to maintain patient confidentiality have legal implications. Mitten has noted:

> Unauthorized disclosure of information about an athlete's medical condition to third parties violates a physician's ethical obligation to maintain patient confidences. In addition, such unauthorized disclosure may expose the physician to legal liability for invasion of privacy . . . [and] for the independent tort of unprivileged revelation of medical information to third parties.[22]

In summary, legal and ethical guidelines make it clear that the team physician is not exempt from the normal obligations placed upon physicians as part of the doctor–patient relationship. In practical terms, this means: (a) the team physician should respect the confidentiality that is a normal part of the doctor–patient relationship; (b) the team physician's judgment (e.g., in relation to return-to-play decisions) should be governed only by medical considerations, rather than by the team's need for the services of the player;

and (c) the team physician has a duty to fully inform the player-as-patient of any medical risks associated with playing with injury or with any pre-scribed treatment. Of course, these codes of ethics and legal considerations describe how, in an ideal world, club doctors and related medical staff *ought* to behave. To what extent, then, do team physicians actually meet these ethical standards in their day-to-day practice? In order to answer this question, the following sections review the available data relating to the ways in which team medical staff members handle these key problems in the practice of sports medicine.

PATIENT CONFIDENTIALITY

Waddington and Roderick found that there is, among medical staff in Eng-lish professional football clubs, no commonly held code of ethics governing the management of confidential issues, and that there are considerable varia-tions in terms of both the amount, and the kind, of information about play-ers doctors and physiotherapists pass on to managers/coaches.[23] Whereas some physiotherapists emphasized their primary responsibility toward the player-as-patient, others saw their primary responsibility as being toward the club. Several physiotherapists emphasized that they were employed by the club and saw this as sufficient justification for passing on information that would normally be considered confidential, such as aspects of a play-er's off-the-field lifestyle. Typical of the responses of physiotherapists who took this position were comments such as, "I think it's my duty to tell the football club. I work for the football club" or "I'm employed by the football club . . . if it was beneficial that the manager should know [something]—or essential that the manager should know—then I would tell him."[24]

Most club doctors were general practitioners and many indicated that they tried to deal with players' problems on the same confidential basis as with patients in general practice. However, Waddington and Roderick also identified serious breaches of medical ethics among doctors. The most flagrant breach occurred in a case in which a club doctor clearly used con-fidential medical information about a player to advance the interests of the club over and against those of the player. In this case, the club doctor threatened to make public medical information about a player—informa-tion that was actually false—to undermine the player's desired transfer to another club.[25]

Given the considerable variation in terms of the ways in which club med-ical staff deal with issues involving confidentiality, it is not surprising that some players expressed considerable reservations about revealing confiden-tial information to club medical staff. As one player starkly put it: "There is no such thing as confidentiality at a football club." One ex-player explicitly drew a contrast between the situation of a physiotherapist in private prac-tice and the club physiotherapist, pointing out that in the case of the former "of course he wouldn't mention things his patients had said" whereas in a football club "the manager's his boss and if the manager asks him something he might feel duty bound to tell him."[26]

The study of sports physicians in New Zealand revealed a similar lack of consistency. Some had contracts that obliged them to share medical information with coaches and team management and five said that they were prepared to disclose information, *even against the wishes of the athlete*, but in line with their contractual obligations. Ten physicians indicated they would keep such information confidential, citing a commitment to traditional obligations to confidentiality, and one practitioner was unsure of what s/he would do in these circumstances.[27] Writing from an American perspective, Mellion and Walsh have similarly noted that confidentiality is "often compromised" by the doctor's relationship to the club and that "information is seldom held in the strict doctor-patient confidentiality."[28]

Although there is clearly a need for more studies in this area, there is enough evidence to suggest that breaches of patient confidentiality may not be unusual within the sports medicine context.

MANAGING INJURIES: RETURN-TO-PLAY DECISIONS AND INFORMED CONSENT

In his book *You're Okay, It's Just a Bruise*, in which he details his work as a team physician with the Los Angeles Raiders between 1983 and 1990, Huizenga describes his job interview with the Raiders' owner. The interview was extraordinarily cursory, consisting of just five questions, three about Huizenga's own participation in sport and one about where he went to college, before the final and most significant question: "Have you ever played hurt?" The significance of this question lies in the unambiguously conveyed message that the team doctor was expected to "buy into" the culture of "playing hurt."[29]

Huizenga describes medical practice in the National Football League (NFL) as a system based on "the dominating owner or coach selecting and paying for the team doctor—who is then magically expected to have the player's best interest at heart."[30] The owner's influence, he suggests, can be all-pervasive and can impact on all aspects of the team doctor's role, including clinical decision making. In this context, Huizenga documents the regular occurrence of malpractice and unethical behavior by team physicians, including a senior Raiders' team physician who did not use a stretcher to move a player with a possible neck injury—thereby, says Huizenga, playing "Russian roulette" with a player's spinal system—because the club owner felt that "the team gets demoralized and plays less aggressively when they see a teammate getting carted off the field on a stretcher"[31]; the prescription of anabolic steroids; the nondisclosure and knowing misrepresentation of information to players about their injuries because the owner wanted the players to continue playing; and doctors coaching young players to feign injury, against the rules of the NFL, so that they could deliberately fail an independent medical examination and thereby be placed on the injured reserve list (this allowed young players to develop their skills at the club while "hiding" them from other clubs who might seek to sign them). Huizenga cites one other revealing practice. The contracts of NFL players cannot be terminated while they are injured and Huizenga notes: "Currently when a dispute arises, team orthopedists testify against the player—their patient. It's unheard of for a doctor in any other situation to testify against his own patient, unless that patient has literally committed murder."[32] These incidents suggest that it may not be unusual for club medical staff to breach medical ethical guidelines, NFL rules and/or the law by subordinating the interests of the individual player-as-patient to those of the club. Huizenga eventually resigned in protest when the club owner supported a team doctor who deliberately withheld information from a patient about a potentially serious spinal problem.

There are some important similarities—though also important differences—between English professional football and the NFL. In both there is a strong culture of "playing hurt." In English football, players learn from a young age to "normalize" pain and to accept playing with pain and injury as a normal part of the life of a professional footballer.[33] Within this situation, doctors and physiotherapists may be subject to pressure from players who wish to return to play before they have fully recovered from injury. However, this does not, in itself, present any special ethical problems, for although players may return to play earlier than the medical staff feel advisable, if the club doctor has provided the player with full information about the possible long-term effects of playing with injury, then the doctor may legitimately feel that s/he has properly discharged her/his responsibilities to the player-as-patient.

In the study by Roderick, Waddington and Parker, some players indicated that their decision to continue playing through injury had been taken under just such conditions. However, Roderick, Waddington and Parker also found that relevant information about their medical conditions may not be conveyed to players, or may even be deliberately withheld as a matter of club policy.[34] The former Chelsea, Everton and Tranmere Rovers player, Pat Nevin, has also noted that managers may seek to withhold information from players about the extent of their injuries and may encourage their physiotherapists to do the same.[35] Such situations clearly raise serious ethical concerns.

In relation to return-to-play decisions in English football, the need to get players playing again as quickly as possible after injury constitutes a major constraint on club doctors and physiotherapists and also has potentially important implications for the quality of care players receive. One club physiotherapist characterized the culture of football, and the associated constraints on club medical staff by saying: "Everything has to be done yesterday. The players have to be fit yesterday. If they miss a week, it's like a month to anyone else." He added: "You tend not to get the player injury-free. You . . . manage the level of injury irritation to play 90 minutes of football."[36]

This physiotherapist, who also worked in a private sports medicine clinic, pointedly described the key difference between his private practice and his practice in football as follows:

> In private practice, the client isn't desperate to be fit by Saturday. The client wants to be cured of the injury so it doesn't come back . . . In private practice, my *modus operandi* is to cure the injury. In professional football, my *modus operandi* is to get the player on the pitch as quickly as possible.

Being a physiotherapist in a football club was, he continued, "a different job" from being a physiotherapist in private practice, or in the National Health Service. Asked about the quality of care he provided in the two contexts, he answered: "Unequivocally, non-negotiable fact . . . my private clients will get better quality treatment than the players . . . Don't doubt this. Yes, a fact."[37]

The need, as this physiotherapist to put it, to "get players fit yesterday" leads to what one doctor called the "unfortunate" need to make medical compromises and return players to competition before they were fit:

> In this game, there's always compromise, unfortunately. If a player says, "Well, I want to get on," we say to the manager: "He's not quite ready, he could do with another week or two weeks rest" and the manager is under pressure because he hasn't got a depth of staff to play or he's got other injuries and he needs this particular player, then sometimes we're overruled.[38]

Even in those situations which would, at least within the context of football, probably be regarded as "good practice" models—in the sense that doctors are working with managers whom they regard as "reasonable," and where they do not feel under strong or direct pressure from managers—there is a clearly felt need to make medical compromises. However, Waddington, Roderick and Parker found that, in other situations, managers may seek to have a much more direct involvement in the management of injuries, and, in such situations, the clinical autonomy of doctors and physiotherapists is much more directly threatened.[39] For example, one physiotherapist cited an example of an injury that left the club without a goalkeeper for the following day's match. The manager refused to accept the judgment of the medical staff and made them subject the player to a fitness test, "which we were forced to do—I mean other than actually saying 'No, I am not doing it,' and losing your job possibly." The physiotherapist said that he "strapped [the player] up and told him that whatever I did just fall about in agony, basically, so the fitness test would end quickly. And so he did that." He added, "You know he's not fit and you shouldn't be doing that but you've been told to do it by the manager." Another physiotherapist described his difficulties working with a manager who regularly sought to intervene in relation to injured players. He described a series of disagreements he and the manager had about whether players were fit to play, and said that on occasions the manager independently conducted fitness tests on players. A club doctor similarly described what he called a "tainted" relationship with a manager who regularly played injured players against his advice; as he put it, "I began to find it difficult to continue . . . My recommendations were not being considered." The doctor indicated that, had the manager not left the club due to the team's lack of success, the doctor may well have chosen to resign.[40]

The precise nature, as well as the strength, of the perceived need to get players playing again as quickly as possible after injury varies considerably from one club to another. In some situations, medical staff may be allowed a significant degree of professional autonomy in their relationship with the player-as-patient. However, Waddington, Roderick and Parker found clear evidence that in other situations—and particularly where the manager insists on being involved in the management of injuries—the doctor's autonomy may be severely restricted and players may be regularly returned to play before medical staff declare them fit. Under these conditions, club doctors and physiotherapists appear to have two choices, both of which are problematic. They may simply adapt to and accept the situation, *in which case the quality of care they are able to offer will be compromised to a greater or lesser degree.* Alternatively, they may come to feel that their professional autonomy has been so circumscribed that they are unable to do their job in what they consider a properly professional manner. In the latter situation, doctors and physiotherapists are likely to find themselves in recurring conflict with the manager, a situation that may be ended only when one or the other leaves the club. Huizenga's book suggests that physicians in the NFL may find themselves with a similar dilemma.

Malcolm's analysis of the diagnosis and treatment of concussion provides a detailed and revealing example of how rugby club doctors may compromise their clinical practice in order to avoid conflicts with the coach.[41] In recent years, there has been growing concern about the long-term health risks associated with concussion. In order to protect players' health, the International Rugby Board (IRB) has adopted a precautionary policy that requires that players sustaining a concussion must abstain from playing and training for a minimum of three weeks, and only resume when declared symptom-free following medical examination. One consequence of the IRB rule is that any diagnosis of concussion automatically deprives the club of the player's services. Malcolm notes that, within this situation, the resistance of players and coaches to a diagnosis of concussion has led "to a rejection of treatment protocols," the IRB guidelines and their underlying precautionary philosophy. Many doctors go to considerable lengths to avoid offering a diagnosis of concussion, with the loss of the player's services this would entail. One doctor said, "It's best not to diagnose it," and a physiotherapist said "you take them off if you suspect it [concussion], but we don't use the c-word unless we have to."[42] Doctors referred to concussion as a "dodgy" or "gray" area but, significantly, Malcolm noted that "the diagnostic examples doctors gave . . . indicated that when called upon to make a clinical judgement, symptoms within the so-called 'grey areas' did *not* lead to a diagnosis of concussion."[43] Thus players might be described in euphemistic terms as "woozy," "woolly headed" or "just sort of bashed," whereas some doctors even argued that loss of consciousness—traditionally regarded in the medical literature as the most serious symptom of concussion—was not, on its own, sufficient to diagnose concussion.[44]

Malcolm highlights the unintended consequences of a rule that was designed to protect players' health, and he concludes that clinicians "come to diagnose concussion in a way that they know will be acceptable to others," i.e., to coaches and players. He describes this as a "compromise," though it is no exaggeration to say that club doctors appear, in this situation, simply to have abandoned altogether a medical definition of concussion and to have substituted for it the lay understanding of coaches and players. As Malcolm notes, "Allowing sporting performance criteria to override medical guidelines . . . enables the diagnosis to become consistent with rugby players' (and coaches') own definitions of what constitutes an injury," thus allowing clinicians to "minimize interpersonal conflicts" by replacing "medically based diagnostic and treatment procedures . . . by the understanding and definition of concussion dominant in the sport subculture."[45] Clearly the professional autonomy of physicians is seriously undermined in a situation in which diagnosis and treatment come to depend on lay, rather than clinical, criteria.

Perhaps the most striking recent example of unethical medical practice in rugby was provided by the so-called "Bloodgate" scandal involving Harlequins Rugby Club in 2009. Trailing in an important match, Harlequins wanted to bring on a specialist kicker, Nick Evans, but Evans had previously been substituted and could only return to the game as a temporary substitute for a player with a blood injury. Another player, Tom Williams, had been given a sachet of fake blood, which he used to produce the effect of a bleeding mouth injury. He was led off the field by the club physiotherapist—who had agreed to the plan—but the club doctor on the opposing side was suspicious and asked to examine the "injured" player. In the dressing room, the Harlequins' club doctor then made a small incision in Williams's mouth to produce genuine blood. Following a disciplinary hearing at the Health Professions Council, during which the physiotherapist admitted using fake blood on four previous occasions, he was struck off the register. A GMC disciplinary hearing held that the doctor's action had "not been in the best interests of her patient" and she was given a formal warning that her actions had been "unacceptable."[46] Clearly the medical staff allowed their commitment to the club's sporting success to override their commitment to the ethics of medical practice.

What appears to be a more common, although less extreme, situation that compromises the position of club medical staff in rugby has been pointed out by Devitt and McCarthy, who have noted that the doctors' privileged position, which gives them access to injured players on the field of play, is frequently misused to convey tactical information to the team. They argue:

> This practice should be not be tolerated. It is imperative, both in the eyes of the players, and in terms of focus, that the physiotherapist and doctor are seen to have sole responsibility for the treatment of injuries while on the field of play. [47]

They suggest there should be a clear understanding of appropriate communication between medical staff and coaching staff—which should not include the passing on of tactical information—and that it is necessary to set appropriate boundaries "with respect to professional conduct and moral obligations."

Much of the data generated by these studies suggest that one implication of Nixon's analysis—that the nonsport world is, as Walk puts it, "more medically prudent than the sport world"—may have a good deal of substance.[48] Thus whereas the currently available data are limited, the existing studies of professional sport do suggest that breaches of confidentiality are not unusual and, indeed, may even be commonplace; that it is by no means rare for information about their injuries to be withheld from players, and that, on occasions, this may be done routinely as a matter of club policy; that club medical staff routinely make medical compromises in their diagnosis and treatment of players' injuries, and that, in some cases, they may, in effect, simply abandon a medical understanding and substitute a lay understanding; and that club doctors may be subject to pressure to deviate from good medical practice in other ways described in the preceding. All these findings are consistent with Nixon's characterization of sportsnets as networks of people—coaches, doctors and others—who provide "biased social support" to athletes in relation to the management of pain and injury.

NIXON'S FRAMEWORK REVISITED

However, it has also been claimed that other research is less consistent with Nixon's framework. Walk's study, based on interviews with student athletic trainers (SATs) at a university in the American Midwest, led him to suggest that the situation is more complex than that described by Nixon. Walk found that many SATs developed close relationships with the student athletes and that this "often resulted in resistance to the intentions of the sportsnet."[49] Thus Walk noted that, although some coaches put pressure on athletes to continue training and competing with injury, most SATs reported that they resisted these pressures. He concluded that there was "little evidence that SATs participated in attempts to return an athlete to play before medically indicated."[50]

A broadly similar picture was described by Safai in her study of the provision of sports medical care in a Canadian university. Safai notes that although a "culture of risk" exists in university sport and that this "frames the negotiation between clinician and patient-athletes, a 'culture of precaution' seems to temper the acceptance and tolerance of pain and injury." Thus although the "culture of risk" is "dominant," she suggests it is "tempered by a concern for the health and safety of student-athletes in sport."[51]

On the basis of their data, both Walk and Safai are critical of Nixon's approach. Walk suggests that his own study offers "a far different picture than that suggested by Nixon, wherein medical personnel, in concert with similarly inclined others, compel athletes to play with injuries, do not relay accurate medical information, and withhold proper care."[52] He argues that Nixon's "model of an insulated, culturally homogeneous, and "conspiratorial" sportsnet is both intuitively suspect and without empirical support," adding:

> Even a sportsnet may be characterized by flaws in its systems of control, related negotiation and conflict, and some measure of freedom for its members, even those with the least power—in the present case, student athletes and student athletic trainers.[53]

Safai similarly suggests that the "culture of risk" in sport is "far more complex than Nixon implies" and that, whereas Nixon argued that an institutional alliance, which includes sports medicine personnel, helps to perpetuate the acceptance of a "culture of risk" by athletes, "more recent research shows that such structures are not monolithic."[54]

The empirical work of Walk and Safai makes a useful contribution to the subject; however, their critique of Nixon appears to be based, at least in part, on an oversimplification of his argument. Walk and Safai are correct to point out that sportsnets are not monolithic, are not equally closed or insulated and are not culturally homogeneous. It is clear, for example, that there may be considerable variations from one situation to another in terms of the degree to which athletes are constrained to continue playing with pain and injury, or in terms of how much information sports physicians convey to—or withhold from—athletes about their injuries and the associated risks of playing while injured. However, such empirical variations in the structures of sportsnets do not undermine Nixon's argument, for not only does he not

imply that sportsnets are monolithic, but, on the contrary, he explicitly recognizes that they are likely to vary in significant respects. Nixon identifies a
number of processes that are likely to account for such variations, suggesting
that sportsnets are "relatively more likely to entrap athletes in the culture of
risk and foster a self-abusive pattern of pain and injury" when the networks
are larger, denser, more centralized, more closed, more homogeneous and
stable and where athletes are more accessible to coaches and others with
authority or control within the sporting context;[55] by implication, they are
less likely to "entrap" athletes where they have the opposite characteristics.
Taking these variables into account can help to explain not only what Walk
and Safai take to be the inconsistencies between Nixon's model and their
own findings, but also some of the variations between their findings and the
findings in relation to professional sport, reviewed earlier.

If it is the case, as Walk and Safai suggest, that clinicians in North American
college sport are less likely than are clinicians in professional sport to deviate
from what is considered good medical practice, this may well be because college sports clinicians are less highly integrated into the sportsnets than is the
case in professional sport, whereas the sportsnets themselves are, in Nixon's
terms, smaller, less dense, less centralized, less closed, less homogeneous and
less stable. For instance, Walk's SATs were all full-time university students
involved in temporary internship programs; their involvement in, and their
commitment to, the university sportsnet was therefore a transitory phenomenon rather than a long-term commitment. And they received either no pay
or a very small income for their work, which led to some students "harbor-
ing strong resentment toward the program as a result."[56] Walk argues that
these "considerations of unpaid, time-consuming labor, [and] gender-based
discrimination and harassment . . . indicated strong bases for the student
trainers to resist the demands that were placed on them." Indeed, it was this
sense of grievance against, and perhaps exploitation by, senior members of
the sportsnet that led to the formation of strong friendships between SATs
and athletes that, as Walk emphasized, "undermined . . . the intentions of the
medical and coaching staff" within the university.[57]

The sportsnet depicted by Walk is characterized by young, inexperienced
SATs working on a temporary basis and with a strong sense of resentment
toward key people; given this situation it is perhaps not surprising that
the relationships that developed between the "transitory members" of the
sportsnet—that is, the student trainers and the student athletes—should
have "worked to undermine a number of totalizing and exploitative tendencies the . . . sportsnet may have had."[58] On a more theoretical level, the
existence of transitory members with a strong sense of grievance would
suggest that the university sportsnet described by Walk is characterized by,
in Nixon's terms, a relatively low level of centralized control, homogeneity
and stability. Nixon's framework would lead us to predict, as Walk's data
indicate, that sports clinicians working in such settings are less likely to be
implicated in health-threatening practices.

It is also clear that there are important differences between college sport in North America and professional sport, whether in the US or the UK. One key difference relates to the levels of competitiveness and, associated with this, the different emphasis placed on, and the rewards associated with, sporting success. Thus Safai notes that many teams in Canadian interuniversity sport "tend to play with less pronounced pressures on success and revenue" than is the case with professional sport or some sports in the NCAA Division I-A in the US.[59] Significantly, she points out that whereas some programs within the NCAA Division I-A value *athlete-students*, the institution in which her study was carried out "positions sport participants primarily as *student-athletes*."[60] She notes that while a few students aspire to compete at the national or professional level, for most students intercollegiate sport is, as one clinician put it, "the icing on the cake, it's not the cake." She also notes that the institutional climate of the unit within which sports medicine unit is located "emphasizes both physical education *and* health" (emphasis in original), and that the behavior of clinicians is "influenced by the clinic's location in an educational and health-oriented administrative unit."[61] Safai's description of the context within which the clinic is located suggests that the clinic is, in Nixon's terms, not highly closed and is not well insulated from the university's broader policy goals relating to the promotion of education and health. In this key respect, it differs radically from the position of sports clinicians in professional sport where sporting success is the overwhelming goal.

Given the preceding comments, it may be appropriate to conclude that the implication of the studies by Walk and Safai is not that Nixon's framework is fundamentally flawed but, rather, that more attention needs to be paid to the dimensions identified by Nixon—size, density, centralization, etc.—in terms of which sportsnets vary. Where sportsnets are relatively large, dense, more centralized, more closed and more stable—as appears to be the case in professional sport—then the constraints on sports medicine practitioners to deviate from what is generally considered good medical practice are likely to be relatively strong; however, where sportsnets are smaller, less dense, less centralized, less closed and less stable—as appears to be the case in the college sport described by Walk and Safai—then the constraints on sports medicine practitioners to make medical compromises and to engage in health-threatening practices are likely to be less strong.

But if Nixon's framework remains of value, might that framework not yield even greater explanatory power if another dimension is added? In order to explore this matter further, let us examine the work of Eliott Freidson.

CLIENT CONTROL AND MEDICAL PRACTICE

In a classic essay originally published in 1960, Freidson pointed out that medical professionals cannot exist without clients, but that clients "often

have ideas about what they want that differ markedly from those suppos-
edly held by the professionals they consult."[62] As a result, consultations
between practitioners and clients often involve a clash between "two different, sometimes conflicting, sets of norms," based on differing understandings of health and illness.[63] Freidson noted that there may be more or
less congruence between the lay cultural understanding of the client and
the professional understanding of the physician and that, to understand
what takes place in medical practice, it is necessary to examine the relative
sources of power of doctor and patient. This led Freidson to propose two
polar types of medical practice:

1. Colleague-dependent practice, in which interaction is primarily
   dependent on the professional evaluations and decisions of the doctor
   and his/her professional colleagues.
2. Client-dependent practice, in which interaction between doctor and
   client is largely dependent on the lay evaluations and decisions of
   clients.

A critical determinant of the type of practice, suggests Freidson, is the
setting within which the practice is located. In this regard, the "authoritative source of professional culture" is located in professionally controlled
organizations such as hospitals and medical schools, for professional
"prestige and power radiate out from the latter and diminish with distance from them."[64] Of critical importance is the fact that the further this
professional system is penetrated, the more free it is of the lay influence
of patients. Thus:

> A layman seeking help finds that, the further within it he goes, the
> fewer choices can he make and the less can he control what is done to
> him. Indeed, it is not unknown for the "client" to be a petitioner, ask-
> ing to be chosen: the organizations and practitioners who stand well
> within the professional referral system may or may not "take the case,"
> according to their judgement of its interest.

As a result:

> Choice, and therefore positive control, is now taken out of the hands
> of the client and comes to rest in the hands of the practitioner, and the
> use of professional services is no longer predicated on the client's lay
> understandings—indeed, the client may be given services for which he
> did not ask, whose rationale is beyond him.[65]

At the other extreme, suggests Freidson, is the position of practitioners
located in the local community. Unlike hospital doctors, who receive their
patients by referrals from other professionals, doctors who practice in the

community are dependent on attracting their own lay clientele, and, in order to do so, are constrained to behave in ways that are in closer accord with lay expectations. As Freidson notes in relation to community-based practice, to "survive without colleagues, it must be located within a lay referral system and, as such, is *least* able to resist control by clients, and *most* able to resist control by colleagues."[66] Thus whereas the hospital-based doctor is surrounded by professional colleagues, is subject to their evaluation and is expected to be responsive to the clinical and ethical professional standards they all share, the community-based practitioner (especially the isolated solo practitioner) is much more subject to evaluation by, and is therefore required to be more responsive to, the lay demands of clients for it is they, rather than professional colleagues, who will determine the success or otherwise of the community-based practice. Lay influence may more or less control not only the practitioner's success in attracting clients, "but, to some extent, also his professional technique and manner."[67]

The peculiar features of the situation of the club doctor in professional sport mean that this type of practice is characterized by an even higher degree of client control than is normally the case in community-based practice. In this regard, the contrasts between the position of the hospital-based doctor and the club physician are quite striking. The club doctor works within an organization in which the key values are not professional values relating to health, but lay values relating to sporting success. And if hospital doctors are the highest-status workers—the "stars," as it were—within the hospital, the "stars" within sports clubs are the players and coaches, and the doctors are reduced to the role of lower-status, "bit part" players, mere "service workers" whose job it is to look after the "stars." Significantly, doctors' remuneration and status within the clubs is often consistent with their position as service workers. Huizenga, for example, records that he "apologetically" raised the issue of his salary with the owner of the Los Angeles Raiders, who offered him, in a "take it or leave it" manner, an annual salary that was less than many players received for a single game.[68] A similar point was made by a doctor at an English football club, who said that the club quibbled about his bill, even though it was "peanuts"; another club doctor indicated that he received just £5,200 per year for his services, even though he had calculated that, applying the BMA's recommended scale of charges, he should have been receiving £25,000.[69] Their role as service workers is also reflected in their nonfinancial status within clubs. Malcolm recorded "a number of incidents where medical staff were demeaned by the behaviour of others within the rugby club setting" and he noted:

> The level of respect afforded to some medical staff in some rugby club contexts . . . marks out sports medicine as being . . . characterized by social rules quite different from those of other, "normal," forms of medical practice, where great respect is usually accorded to medical practitioners.[70]

And far from respecting their status as medical experts, some managers in English football, as noted earlier, simply disregarded the advice of their own club doctors and physiotherapists.

Not only do club doctors work in a situation dominated by lay sporting values, but, unlike many doctors, they are frequently professionally isolated. Thus Malcolm noted that rugby club doctors "tend to work in isolation from other professional colleagues,"[71] and a football club doctor complained that his position was difficult because he was, as he put it, "a single voice and if I disagreed with what was going on, then there were a lot more people around . . . to perhaps try to persuade me to change my mind."[72] There were also relatively few opportunities for club doctors to meet professionally with colleagues from other clubs.[73] As Freidson noted:

> All else being equal in this situation of minimal observability by colleagues and maximum dependence on the lay referral system, we should expect to find the least sensitivity to formal professional standards and the greatest sensitivity to the local lay standards.[74]

This is, it is suggested, what we frequently find in the case of sports medicine, especially in the situation of club medical practice in professional sport.

It has been suggested that the situation of club medical practice is one that constrains doctors to orient themselves primarily toward the demands of the lay clientele—which in this case consists of other members of the sportsnet—rather than toward the community of medical practitioners, and that this in turn is likely to constrain practitioners to make both ethical and clinical compromises that they would not be required to make in other practice situations. But if club doctors are constrained to make such medical compromises, and also to accept relatively poor working conditions, then we need to ask why: why do doctors accept such forms of employment?

By far the most common motivation that leads doctors to accept employment as club doctors relates not to professional goals, such as improving clinical expertise or qualifications, or moving into sports medicine as a full-time career, but derives from their long-standing love of sport and, in many cases, their commitment to a particular team. One English football club doctor, whose father had been the previous club doctor, explained: "I did medicine so that I could be the team doctor—I wasn't interested in any other team." Another club doctor said: "Basically although I'm 46, there's a ten year old boy inside saying 'Fantastic! Fantastic! It's great'"; a third simply described the role of club doctor as "the next best thing to playing."[75] In rugby, Malcolm has noted that the most commonly cited motivations for acting as club doctor were "support for the team" and a "general interest in sport"—few cited "occupational experience" or "interest in sports medicine" as major motivational factors.[76] Huizenga similarly describes a visit to the office of Dr. Rosenfeld, who was a senior doctor with the Los Angeles Raiders:

> Once I stepped into his office, I could see what made him really proud. His walls were plastered with Raider memorabilia . . . and multiple shots of Dr. Rosenfeld assisting dazed athletes off the field with thousands of spectators serving as a blurry backdrop.[77]

Most club doctors have a strong and prior commitment to sport before they enter club medical practice. As Freidson has noted, there may be a marked discrepancy between the professional culture of doctors and the lay culture of their patients; however, in the case of club medical practice, it might be suggested that this gap is bridged, not by the fact that the patients share the professional culture of the doctor but, on the contrary, by the fact that the club doctor shares the sporting culture of his/her clientele. What are the key elements of this sport ethic?

Coakley has noted that the key aspects of the sport ethic are a dedication to "the game" above all else, a relentless striving for improved performance, an acceptance of risk and a willingness to play through pain and injury and an unwillingness to accept obstacles in the pursuit of sporting success.[78] He also suggests that many forms of deviance within sport, such as drug use and violence, may be understood as arising not from a rejection of these norms of sport, but as a result of overconformity—that is, an unquestioned acceptance of, and extreme conformity to, this sport ethic. This type of "overdoing-it deviance," he suggests, involves an overcommitment to the goal of sporting success, which may lead, for example, to the willingness to risk serious injury in order to continue competing and to an acceptance of unfair means if these enhance the likelihood of sporting success.

Coakley's concept of overconformity is, it is suggested, also helpful in understanding those aspects of the behavior of sports physicians that deviate from what is generally considered good medical practice. Many club doctors, it is clear, have a long-standing and real commitment to the sport ethic. However, key aspects of the sport ethic sit uncomfortably alongside the key values of medical ethics. And just as some athletes develop an overconformity to the sport ethic, so too, it is suggested, do some club doctors. Thus whereas most club doctors will have a dual allegiance to medical ethics and to the sport ethic, the work situation of club doctors constrains them to pay greater attention to the latter at the expense of the former; in short, the work situation of club doctors constrains them to "buy into" the sport ethic and to the key goal of sporting success and, at least to some degree, to "buy out of" medical ethics. The clearest example of this process of overconformity to the sport ethic and the associated "buying out of" medical ethics is provided by a process that has only been referred to briefly in this chapter but has been extensively analyzed elsewhere; it constitutes the clearest and perhaps most serious breach of medical ethics within the sporting context: the widespread involvement of sports physicians in the development and use of illicit performance-enhancing drugs (see, for instance, Hoberman's contribution in this collection).[79] If the deviations from good medical practice that have been the focus of this chapter are less extreme, they nevertheless have their origins in broadly similar processes.

CONCLUSION

It has been argued that the work situation of sports medicine practitioners—and, in particular, of club doctors—is one that is likely to constrain them to make ethical and clinical compromises that they would not be required to make in other practice situations. The UK's Faculty of Sports and Exercise Medicine has recently published a professional code containing ethical guidance for sports physicians,[80] but it may be argued that what is required is not a call for more ethical behavior but, rather, a change in the structural location of sports physicians vis-à-vis other people within the sportsnet. Nixon has suggested that the physical welfare of athletes could be protected by partitioning the "networks of influence over medical and sports decisions," such that the influence of coaches and others over medical decisions is reduced:

> What this means in concrete terms is that the positions of doctors and trainers are not directly connected to those of coaches, athletic directors, boosters, or other members of sportnets who might be tempted to sacrifice the welfare of athletes for the benefit the team.[81]

Similar considerations underlie Huizenga's recommendation that team doctors should, like the doctors who supervise boxing in California, be appointed "to a set term not unlike a judge, perhaps by consensus of owners and players, but then supervised solely by an impartial medical board or state commission."[82] The need to increase the professional autonomy of sports physicians was also one of the key recommendations of the study of English football by Waddington, Roderick and Parker. They wrote:

> Urgent consideration needs to be given to defining the respective rights and responsibilities of the club doctor, physiotherapist and manager in relation to the management of injuries and other health-related issues. A central object of this exercise should be to define the roles of the respective parties in such a way as to maximise the clinical autonomy of doctors and physiotherapists, and to minimise the day-to-day involvement of managers in the management of injuries.

They suggested that this will "make a major contribution towards creating the conditions conducive to good clinical practice, and to protecting the health of players."[83]

NOTES

1. Nixon, "Social Network Analysis"; "Accepting the Risks"; "Coaches' Views"; "Relationship of Friendship Networks."
2. Walk, "Peers in Pain," 24.
3. Young, "Violence, Risk and Liability."
4. Freidson, "Client Control"; *Profession of Medicine.*
5. Mitten, "Emerging Legal Issues," 8.
6. BMA, *Medical Ethics Today*, 595.
7. Roy and Irvin, *Sports Medicine*, 3.
8. Nixon, "Social Network Analysis"; "Accepting the Risks"; "Coaches' Views"; Young, "Violence, Risk and Liability"; Roderick, Waddington and Parker, "Playing Hurt."
9. Young, White and McTeer, "Body Talk," 190.
10. Crane, "Association Football," 332 (emphasis added).
11. Graf-Baumann, "Law and Ethics," 31.
12. Anderson and Gerrard, "Ethical Issues," 89.
13. BMA, *Medical Ethics Today*, 596.
14. GMC, *Confidentiality*, 2.
15. Faculty of Occupational Medicine of the Royal College of Physicians of London, *Guidance on Ethics.*
16. BMA, *Medical Ethics Today*, 596.
17. Devitt and McCarthy, 'I Am in Blood," 175–176.
18. "Team Physician Consensus Statement," 877.
19. Mitten, "Emerging Legal Issues," 8–9.
20. Ibid., 26–27.
21. Junge, "Obligations of Team Physicians," 3.
22. Mitten, "Emerging Legal Issues," 30.
23. Waddington and Roderick, 'Management of Medical Confidentiality."
24. Ibid., 120.
25. Ibid., 120–121.
26. Ibid.
27. Anderson, "Writing a New Code," 1080.
28. Mellion and Walsh, "Team Physician," 1.
29. Huizenga, *You're Okay.*
30. Ibid., 315.
31. Ibid., 124–125.
32. Ibid., 316.
33. Roderick, Waddington and Parker, "Playing Hurt."
34. Ibid., 175–176.
35. Nevin and Sik, *In Ma Head*, 83.
36. Waddington, "Ethical Problems," 189.
37. Ibid., 189.
38. Ibid., 190.
39. Waddington, Roderick and Parker, *Managing Injuries.*
40. Waddington, "Ethical Problems," 194.
41. Malcolm, "Medical Uncertainty."
42. Ibid., 204.
43. Ibid., 202 (emphasis in original).
44. Ibid.
45. Ibid., 191.
46. Carter, '"Bloodgate" Rugby Scandal: Doctor tells General Medical Hearing of Deep Shame'.
47. Devitt and McCarthy, "I Am in Blood," 178.
48. Walk, "Peers in Pain," 24.

49. Ibid., 50.
50. Ibid., 36.
51. Safai, "Healing the Body," 139.
52. Walk, "Peers in Pain," 46.
53. Ibid., 50.
54. Safai, "Healing the Body," 128, 138.
55. Nixon, "Social Network Analysis," 132.
56. Walk, "Peers in Pain," 31.
57. Ibid., 32.
58. Ibid., 50.
59. Safai, "Healing the Body," 131.
60. Ibid., 138 (emphasis in original).
61. Ibid.
62. Freidson, "Client Control," in *Medical Care*, 260.
63. Ibid. 262
64. Ibid., 267.
65. Ibid., 267–268.
66. Ibid., 268 (emphasis in original).
67. Ibid., 266.
68. Huizenga, *You're Okay*, 63.
69. Waddington, Roderick and Parker, *Managing Injuries*, 9–10, 13–14.
70. Malcolm, "Sports Medicine," 176–177.
71. Malcolm, "Unprofessional Practice?" 383.
72. Waddington, *Sport, Health and Drugs*, 77.
73. Waddington, Roderick and Parker, *Managing Injuries*, 14.
74. Freidson, "Client Control," in *Medical Care*, 269.
75. Waddington, Roderick and Parker, *Managing Injuries*, 10.
76. Malcolm, "Sports Medicine," 170.
77. Huizenga, *You're Okay*, 8.
78. Coakley, *Sport in Society*.
79. Waddington, *Sport, Health and Drugs*; "Doping in Sport"; Waddington and Smith, *Introduction*.
80. Faculty of Sports and Exercise Medicine, *Professional Code*.
81. Nixon, "Social Network Analysis," 133.
82. Huizenga, *You're Okay*, 316.
83. Waddington, Roderick and Parker, *Managing Injuries*, 68.

BIBLIOGRAPHY

Anderson, Lynley. "Writing a New Code of Ethics for Sports Physicians: Principles and Challenges." *British Journal of Sports Medicine* 43, no. 13 (2009): 1079–1082.
Anderson, Lynley, and David Gerrard. "Ethical Issues Concerning New Zealand Sports Doctors." *Journal of Medical Ethics* 31 (2005): 88–92.
British Medical Association. *Medical Ethics Today: The BMA's Handbook of Ethics and the Law*. London: BMJ Books, 2003.
Carter, Helen. "'Bloodgate' Rugby Scandal: Doctor tells General Medical Hearing of Deep Shame." http://www.guardian.co.uk/sport/2010/aug/24/bloodgate-rugby-scandal-doctor-shame. Accessed 23rd April 2012.
Coakley, Jay. *Sports in Society*. 9th ed. New York: McGraw-Hill, 2007.
Crane, John. "Association Football: The Team Doctor." In *Medicine, Sport and the Law*, edited by S.D.W. Payne, 331–337. Oxford: Blackwell Scientific Publications, 1990.

Devitt, B.M., and C. McCarthy. "'I Am in Blood Stepp'ed in so Far . . . ': Ethical Dilemmas and the Sports Team Doctor." *British Journal of Sports Medicine* 44 (2010): 175–178.

Faculty of Occupational Medicine of the Royal College of Physicians of London. *Guidance on Ethics for Occupational Physicians*. London: Faculty of Occupational Medicine, 1999.

Faculty of Sports and Exercise Medicine. *Professional Code*. London: FSEM, 2010.

Freidson, Eliot. "Client Control and Medical Practice." *American Journal of Sociology* 65 (1960): 374–382.

———. "Client Control and Medical Practice." In *Medical Care*, edited by W.R. Scott and E.H. Volkart, 259–271. New York: Wiley, 1966.

———. *Profession of Medicine*. New York: Dodd, Mead and Co., 1970.

General Medical Council. *Confidentiality*. London: GMC, 1995.

Graf-Baumann, T. "The Law and Ethics of Football Injuries." *FIFA Magazine*, February 1997, 31

Junge, M. "Obligations of Team Physicians." *Virtual Mentor* 6, no. 7 (2004). http://virtualmentor.ama-assn.org/2004/07/hlaw1–0407.html (accessed 7 July 2010).

Huizenga, R. *You're Okay, It's Just a Bruise*. New York: St. Martin's Griffin, 1995.

Malcolm, Dominic. "Medical Uncertainty and Clinician–Athlete Relations: The Management of Concussion Injuries in Rugby Union." *Sociology of Sport Journal* 26 (2009): 191–210.

———. "Sports Medicine: A Very Peculiar Practice? Doctors and Physiotherapists in Elite English Rugby Union." In *Pain and Injury in Sport: Social and Ethical Analysis*, edited by Sigmund Loland, Berit Skirstad and Ivan Waddington, 165–181. London: Routledge, 2006.

———. "Unprofessional Practice? The Status and Power of Sport Physicians." *Sociology of Sport Journal* 23 (2006): 376–395.

Mellion, M., and W. Walsh. "The Team Physician." In *Sports Medicine Secrets*, edited by M. Mellion, 1–4. Philadelphia: Hanley and Belfus, 1994.

Mitten, M.J. "Emerging Legal Issues in Sports Medicine: A Synthesis, Summary, and Analysis." *St. John's Law Review* 76, no. 5 (2002): 5–86.

Nevin, P., and G. Sik. *In Ma Head, Son*. London: Headline, 1997.

Nixon, Howard L., II. "Accepting the Risks of Pain and Injury in Sport: Mediated Cultural Influences on Playing Hurt." *Sociology of Sport Journal* 10 (1993): 183–196.

———. "Coaches' Views of Risk, Pain, and Injury in Sport, with Special Reference to Gender Differences." *Sociology of Sport Journal* 11 (1994): 79–87.

———. "The Relationship of Friendship Networks, Sports Experiences, and Gender to Expressed Pain Thresholds." *Sociology of Sport Journal* 13 (1996): 78–86.

———. "A Social Network Analysis of Influences on Athletes to Play with Pain and Injuries." *Journal of Sport & Social Issues* 16, no. 2 (1992): 127–135.

Roderick, Martin, Ivan Waddington and Graham Parker. "Playing Hurt: Managing Injuries in English Professional Football." *International Review for the Sociology of Sport* 35, no. 2 (2000): 165–180.

Roy, S., and R. Irvin. *Sports Medicine: Prevention, Evaluation, Management and Rehabilitation*. Englewood Cliffs, NJ: Prentice Hall, 1983.

Safai, Parissa. "Healing the Body in the 'Culture of Risk': Examining the Negotiation of Treatment between Sport Medicine Clinicians and Injured Athletes in Canadian Intercollegiate Sport." *Sociology of Sport Journal* 20 (2003): 127–146.

"Team Physician Consensus Statement." *Medicine and Science in Sport and Exercise* 32, no. 4 (2000): 877–878.

Waddington, Ivan. "Doping in Sport: Some Issues for Medical Practitioners." In *Doping and Public Policy*, edited by John Hoberman and Verner Møller, 31–44. Odense: University Press of Southern Denmark, 2004.

———. "Ethical Problems in the Medical Management of Sports Injuries: A Case Study of English Professional Football." In *Pain and Injury in Sport: Social and Ethical Analysis*, edited by Sigmund Loland, Berit Skirstad and Ivan Waddington, 182–199. London, Routledge, 2006.

———. *Sport, Health and Drugs*. London: Spon, 2000.

Waddington, Ivan, and Martin Roderick. "Management of Medical Confidentiality in English Professional Football Clubs: Some Ethical Problems and Issues." *British Journal of Sports Medicine* 36, no. 2 (2002): 118–123.

Waddington, Ivan, Martin Roderick and Graham Parker. *Managing Injuries in Professional Football: The Roles of the Club Doctor and Physiotherapist*. Leicester: Centre for Research into Sport and Society, 1999.

Waddington, Ivan, and Andy Smith. *An Introduction to Drugs in Sport: Addicted to Winning?* London: Routledge, 2009.

Walk, Stephan. "Peers in Pain: The Experience of Student Athletic Trainers." *Sociology of Sport Journal* 14 (1997): 22–56.

Young, Kevin. "Violence, Risk and Liability in Male Sports Culture." *Sociology of Sport Journal* 10 (1993): 373–396.

Young, Kevin, Philip White and William McTeer. "Body Talk: Male Athletes Reflect on Sport, Injury and Pain." *Sociology of Sport Journal* 11 (1994): 175–194.

11 Making Compromises in Sports Medicine

An Examination of the Health–Performance Nexus in British Olympic Sports

Andrea Scott

In his historical examination of the development of sports medicine and its growing prominence in elite level sport, Hoberman asserts that a drive for performance enhancement is "the inherent logic of high-performance sport" and offers an insight into the scientific and medical practices (and some of the associated dilemmas) of practitioners involved in this performance-centered work setting.[1] In a similarly developmental approach, Waddington contends that the association of sports medicine with athletic performance has arisen from its development within both an increasingly "medicalized" society and a contemporary sporting context driven by a "win at all costs" ethic.[2] Thus, for Waddington, practitioners are willing to make their skills available to those who simply request their services as well as those eager to improve their level of performance. Both analyses provide well-documented accounts of sport medicine's development and its association with performance enhancement.

These conclusions essentially stem from the analysis of the development of performance-enhancing drugs than from a wider interest in the orientation of sports medicine practitioners to performance-related concerns. Subsequent sociological research has, however, acknowledged the balance between health and performance in the everyday practices of sports medicine clinicians. In her study of sports medicine, health and the culture of risk among doctors, physiotherapists and administrators in Canadian high-performance sport, Theberge asserts that performance concerns are at the center of medical practice,[3] and that this performance-driven model of athlete care is an example of the consumer-oriented model of professional practice where consumers are able to "define their own needs and the manner in which those needs are catered for."[4] Yet, whereas Theberge contends that performance enhancement is a defining feature of the treatment negotiations between athletes and clinicians (see also Theberge's contribution in this collection), she maintains that this is often tempered by clinicians' "professional obligation to safeguard athletes' health and well-being."[5] Such obligations are also evident in Safai's research into the dialogue between health care providers and injured athletes in Canadian intercollegiate sport.[6] She argues that the work of sports medicine clinicians is characterized, on the one hand, by accepting a "culture of risk" in sport and, on the other, a "culture of precaution" where sports medicine clinicians put the longer-term health of athletes first.

Drawing upon the perspectives of doctors and physiotherapists working in British Olympic sport, this chapter endeavors to expand our understanding of how clinicians balance concerns about health and performance. Initial discussion examines some of the pressures that emerge from a context in which performance is a defining feature and highlights how clinicians are constrained to mold their medical practice to suit the demands of their working context and satisfy their clients. It also considers the consequences this performance focus has for doctors and physiotherapists' *respective* clinical autonomy.

The ambivalence over sports medicine clinicians' involvement within performance enhancement has led some academics to question the moral and ethical convictions of these practitioners in comparison to their colleagues in other medical contexts (see Waddington's contribution in this collection). Discussing the role of sports medicine doctors specifically, McNamee and Edwards argue that doctors have a clear code of practice that is concerned with health promotion and contend that "for a practice to fall within the class of medicine it is necessary that it possess the attribute of aiming to relieve suffering. This goal is a necessary condition of medical practice."[7] For them, sports medicine's apparent commitment to enhancing human performance negates the traditional goals of medicine and thus means that it cannot be considered a part of the broader profession. Whereas it is not the intention of this chapter to discuss the "place" of sports medicine within its broader profession, the analytical focus is upon the way in which concerns about health and performance *differ* between doctors and physiotherapists as a consequence of their membership within their broader professional bodies. Data reveal that such membership both enables and constrains doctors and physiotherapists as they attempt to balance concerns about the longer-term health of athletes with more immediate concerns over sporting performance.

METHODS

Data were derived from semi-structured interviews undertaken between January and May 2008 with fourteen doctors and fourteen physiotherapists who were then members of the British Olympic Association's (BOA) medical and physiotherapy committees (each Olympic sport National Governing Body nominates one doctor and one physiotherapist to the respective committees). These individuals were considered to be the most appropriate sports medicine professionals to target as they were likely to be most centrally involved in the delivery of health care to Olympic athletes and thus able to provide considered reflections on their involvement in sports medicine. Targeting the committees was also the easiest way of identifying contacts and guaranteed a breadth of coverage across all Olympic sports. Interviews lasted between thirty and ninety minutes and were recorded and transcribed verbatim. Interviewees were asked about how they became involved in sports medicine, their typical routines when treating athletes at home and at competition events such as the Olympics and any difficulties they experienced within their role. They were also asked about their working relationships with athletes, coaches and other medical staff and how these relationships impacted upon their medical decision making.

ATHLETE PRESSURE: TIME AND WINNING

One of the defining features of the performance model of medical care in British Olympic sports is the way in which clinicians' prioritize the competitive interests of athletes. In this context, athletes' interests center on winning and, in particular, winning Olympic medals. Thus, the timing of particular competitions and the centrality of these competitions for athletes' careers became one of the principal considerations by which sports medicine clinicians decide on athletes' treatment programs and, during competition, on whether or not they would take measures to allow the athlete to compete despite being injured (for example, providing athletes with a painkilling injection).

The primacy of the performance model for sports medicine practice was clearly demonstrated in the descriptions doctors and physiotherapists provided of their initial consultations with injured athletes. Rather than clinicians inquiring about injury in the first instance, questions were most often about the time-tabling of competitions. One doctor stated, "You always have to ask people 'what's the next competition coming up, what's the next event?'" Similarly, another doctor noted, "The first question I will ask somebody is 'what have you got coming up?'"

Respondents also discussed some of the medical compromises they felt obliged to make when athletes became injured during, or in the run-up to, a major competitive event. Clinicians were aware that athletes working toward competing in an Olympic Games were constrained by particular time pressures, and respondents described how they felt compelled to take greater medical risks because of how significant the Olympics are for athletes. One physiotherapist stated:

> If it's an Olympic Games you would probably say, "Okay, you might make it worse but we will do x, y and z, we will tape it [and] the doctor might put a painkilling injection in." You would do anything that you possibly could to get the athlete out there and to give them a chance.

The majority of respondents recognized that the Olympics was an "extraordinary" event and discussed the pressures on athletes to compete, which stemmed from the event only occurring once every four years. Clinicians described how they did not want to deny an athlete what might be their only chance at being successful at such a mega-event, and this became one justification for decisions to be focused on athletes' performance goals. One doctor said:

> There is no doubt that the Olympics is an extraordinary four-yearly event and, you know, excuse the pun or the phrase but it's "shit or bust" for some people. Therefore, there may be some extraordinary decision making that takes place.

In a similar way, a physiotherapist clearly described her rationale for making medical judgments during an Olympics:

> The Olympics comes every four years and if you're two months out and you have trained for three years and ten months what are you going to do? You're going to take a risk and get everything as good as you can.

Although it was not clear if the respondents themselves felt that the Olympics were "extraordinary" or if they were referring to the significance of this event for the athletes they cared for,[8] it is clear that such external factors impacted upon doctors' and physiotherapists' judgments on the balance between health and performance. The four-yearly cycle of the Olympics was a central rationale for performance-oriented clinical practice.

Clinicians were generally open about discussing some of the medical risks they would take during an Olympic Games, which reinforces the depiction within previous pain and injury literature that members of the "sportsnet" have normalized their work within a culture of risk.[9] One physiotherapist acknowledged:

> We might put them [athletes] at more risk depending on the level of competition they are at. If it's an Olympics as opposed to a regular domestic race obviously you try to get them to the start line in whatever circumstances that you can.

A similar point was made by one of the doctors:

> If they are at an Olympic Games and they have got a really good chance then you will patch them up to let them perform and give them the guidance and the knowledge that you know is probably not good for them but this is how you are going to get through whatever event that you have got.

Another physiotherapist described how medical treatment was simply about "patching up and pushing on" when athletes were injured and/or in pain during these events. Likewise, one physiotherapist said, "If this was an Olympic final then we would strap them up, give them some tablets and send them on."

Whereas these excerpts depict the "compete at all costs" attitude accepted by physiotherapists and doctors as a central feature of the culture of Olympic sport, the following quote illustrates the difficulties clinicians have in negotiating these risky decisions with athletes. For this doctor, debating with an athlete about whether to compete while injured is futile as it is the Olympics rather than longer-term health that will be at the forefront of an athlete's mind.

> It's fairly difficult basically because if you try to rush a decision with someone about whether they should take part in an Olympic final where they have qualified and they have trained for sixteen years or something to get there and you are saying, "Well, I don't think you should run because you have got arthritis in your knee." They are going to say, "That's fine; I don't care. I want to get a medal." You could debate further whether that is a rational decision or not. But if you said to them, "Would you have given up an Olympic final?" they would say, "Absolutely not."

Pressures associated with the timing of Olympic competition and the significance of Olympic competition for athletes are vital to explaining the way a performance rationale influences sports medicine practice. Sports clinicians need to be aware of time-related constraints in order to meet the demands of athletes who are training and competing at this level.

Alongside pressures associated with the timing of Olympic competition, a number of interviewees also described how the ages and career stage of athletes constrained them to take different risks with athletes' longer-term health. One respondent said that "you often take shortcuts depending on where people are and the stage of career they are at." Another made explicit reference to how the age of the athlete was an important consideration in his decision to allow an athlete to compete while injured:

> If someone had a stress fracture and they were thirty-five and coming up to the Olympic final and it was their last event and then they were going to retire, you would probably say, "Get on with it." But if it's a seventeen-year-old who has got twenty years [of competing] and they are going to go to lots of different Olympics then you might say they are better off not taking a risk. So you have to tailor your treatment to what is going on for the athlete.

Thus, like the clinicians in Safai's research, interviewees balanced cultures of risk and precaution. Moreover, conceptions of time centrally underpin the way sports clinicians tailor their treatment to athletes' performance-dominated interests. As a consequence of their social situations, sports clinicians are conscious that athletes participating at the Olympic level are constrained by time in numerous ways. In the interviews, this was emphasized in two ways. First, clinicians recognized the needs of athletes to be fit for major competitions (particularly Olympic competition) and how this constrained them to provide "quick-fix" treatments during these major events because of the significance of the Olympics for athletes. Second, interviewees discussed how the four-yearly cycle of Olympic competition impacted upon the "shelf lives" of athletes' careers. Clinicians were aware that athletes were under increasing pressure to be fit for the Olympics because they may only have "one shot" at being successful.

SUPPLY AND DEMAND: THE CONSUMERIST
MODEL OF SPORTS MEDICINE

Over the course of the interviews it became clear that sports medicine practice at the Olympic level was premised on a consumer-focused model of medical care and that sports clinicians regarded athletes as their customers. A succinct description of this customer focus was provided by a doctor who had extensive experience of practicing in sports medicine in a number of different Olympic sports. This doctor compared his role as a sports medicine physician to a project manager and indicated that the treatment approach was always concerned with the customer's wants and needs. He stated, "You have to advise the customer on what are the available products, how do they administer the product and so forth. At the end of the day the customer is still first and they are ultimately the end game." Another way that clinicians highlighted the client-centered approach was in the ways they expressed how their competence was assessed. Doctors and physiotherapists were acutely aware that their "success" as sports medicine practitioners relied upon the evaluation of athletes and other members of their working context (for example, performance directors and coaches). Such evaluations were not based on the athlete's long-term health, but on the competitive success of athletes. This was particularly important during an Olympics. One doctor acknowledged:

> Your success or failure in the management of a condition in the Olympics is basically measured in the performance of that athlete. So it's measured in medals or it's measured in finalists or semifinalists or through to the next round or measured in whatever the relative level of success is expected of that athlete.

Likewise, when discussing the negotiated balance between health and performance, one physiotherapist explained how success in the market for sports medicine was dependent upon the clinician's acceptance of the client's performance-motivated demands:

> It doesn't matter how good you are as a clinician, if you haven't got the ability to do all of that and understand all of that, you won't make it as a sports physiotherapist or physician because that's what you will build or lose your reputation on.

In this excerpt, the physiotherapist also highlights the relative marginalization of the clinician's knowledge as a medical "expert" ("It doesn't matter how good you are as a clinician"). Instead, this physiotherapist emphasizes how expertise is concerned with and judged on clinicians' collusions to the performance goals of sport. The complicity of clinicians to the performance motivations of athletes was reinforced by a doctor who explained the constraints on him to say "what the athlete wanted to hear." In this example, the doctor described a situation where he felt compelled to provide what he saw as a "quick-fix" injection treatment to an athlete.

> In the end I am helping them as much as possible and I will rationalize it to myself like I did [on a particular occasion] and I did give the injection . . . So I said to him, "Well, if we fix this then the deal is you need to get the rest sorted out." So we gave him the quick fix and then there is no excuse as he has got to do the rest. I know it is slightly the wrong way around but it *keeps them happy* and if you turn around and say no, you know the traditional consultant attitude of no, no, no, then *they will just bounce off to someone else* and get someone else to get their injection. (Emphasis added)

Johnson's concept of patronage is useful in this regard as this respondent clearly demonstrates the power of the athlete-consumer in the negotiation between him/herself and the clinician. For Johnson, systems of patronage arise when consumers have the ability to define their own needs and how those needs might be catered for. This doctor recognized that the athlete-consumer had the right to define the best service for his/her needs and was aware that if these needs are not met, the consumer would simply go elsewhere. For Johnson, this form of consumer power is a "systematic source of pressure upon practitioners,"[10] and this is demonstrated in the doctor's decision to provide the athlete with a "quick-fix" treatment with which the doctor was not completely comfortable. The negotiation of conditions ("the deal is") also illustrates clinician–athlete interdependency whereby the doctor needs the continuation of consultations with the athlete to retain career status and the athlete needs the doctor to enable participation.

Also typified in this quote ("the traditional consultant attitude") is the enduring assumption in medicine that the "doctor knows best" by virtue of his professional status. In recognition of this, Freidson examined how doctors seek to control their clients by attempting to persuade them that their advice is correct and that it should be followed.[11] The previous extract demonstrates how this assumption may not be wholly applicable in the context of sports medicine. Here, not only are athletes able to "bargain" their treatment with clinicians, they are also able to choose whether or not to follow the advice provided and are able to seek the help they wish elsewhere. In this way, the legitimacy of the doctor's position as medical "expert" is undermined. Following Johnson, those with esoteric knowledge (such as doctors) become "clients" themselves because of their limited responsibility for the information or medical services that they provide. The current data reveal that clinicians were often relatively subservient to their athlete-consumers.

SECOND OPINIONS

Another indication of the consumer-driven focus of sports medicine was reflected in clinicians' acceptance that athletes consulted multiple practitioners for second opinions and/or alternative treatments for their injuries. Unlike in professional football where footballers would usually seek second opinions without informing their club or the medical staff at the club for fear of undermining their authority or being regarded as "bad-patients,"[12] British Olympic clinicians described how this was a normal aspect of athletes' behavior and was openly discussed between them and the athletes who were under their care. Doctors and physiotherapists described how they normalized this behavior and discussed how this was not to be seen as an attack on their clinical competence. When asked how he felt when athletes wanted second opinions, one doctor explained:

> Oh, they can do for sure, absolutely, and at the end of the day you are there to only advise and if they don't like the advice they are perfectly entitled to go elsewhere . . . At the end of the day if a doctor tells you that you have done something wrong and you can't go to the games because of it you know there is a very bright light burning in that brain that's going to not accept that. And why shouldn't they? I think that doctors shouldn't get upset about people going to see other people.

Not only did the majority of interviewees reflect on athletes' use of second opinions in a largely positive light; they further stressed how they could utilize second opinions to facilitate their own practice. For instance, when asked if second opinions were encouraged, one physiotherapist clearly stated, "Yeah, at times absolutely, if we are really not sure of the diagnosis." Similarly, one doctor considered how receiving second opinions from other sports medicine doctors where he worked was beneficial:

Everyone is a bit precious naturally about their athletes and they don't want to be looking after someone and think what if I sent them off to see [clinician's name] next door then am I admitting failure and defeat and all the rest of it because you are not. And actually, since I started doing it more and more you actually realize how much it strengthens [your practice]. The coaches and athletes then trust you even more, and it is really good with your relationships with other doctors as well so it is very good.

Discussions of athletes' use of second opinions and clinicians' perspectives on the consumer-focused nature of medical practice reveal the ways in which athletes' demands are central to decisions about treatment. Moreover, these data shed further light on clinicians' performance-driven treatment rationales. Athletes are relatively autonomous in their negotiations with clinicians and, in particular, are able to define their own needs and define the best ways for those needs to be met.

EXTERNAL PRESSURES: COACHES

Alongside the documented constraints from athletes, a number of clinicians indicated that pressures to conform to performance goals can also arise from the motivations of the coaching staff. This is perhaps surprising because, in comparison to team sports such as professional football, where managers and coaches are relatively dominant and the employment of doctors and physiotherapists may be under the jurisdiction of these staff,[13] sports medicine clinicians in Olympic sports are less likely to be solely employed by one sport and coaches are less likely to be directly involved in the appointment of these clinicians.[14] Nevertheless, clinicians described how their relationships with coaches are central to their sports medicine practice. This was reinforced by one physiotherapist who said "coaches are always in the equation" when clinicians discussed the medical management of athletes. In addition, a doctor acknowledged the coach's influence over medical decisions during medical consultations with injured athletes. He said, "I think if you said on medical grounds that this person shouldn't train and the coach said that they had to train then, you would just have to say 'fine.'"

Clinicians also described how, in some situations, coaches "sided" with the athletes, making it even more difficult for the clinician to gain compliance. One of the doctors noted:

They [the coach] desperately want someone . . . and then you just have to [put them in the team]. And often the other thing is the athlete is often desperate to get in [the team], too, so you get it from both ends.

To this end, clinicians explained how they were always likely to involve the coach after the initial consultation had taken place with an athlete. Clinicians also encouraged athletes to discuss their injuries with their coach (even if the athlete was reluctant to do so) as clinicians felt that this was better for the athlete in the longer term. One physiotherapist said:

> We have had situations where athletes want situations to be confidential but normally, if it is going to affect the performance, you normally say to the athlete, "Look, this is affecting the performance of the team; you have to discuss this with the coach." And they do. We have never had a situation where they have refused to do that.

This was echoed by another physiotherapist:

> We will always discuss with athletes what they want to share. We have had some instances when we have been away where we have had confidential information about an athlete's health but if it became detrimental to that athlete's situation in that environment then we would have to consider discussing but not divulging all of the information, but discussing the situation.

These two quotes demonstrate physiotherapists' prioritization of performance and how, here, it takes precedence over client confidentiality. The examples indicate that clinicians do not actually break confidentiality, but persuade athletes not to put them in a position where they feel compromised. These excerpts also reveal how physiotherapists see the coach as a central figure who should be informed about the athlete's health. Clinicians' rationales for involving coaches in medical decisions are a consequence of clinicians' needs to be seen as effective in the context of Olympic sport. The current data reveal that clinicians were under pressure to be seen by coaches as "good" clinicians. Being regarded as a good clinician was usually assessed on whether or not the coaches felt they had made the "right" decisions about an athlete's injury. If their advice was not regarded as effective, this had implications for how they were judged and respected.

> Some of them [coaches], because you are never going to be right all of the time, but if you make a wrong call they will never forgive you for that. So that puts you under a lot of strain.

The power of coaches and the influence they have over clinicians' status in the sports context was also demonstrated in a discussion with a doctor who described his experiences of starting out in sports medicine and the importance of gaining the respect of the coach:

> One of the things that you need is to treat one of the good players early on. If they get better then it's like, ooooh, this guy knows what he is

talking about. And you need that. You need to be able to, when you first start, to gain their respect and it's as simple as that. If you can do that then you have less problems. If you do have some difficult cases early on then you're flummoxed and you really have a great difficulty in gaining their respect.

The position of doctors and physiotherapists is dependent, to a greater or lesser extent, on the satisfaction of the client as athlete as well as the client as coach. In order to establish themselves in their workplace, clinicians demonstrated a commitment to the needs and demands of coaches even if this meant compromising their professional medical opinions and/or ethical conventions.

DECISION MAKING, INFORMED CHOICE AND THE IMPACT ON CLINICIAN AUTONOMY

In contrast to professional football, where information about athletes' injuries was occasionally withheld from players and the implications of certain procedures not fully discussed,[15] clinicians in Olympic sports took satisfaction from their belief that they had provided athletes with all of the relevant information about particular treatments so that athletes could make informed choices about competing while injured. The evidence from interviews confirmed clinicians' recognition of athletes' centrality in decision making about their bodies, and that clinicians avoided taking complete responsibility for athletes' longer-term health and allowed athletes to make final decisions about training and/or competing while injured and in pain. For these clinicians, their only viable role in the treatment of pain and injury was as "wielders of advice" rather than as wielders of authority. This is not to suggest that the clinician left the decision solely with the athlete. Rather, many argued that once they had provided all of the appropriate information to the patient, in effect, their job was complete.

It was very rare for a clinician to prevent an athlete from competing when injured, and this most often occurred when an injury was "clear-cut," such as a broken leg. Clinicians stated that their justifications for allowing athletes to make the final decisions about their medical treatment, and whether or not they competed while injured, was because they felt athletes should have ownership of their bodies. When discussing the ways in which this was managed, one physiotherapist described how making a decision for an athlete would be akin to robbing the athlete of their freedom:

> If the player really wanted to play and the coach really wants them to play and I have said if he plays this [a more serious injury] might happen, he is playing a game with some responsibility and I don't see or think anyone should rob themselves of the responsibility for their own

body. I think we are all responsible for ourselves and I think it's really important for them to take control.

The belief that athletes should have ultimate responsibility over "risky" decisions was also evident in interviews with doctors:

> These guys have trained since kids and this is the biggest moment in their life and to say they can't perform . . . I think it's very important as much as you can to get the athlete to make that decision. They will always want to [compete] but I think you have to put to them what the dangers are.

The preceding examples demonstrate how clinicians recognize their limited scope of influence in the context of Olympic sport. Rather than understanding clinicians as part of "conspiratorial" networks designed to cajole athletes into accepting the culture of risk and playing/competing with injury,[16] the evidence demonstrates clinicians' personal need to remain useful and valid in their workplace, which may best be achieved by allowing athletes to define and demand their own needs. In Freidson's words, the clinician "is chosen on the basis of lay conception of what is needed, not by professional criteria"[17] The fact that doctors and physiotherapists do not see themselves as autonomous in their workplace is demonstrated in their belief that the subjective desires of others are more significant, and thus they argue that any final decision concerning an athlete's health is not within their jurisdiction. One way in which clinicians emphasized this belief was in their communications with other health care providers for support about particular decisions and in the documentation of their consultations with athletes. These methods were most often used when clinicians encountered difficult situations that compromised their professional medical opinion and were used to protect their credibility as clinicians. One doctor stated:

> If they insisted they were [competing] then I would write that advice down, and I always do write proper notes and I would tell them [the athlete] that I had advised them not to continue and that they were going to continue nevertheless and just document it.

Similarly, a physiotherapist explained:

> If I was really concerned I would probably get them to sign something to the effect that they fully understood the potential implications of doing something.

Alongside the documentation of consultations with athletes, clinicians also described how they would discuss difficult situations with other doctors or physiotherapists for backup and approval. One of the clearest examples of this was in a discussion with a doctor who was recounting his (and his colleagues') fear of being sued for some of the "strange" things that had to be done while practicing in sports medicine. He explained:

> We worry about being sued and all the rest of it but if you think, "Can I stand up and justify this in court and would a reasonable number of my peers support me?" and if they would then that's fine.

These examples illustrate that clinicians recognize their medical practice within Olympic sports is not straightforward and/or "normal," but structured by the specific context in which they practice. Clinicians also recognize that their working practices and, in particular, decisions about athletes' injuries are constrained by the social relationships (e.g., with athletes, coaches, governing bodies) in which they are enmeshed. These data demonstrate that, in Olympic sports, clinicians are relatively weak compared to athletes and coaches. Given their lack of autonomy relative to athletes and coaches, clinicians need to assert themselves in other ways so as to maintain their professional status and remain respected by their clients. Thus, doctors and physiotherapists choose to conform to the desires of more powerful agents in the Olympic sport figuration over their need to be seen as medically "correct" so as to gain social validation and security, uphold their identity as medical "experts" and ensure that their interdependent relationships with athletes and coaches continue. In contrast to Nixon, who portrays clinicians as standing alongside coaches, team owners, etc., and in opposition to athletes, it is more accurate to depict these relations as multipolar and fluid, with clinicians aligning themselves with various actors at various times. The illustration in these data that clinicians may sometimes prioritize self-esteem within their workplace over more orthodox medical concerns highlights the importance of interdependence to the understanding of human relations.

DOCTORS' AND PHYSIOTHERAPISTS' VIEWS ON PERFORMANCE VERSUS HEALTH

The contextual constraints of working within Olympic sport, coupled with the pressures from coaches and athletes on practitioners to adopt the performance orientation of their clients, lead physicians to recognize that the kind of treatment they provide for patients in the sports context is, in some ways, different from the treatment they provide as GPs or hospital practitioners. While recognizing that their primary role in the treatment of athletes is to ensure the continuation of performance, a number of doctors also made reference to the importance of viewing the athlete's longer-term health above such performance motivations. One doctor stated:

As the doctor for an athlete you are the patient's doctor, you are their advocate for health. It is your duty to provide them with as much knowledge as you are able about their condition to allow them to make an informed choice as to what to do. I think it is very dangerous when, as a doctor, you end up working in effect for an organization, a team, and those clear boundaries of duties of care become in any way blurred. I think that is poor medicine and poor practice.

Understanding his medical position as compromised within the sports context, another doctor described the reservations he had for giving an athlete a local anesthetic injection before an important event and drew a distinction between his everyday practice as a GP and his role in sports medicine. He explained: "I had grave reservations about doing it but [the athlete] came through it. There have been instances where you do things where you feel you probably wouldn't otherwise." The justification for this doctor's decision to inject was associated with the importance of the event and the desires of the athlete. This was echoed by another experienced sports medicine doctor who described the actions of one of his colleagues:

One colleague injected on three occasions for a [serious injury] and it ended up that the athlete won a [medal] but couldn't train for eleven months. Although the athlete would have thought the doctor had done the right thing because it is once every four years, undoubtedly, he would have normally rested that. And he probably had a stress fracture but they didn't want to scan it because *they didn't want to know.*

The doctor in this extract clearly demonstrates the tensions between doctors' commitment to the longer-term health of the patient-athlete and the constraints on them to allow the athlete to compete in a major event. Rather than being seen by the athlete (and possibly the coach) as responsible for denying the athlete his/her chance to be successful at the Olympics, the doctor chose not to find out the extent of the patient's injury. The importance of competition also featured in the following doctor's rationale for stitching an athlete's injury and allowing him/her to compete in an event without allowing the injury time to heal. Although he justifies his actions in this way, this doctor also expresses, on reflection, his discomfort with making this decision:

I patched someone up knowing that I had done it, knowing that I was going to be at their next event and I would perhaps say, "Right, that's an important event." And it was, it was an Olympic qualifier. So someone [competed] twenty-four hours after having [their injury] stitched up. *It should never have been allowed.*

Whereas these examples highlight doctors' *concerns* for athletes' longer-term health, in every case, the doctors made decisions that erred on the side of performance. Doctors are aware that the demands on their services are different and contradict some of the conventions of medical practice and thus parts of the ideology on which the professional status of medicine is based. However, all of these decisions were essentially driven if not by patient demand, then in collusion with the injured athlete.

The notion that doctors tend to err on the side of performance rather than being fully committed to athletes' longer-term health may therefore emerge from their ideological commitment to the pledges of the medical profession and not from their work within sport. Given their interdependence with the broader medical profession and the associated assumption that doctors are the primary advocates for the health and well-being of their patients, doctors perceive themselves as having a duty to talk about health issues. Moreover, the legitimacy of the medical profession is premised on ethical guidelines and a commitment to moral responsibility. To be seen to be part of that broader profession, and to enjoy the associated status, sports medicine doctors are constrained to demonstrate those ethics in their practice. However, doctors in the current study have demonstrated the difficulties in making the "right" moral and ethical choices given that what is "right" has a specific definition in the context of their work or, to use Freidson's terminology, their "everyday work settings."[18]

Doctors' claims to be cognizant of athletes' health concerns may be a reflection of their need to establish their legitimacy through abiding by the conventions and traditions of medicine. Whereas sport and exercise medicine has been successfully awarded specialty status, established medical bodies maintain some control over the role and format of this medical subdiscipline. Although sport and exercise medicine physicians recognize their role in Olympic sport as different from "orthodox medicine," there is an implicit acknowledgment that their work is only going to be seen as legitimate if what they do is seen to abide by the broader conventions of the medical profession.

Interviews with physiotherapists, on the other hand, reveal that they were less constrained by health concerns and more centrally motivated by performance orientations. In the interviews, physiotherapists were more likely to discuss their involvement in the performance outcomes of athletes than were their doctor counterparts. For example, one physiotherapist described how he felt he had a vital role in the performance success of the British Olympic team. He described his work thus: "Our mission is mission 2012. Gold medals. And we want to be fourth on the medal table." Indeed, the majority of physiotherapists described how their motivations for being involved in sports physiotherapy revolved around being part of an elite sporting network. The emphasis on being part of the team was also expressed by one respondent when describing his motivations for being a sports physiotherapist:

> To be involved at that sort of level is something that you think, yeah, I would really like to be involved in that. I love the competition element;

> I love the whole team aspect, the team approach, team bonding, if you like. You're part of the team when they win medals . . . and just to be part of that, that is the reward.

The perception of physiotherapists that they were working alongside Britain's Olympic sporting elite also had implications for the way in which they identified with their profession. The physiotherapists in this study, like those in elite rugby,[19] believed that their work within Olympic sports places them at the "cutting edge" of the physiotherapy profession. Sports physiotherapists in the current study believed that their job required practitioners with particular personality characteristics. In the following example, one physiotherapist distinguished between successful and unsuccessful sports physiotherapists in terms of the personality traits he considered to be central to this area of practice:

> We have cases of people who are very good technically, very good clinically but don't fit into an elite sporting environment because they simply don't have the competencies in terms of the communication skills, the ability to take the right information at the right time and make the right decisions.

However, the belief that they are at the cutting edge of their profession was most clearly expressed by physiotherapists when they compared their work in Olympic sport to their previous positions within the UK's National Health Service (NHS) or when they compared themselves to others who worked outside of Olympic sport. The majority of physiotherapists interviewed believed that one of the main distinctions between themselves and physiotherapists working within the NHS was in terms of the quality of care that they provided to their athlete-patients and, in particular, the time they spent with them during treatment. This contrasts to Waddington's research in professional football, where he argued that the quality of treatment provided by football club doctors and physiotherapists was compromised because they were primarily employed in a sports, and not a health care, context.[20] Discussing the NHS, one physiotherapist made the following comment:

> The main focus is on their waiting lists. It's all about getting their waiting lists down. So, it's the amount of people through the door and the amount of people through the door at the other end. They are not concerned about getting people better generally, they are concerned about getting people through the door and off the waiting list whereas here, what we are concerned about more so is actually, no matter what is happening, we want to get people better. I think, to a large extent, sometimes that approach within the NHS is damaging to physiotherapy because there are plenty of people that can give out exercises and

say [to a patient] you will get better, go away. Whereas here, we are very hands-on, and we will have people back as many times as needed to get them better.

Not only was sports physiotherapy seen as providing a better level of care, it was also seen as more advanced in terms of its techniques and aims. For example, when reviewing the selection processes and criteria for a physiotherapy post at the Olympic games, one physiotherapist stated:

> They are looking for people who are looking to develop themselves all of the time so if someone has literally just turned up for work at an NHS clinic every day and have [*sic*] not really done anything to extend themselves, they probably wouldn't be the sort of people they were looking for in sport.

Similarly, another respondent explicitly refers to sports physiotherapy as being more involved and more advanced than in the NHS:

> We are very much part of a big team here rather than in the NHS where *physiotherapy is just physiotherapy.* Within the NHS you get them [the patient] so far whereas here we will continue until they are back to 110 percent training again and competing. (Emphasis added)

These excerpts highlight physiotherapists' beliefs that their work within Olympic sport is at the peak of their profession. Data also suggest that this belief is matched by greater autonomy over their practice and, also, a relatively equal status with medical practitioners. This arguably greater freedom over their clinical practice is expressed in the following quote when the interviewee explains the characteristics of her practice as a sports physiotherapist and the practices of physiotherapists who may have an interest in sport but have limited experience and expertise:

> I think a sports physiotherapist has an appreciation of the big picture. They understand the nature of what it is to be an athlete. They understand the concepts of time constraints and they understand that [they] need to push the boundaries because [they] need to get them better in the shortest possible time. A physiotherapist who is interested in sport will follow slightly more traditional, probably slightly more conservative routes where you *do things according to the book.* You know, you're not allowed to stretch until it is pain-free for ten days post muscle tear. Well, if you had said that to an athlete you *would be out on your ear* and you would just not survive as a sports physiotherapist.

From these data, it could be argued that sports physiotherapy has a less clear code of practice regarding helping patients to be "healthy," but that this allows them greater freedom and autonomy over their practice and the capacity to more fully embrace the performance motivations and demands of their "customers" than their doctor counterparts. For example, the missions and aims of the Association of Chartered Physiotherapists in Sports Medicine (ACPSM) do not make any reference to the longer-term health of athletes but are primarily concerned with providing "a specialist service to meet the needs of athletes, coaches, officials and parents."[21] Doctors who, by way of contrast, are in part enabled by the legitimacy and status from their association with the "traits" the medical profession claims for itself, are also constrained by their need to conform to a more explicit code of practice. As a result of their relatively lower occupational status, sports physiotherapists may be able to be more flexible in their practice and thus more able to directly serve the needs of their sporting clients.

The working practices of doctors and physiotherapists may also explain the clearer association of physiotherapists with performance goals. For instance, physiotherapists were more likely to be employed full-time in sports medicine, were more likely to work a greater number of hours than doctors and were more likely to regard their work within Olympic sport (or sports physiotherapy more generally) as their primary source of employment. None of the physiotherapists interviewed were currently employed within the NHS. This has obvious implications for the relative integration of physiotherapists and doctors into Olympic sport and further contributes to the contention that physiotherapists are at the "front line" of athlete health care. The fact that physiotherapists provide the majority of health care to Olympic athletes allows them greater integration into the Olympic sports context and may also be a reason for them to more readily accept and internalize the role of the performance culture of Olympic sport.

CONCLUSION

This chapter has examined the tensions that doctors and physiotherapists working in British Olympic sport experience in relation to health and performance and has outlined the justifications for their practice priorities. The medical decisions clinicians make about athletes' injuries as well as their decision to focus by and large on short-term performance goals are framed by the demands and needs of their athlete and coach clients. As a consequence of their work in high-performance sport, clinicians are constrained to modify their practices in order to uphold their professional integrity and remain useful and valid in their work setting. As a result of a consumer-led focus, athletes and coaches are able to bargain the treatment process more readily, and clinicians' autonomy over medical decisions is compromised. This case study also sheds further light on how structural issues, such as clinicians' membership of their broader professions, has enabled and constrained their position within the health–performance nexus. The practices of sports medicine clinicians cannot be morally judged by the criteria outlined in the conventional medical model, its Hippocratic Oath and its standard ethical procedures. Rather, sports medicine clinicians' work needs to be understood as a shifting balance between their need to adopt a position more closely associated with sports performance in their everyday work at the same time as adhering to the conventions of their broader professional bodies for status and validation.

NOTES

1. Hoberman, *Testosterone Dreams*, 190.
2. Waddington, "Development of Sports Medicine"; *Sport, Health and Drugs*.
3. Theberge, "It's Not about Health."
4. Johnson, *Professions and Power*, 65.
5. Theberge, "It's Not About Health', 177.
6. Safai, "Healing the Body."
7. McNamee and Edwards, "Why Sports Medicine Isn't Medicine," 104.
8. Although there are grounds for believing that there is a considerable convergence in views on such matters. See, e.g., Malcolm, "Medical Uncertainty."
9. Nixon, "Social Network Analysis"; Safai, "Healing the Body."
10. Johnson, *Professions and Power*, 65.
11. Freidson, *Profession of Medicine*.
12. Roderick, *Work of Professional Football*, 63.
13. Waddington, Roderick and Parker, "Playing Hurt"; Malcolm and Sheard, "Pain in the Assets."
14. Scott, "More Professional?"
15. Waddington, Roderick and Parker, "Playing Hurt."
16. Nixon, "Social Network Analysis."
17. Freidson, *Profession of Medicine,* 107.
18. Ibid., 87.
19. Malcolm and Sheard, "Pain in the Assets."
20. Waddington, "Jobs for the Boys."
21. The ACPSM lists a further four missions:
    1. To improve the techniques and facilities available for the prevention and treatment of sports injuries.
    2. To inform all interested individuals and bodies of the existence, skills and availability of chartered and HPC registered physiotherapists.
    3. To encourage the development and publication of research in the field of sports physiotherapy in the UK and abroad.
    4. To encourage continuing specialist education of the membership.
    See www.associationsdirectory.org/Directory/Sports_&_Fitness/Sport_Physiotherapy/2983/ACPSM/. Accessed 25th October 2008.

BIBLIOGRAPHY

Association of Chartered Physiotherapists in Sports Medicine. "Continuing Professional Development." Association of Chartered Physiotherapists in Sports Medicine, 2008. http://www.acpsm.org/cpd.asp (accessed 7 September 2010).

Freidson, Eliot. *Profession of Medicine: A Study of the Sociology of Applied Knowledge.* New York: Dodd, Mead and Co., 1970.

Hoberman, John. *Mortal Engines: The Science of Performance and the Dehumanization of Sport.* New Jersey: Blackburn Press, 1992.

———. *Testosterone Dreams.* Berkeley: University of California Press, 2005.

Johnson, Terry. *Professions and Power.* London: Macmillan, 1972.

Malcolm, D.E., and K. Sheard. "Pain in the Assets: The Effects of Commercialisation and Professionalisation on the Management of Injury in English Rugby Union." *Sociology of Sport Journal* 19 (2002): 149–169.

Malcolm, Dominic. "Medical Uncertainty and Clinician-Athlete Relations: The Management of Concussion Injuries in Rugby Union." *Sociology of Sport Journal* 26 (2009): 191–210.

McNamee, M., and S. Edwards. "Why Sports Medicine Isn't Medicine." *Health Care Analysis. Journal of Health Philosophy and Policy* 14, no. 2 (2006): 103–109.

Nixon, Howard. "A Social Network Analysis of Influences on Athletes to Play with Pain and Injury." *Journal of Sport & Social Issues* 16 (1992): 127–135.

Roderick, Martin. *The Work of Professional Football. A Labour of Love?* London: Routledge, 2006.

Safai, Parissa. "Healing the Body in the 'Culture of Risk': Examining the Negotiation of Treatment between Sports Medicine Clinicians and Injured Athletes in Canadian Intercollegiate Sport." *Sociology of Sport Journal* 20, no. 2 (2003): 127–146.

Scott, Andrea. "'More Professional?' The Occupational Practices of Sports Medicine Clinicians Working with British Olympic Athletes." Unpublished PhD thesis, Loughborough University, 2010.

Theberge, Nancy. "It's Not about Health, It's about Performance." In *Physical Culture, Power and the Body,* edited by J. Hargreaves and P. Vertinsky, 176–194. London: Routledge, 2007.

Waddington, Ivan. "The Development of Sports Medicine." *Sociology of Sport Journal* 13, no. 2 (1996): 176–196.

———. "Jobs for the Boys. A Study of the Employment of Club Doctors and Physiotherapists in English Professional Football." *Soccer & Society* 3, no. 3 (2002): 51–64.

———. *Sport, Health and Drugs: A Critical Sociological Perspective.* London: E & F Spon, 2000.

Waddington, I., M. Roderick and R. Naik. "Methods of Appointment and Qualifications of Club Doctors and Physiotherapists in English Professional Football: Some Problems and Issues." *British Journal of Sports Medicine* 35, no. 1 (2001): 48–53.

Waddington, I., M. Roderick and G. Parker. "Playing Hurt. Managing Injuries in Professional Football." *International Review for the Sociology of Sport* 35, no. 2 (2000): 165–180.

12 Sports Physicians and Doping
Medical Ethics and Elite Performance

John Hoberman

Relationships between sports physicians and elite athletes have been ethically troubling for most of the century that has elapsed since high-performance sport emerged toward the end of the nineteenth century. The extreme demands that are imposed on elite athletes have created two kinds of ethical problem. The first is the implicit mandate to handle injuries in such as way as to keep the athlete functioning; this can mean suppressing pain and thereby running the risk of doing further damage. The second, and more publicized, ethical problem is the focus of this chapter: the participation of doctors in the doping of athletes by means of illicit performance-enhancing drugs. Over the past half century medical officials have consistently opposed doctors' collaborations with athletes who dope. But official disapproval has coexisted with many doping collaborations between physicians and elite athletes. This chapter examines how doctors have rationalized their participation in such arrangements and either addressed or evaded the demands of medical ethics as they are understood by the medical establishment. We will see how the most aggressively nonconformist sports physicians exempt their relationships with athletes from the normal rules of medical practice. Finally, we will briefly examine the careers of five doping doctors from four countries whose declarations of independence from traditional medicine ended in criminal charges and/or disgrace.

It is important to recognize that doctors' roles within elite sport have evolved over this long period of time. As early as the 1890s, the French physician Philippe Tissié was testing a variety of liquids (including rum and champagne) on a long-distance cyclist for the purpose of testing the physiological effects of these "stimulants." As counterintuitive as it may seem to the modern observer, the primary purpose of these experiments was to observe the effects of these substances on the health of his human subject. Neither this pioneering sports physician nor his European contemporaries demonstrated a concern about the enhancement of performance or the ethics of performance enhancement. Prior to his emergence as a celebrity in the not-so-distant era of mass communications, the high-performance athlete of the fin de siècle period offered scientists an opportunity to study the effects of athletic stress on the human organism. Cyclists' use of powerful drugs such as strychnine and cocaine was seen as an acceptable strategy to reduce pain and fatigue. The idea that pharmacological performance enhancement constituted a dishonorable breach of sporting ethics still lay several decades in the future.

The condemnation of "doping" on ethical grounds was publicly discussed in sporting circles during the 1920s and 1930s.[1] Modern readers may be surprised to read the following commentary from a prominent German pharmacologist that appeared as early as 1933:

> The use of artificial means [to improve performance] has long been considered wholly incompatible with the spirit of sport and has therefore been condemned. Nevertheless, we all know that this rule is continually being broken, and that sportive competitions are often more a matter of doping than of training. It is highly regrettable that those who are in charge of supervising sport seem to lack the energy for the campaign against this evil, and that a lax, and fateful, attitude is spreading. Nor are the physicians without blame for this state of affairs, in part on account of their ignorance, and in part because they are prescribing strong drugs for the purpose of doping which are not available to athletes without prescriptions.[2]

This editorial against "doping" leaves unclear whether Dr. Otto Riesser believed these unspecified substances actually worked. Three years earlier, he had cautioned credulous athletes that the pharmacological manipulation of human athletic performance was far more complicated than they believed it to be, and that they should not rely on drugs to improve their performances.[3] The larger point beyond the question of efficacy was whether attempts to dope constituted violations of "the spirit of sport"—a phrase that recurs in the *World Anti-Doping Code* published in 2009. "Doping," the World Anti-Doping Agency (WADA) proclaims, "is fundamentally contrary to the spirit of sport."[4] It is important to recognize that this condemnation of "doping" applies regardless of whether or not the drugs actually work because, from this perspective, what really matter are the intentions of the athletes. After all, Otto Riesser's disapproval of doping on ethical grounds coexisted with his own doubts about the effectiveness of the substances athletes were using. It is significant that the Danish physiologist Ove Bøje, who carefully observed the doping scene of the 1930s, took an opposing position on the ethics of the "doping" issue. The use of ultraviolet rays, he reported in 1939, had been criticized as "unsportsmanlike in spirit . . . although no general agreement has been reached." His own position on such practices was nonjudgmental, because what really mattered was the health of the athlete.[5] Decades would pass before the spread of effective doping drugs, such as amphetamines and anabolic steroids during the 1950s and 1960s, respectively, demonstrated to many athletes (although this was not clear to all doctors) that pharmacological performance enhancement was real.[6] Confirmation of the efficacy of these drugs strengthened the "spirit of sport" argument by confirming what some regarded as the "unfair" advantages created by effective doping drugs. To others, including some sports physicians, the effectiveness of anabolic steroids, in particular, was a compelling rationale for their use by elite athletes; for this reason, the pro-steroid lobby among sports physicians has been evident, although certainly not predominant, since the late 1960s and 1970s.[7] Uncertainties about the ethical status and medical consequences of doping practices have thus survived intact among sports physicians since the interwar period during which Riesser and Bøje published their commentaries.

Medical publications and official medical bodies, on the other hand, have been unanimous in condemning doping and those physicians who expedite the doping practices of athletes. Even before the 1988 Ben Johnson scandal at the Seoul Olympic Games brought athletic doping to the attention of the entire world, some medical groups had already addressed the issue of doping and medical ethics. As early as 1957, at a time when the existence of anabolic steroids was virtually unknown to the general public, the American Medical Association (AMA) passed a resolution in response to "testimony painting a shocking picture of widespread and indiscriminate use of stimulants, such as amphetamine, to improve the performances of athletes in competition. It [is] said that this vicious practice extends to children in our schools."[8] A generation later, the World Medical Association issued the following declaration: "The physician must oppose all methods which are not in accord with medical ethics or which have injurious consequences for the athlete who uses them; this applies, in particular, to procedures which alter the composition of the blood or biochemical processes." More specifically, the declaration prohibits "the use of medications or other substances, irrespective of their type or the manner in which they are introduced into the body, including stimulants or sedatives that affect the central nervous system, or procedures that alter the reflexes in an artificial manner."[9] In a similar vein, the German Sports Physicians Association declared in 1984: "Every type of prohibited performance enhancement in sport" was to be regarded as forbidden, and that any "crossing of the boundary" that separates therapy from performance enhancement was to be condemned.[10] In 2005, the Committee on Sports Medicine and Fitness of the American Academy of Pediatrics issued a policy statement that begins as follows: "Performance-enhancing substance use in young people is a concern to pediatricians and society because of potential adverse health consequences and the effects that such practices have on moral development of the individual and on fair athletic competition for all."[11] Half a century after the 1957 AMA statement on doping, medical officials continued to condemn doping on both medical and moral grounds.

This official disapproval notwithstanding, the fact remains that many doctors have participated in the doping milieu within elite sport. The prominent British medical journal the *Lancet* commented in 1988: "Although evidence of direct involvement of medical practitioners in the procurement and administration of hormones is lacking, their connivance with those who do is obvious and their participation in blood doping is a matter of record."[12] It was not long before evidence of direct involvement of doctors in doping did become a matter of record. The Canadian Dubin Commission report that appeared in 1990 following the Ben Johnson scandal took a broad and detailed look at the doping culture of this era and reached the following conclusion: "Physicians have played an important role in supplying anabolic steroids and other banned drugs to athletes for performance enhancement. Many athletes who testified at this Inquiry received banned substances from physicians, in some cases together with medical supervision and in other cases without any medical care whatsoever."[13] This scenario has been confirmed over and over again in the course of the two decades that have elapsed since the Dubin Commission substituted documentation for speculation regarding doctors' direct involvement in the doping subculture.

Having looked carefully at how doctors function within the world of elite sport, and at the special pressures this subculture exerts on everyone involved, Ivan Waddington has analyzed what he calls the "doctors' dilemmas" that have become an inextricable aspect of this sports milieu. It is important to recognize that these dilemmas involve doctors' own values and individual choices and not merely the structural factors within sports medicine that can make the very term *sports physician* seem like a contradiction in terms. Conflicts of interest within the high-performance sports medicine that serves highly paid professional and Olympic-level athletes are by now widely acknowledged. In this domain, doctors are frequently tempted to de-emphasize the athlete's status as a patient in favor of treating him or her as a commercially valuable asset whose performances take precedence over genuine medical needs. The discounting or superficial treatment of athletes' injuries is the most common form of unprofessional sports-medical conduct. The medical misbehaviors that result from these conflicts of interest can also include physician-assisted doping. This is a more elective type of misconduct than the medically dishonest handling of injuries, because supervising an athlete's doping regimen requires long-term planning that responding to injuries usually does not. As a recent example, a prominent sports-medical official has acknowledged that the world's most popular sport is vulnerable to this sort of misconduct. Michel d'Hooghe, the Belgian doctor who is the head of the medical commission of the Fédération Internationale de Football Association (FIFA), asked the thirty-two national team senior doctors at the 2010 World Cup tournament in South Africa to reaffirm the medical oath they had once taken by signing a statement to that effect. "The doctors have all taken the Hippocratic Oath," he said, "but we must not be so naïve to presume that athletes obtain forbidden medications without assistance. Sometimes, the doctors are guilty."[14]

Many people will react to physician involvement in athletic doping with surprise. Because sport is traditionally associated with good health, those who are unfamiliar with the unique stresses endured by high-performance athletes may mistakenly assume that the medical needs of athletes and nonathletic people are essentially the same. Although this is true in some respects, the constant stress of training often creates special medical problems. As the controversial West German sports physician Heinz Liesen put it in 1988: "The body of a high-performance athlete is no longer comparable to the body of a normal person."[15] Some elite athletes today employ an entire medical support team, consisting of a doctor, a masseur, a nutritionist, a psychologist and other specialists. The mobilization of this kind of medical expertise is clearly aimed at producing athletic productivity rather than good health, and this ethos encourages additional medical support that can take the form of medically supervised doping. Consequently, as Waddington has pointed out, "while part of the ideology surrounding sports medicine suggests that sports physicians are in the front line of the fight against doping in sport, the reality, it is argued, is that sports medicine is actually one of the primary contexts within which performance-enhancing drugs have been developed and disseminated within the sporting community."[16]

The emergence of a steroid lobby among sports physicians was evident in West Germany during the 1980s, even as their public pronouncements were constrained by the international anti-doping norms that became increasingly influential during that decade. During the 1970s, such inhibitions had been largely absent. In the wake of the stunning successes of East German athletes at the 1976 Montreal Olympic Games, four prominent West German sports physicians—Armin Klümper, Herbert Reindell, Wildor Hollmann and Wilfried Kindermann—downplayed the medical risks associated with steroid use and recommended that they be used under medical supervision. "Until 1976 I regarded anabolic steroids as harmless," Hollmann said in 1989.[17] A year later, the conservative politician Wolfgang Schäuble endorsed this view: "We advocate only the most limited use of these drugs and only under the complete control of the sports physicians . . . because it is clear that there are [sports] disciplines in which the use of these drugs is necessary to remain competitive at the international level."[18] Many years later Schäuble would serve two terms as Germany's federal minister of the interior (1989–1991, 2005–2009), a position that includes responsibility for matters of sports policy, including doping. By the time of Schäuble's terms as minister of the interior, anti-doping policies had become mandatory for politicians and sports federations officials around the world. But prior to the emergence of this regime of pharmacological political correctness, conflicts between a small but high-profile cadre of West German sports physicians and their critics became a frequent topic of sports coverage in the serious German press.

During the 1980s, West Germany became the only modern society to produce a small but influential group of celebrity sports physicians. Their rise to prominence was made possible by the belief, shared by a substantial portion of the West German political establishment, that German success in international sports competitions contributed to maintaining national morale.[19] In a society where a member of Parliament (Bundestag) had publicly declared that anabolic steroid use was a requirement for preserving German competitiveness, the celebrity sports physician understood that pushing the envelope on behalf of boosting the performances of German athletes had the tacit support of powerful political actors who would not be inclined to take anti-doping rules too seriously. It is, therefore, not surprising that it took the Bundestag two decades to finally pass the "Law to Promote the Struggle against Doping in Sport" (*Gesetz zur Verbesserung der Bekämpfung des Dopings im Sport*). The law took effect on 1 November 2007 and does not criminalize athletes for their doping behaviors. Given this sort of license, the celebrity sports physicians saw themselves as autonomous and exceptional doctors who were not subject to the normal rules of medical practice.

In retrospect, it is clear that the West German celebrity sports physicians of the 1980s created a sports-medical style that has been inhibited, though not fully eradicated, by the stricter anti-doping regimens that came into effect after the Ben Johnson scandal and subsequent events. The arrival of WADA on 1 January 2000 established both norms and a bureaucracy promoting sanctions that could finally give the global anti-doping campaign a credibility the International Olympic Committee (IOC) and major international federations had failed to create over the previous several decades.[20] But before the creation of this global (and still inadequate) apparatus, the high-profile sports physicians in Germany had many opportunities to argue on behalf of a sports-medical model in which they played the starring role as fearless and determined advocates of their athletic clients.

One characteristic of this sports-medical style is an egocentricity that makes several claims. The charismatic sports physician possesses special powers that allow him to serve elite athletes in ways ordinary doctors cannot. Hans-Wilhelm Müller-Wohlfahrt "spoke of his empathy with his patients, his need to listen to their personal stories, the superiority of sensitive hands to technological diagnosis, and the 'courage' required of the doctor to 'really engage' with his patient." "We are both frontline people, Armin Klümper said of himself and his fellow sports physician Heinz Liesen, who really take care of athletes instead of sitting in the ivory tower of science."[21] One journalist described Liesen as "a man who exerts an inexplicable power of attraction over elite athletes, a psychosomatic magician."[22] The charismatic German sports physician can thus be understood as a modern version of the "magical healer" (*Wunderheiler*) of premodern German medicine. The modern *Wunderheiler* of the 1980s drew his authority from the sportive nationalism of the German people and some political leaders. One of these highly publicized sports physicians, Josef Keul, was hailed for years as "the Doyen of German Sports Medicine." This eventually doping-compromised sports physician was a member of the West German National Olympic Committee, where he served as its anti-doping delegate, and the German Sports Association; in 1990, he was awarded the Federal Order of Merit (First Class) by the German government for his presumed contributions to the campaign against doping in German sport.

The charismatic sports physician therefore regards himself as entitled to go where ordinary colleagues fear to tread on either ethical or medical grounds. "Everything that helps is permitted," Armin Klümper said in 1984. He clearly feels contempt for more cautious medical colleagues who take refuge in "in the ivory tower of science" rather than practicing sports medicine out on the "front lines." One justification for the more daring versions of elite sports medicine was the widely accepted idea that modern high-performance sport had driven the human body to its natural limits. "We have reached the maximum," Wildor Hollmann declared in 1984. "The athletes have entered the biological border zone."[23] "Elite sport has now reached the limits of human performance where extreme physiological events occur," Heinz Liesen said in 1988. "The body of the high-performance athlete is no longer comparable to the body of a normal person."[24] The rhetorical point of this observation was to justify unorthodox medical interventions that sometimes provoked objections from other sports physicians. In 1987, for example, the same Herbert Reindell who had endorsed medically supervised steroid doping in 1976 stated, "Anyone who, like Mr. Liesen, gives injections according to unproven hypotheses violates medical ethics."[25] Responding to what he described as the media spectacle of "Heinz Liesen rushing all over the place giving immunity-boosting injections," the internationally recognized anti-doping scientist Manfred Donike said, "the first word that occurs to me is 'charlatan.'"[26] This conflict between the "frontline people" and their disapproving colleagues, although involving only a small group of professionals, was widely broadcast to the West German public. That the most ambitious (and, perhaps, reckless) sports doctors were attracting the most attention and the most famous athlete-clients was evident to anyone who observed the West German elite sports scene at this time. As we will see, the success of the cutting-edge practitioners in the 1980s prefigured the emergence in the 1990s of a new affinity group of "antiaging" doctors whose numbers were increasing at this time and have been growing ever since. It is not surprising that some of these practitioners have aided and abetted the hormone doping of elite athletes.

The "frontline" German sports physicians of this era thus made a point of refusing to recognize ethical standards as a significant topic for high-performance sports medicine. A corollary of this attitude was their view that the anti-doping campaign was an unjustifiable nuisance or a fraud, or both. "I regard it as better to leave the dishonest doping discussion behind and worry instead about the health of the athlete," Heinz Liesen said in 1999. "There are many people who talk about doping and don't have a clue."[27] The public controversy about steroids, Liesen said in 1985:

> Is the fault of the press, and the sporting press in particular. They should worry about the bodybuilders, who are constantly abusing [these substances]. The world-famous hormone researcher Adlerkreutz from Finland says at every conference that giving testosterone to a man is much less dangerous than giving birth control pills to a woman. Why do we make such a drama out of this? If a body cannot regenerate itself by producing a sufficient amount of hormone, then it is certainly appropriate to help it out, just as one would give vitamin C, B-1 or B-2 or stimulate its immune system, so that it can recuperate rather than remain sick.[28]

Liesen's insistence that anabolic steroids were primarily therapeutic drugs contained an element of truth. Two of these androgenic drugs, testosterone propionate and methyltestosterone, had been introduced into clinical medicine in the US in the late 1930s, several years after the first laboratory synthesis of testosterone was achieved in Europe in 1935.[29] Prior to the gradual stigmatizing of anabolic steroids during the 1980s, the medical profession had for decades regarded these drugs as therapeutic agents with legitimate medical uses and as benign substances that were frequently reported to produce a sense of "well-being."[30] The doping scandals of the 1980s did more than any other factor, such as the unhealthy image of bodybuilding at that time, to drive the anabolic steroid into the domain of the "war on drugs" and the notoriety that entailed. It was the difficult task of the ambitious sports physicians to swim against this current by emphasizing the reparative role of the drug and how much this meant to the athlete-patient. "It is my duty to help athletes with long seasons and a short recovery period to achieve their best performances," Liesen said in 1986.[31] Even Wildor Hollmann, a prominent sports scientist and sports physician who served as the unofficial ethicist of sports doping in the German media at this time, argued that ethical objections to the use of steroids "do not change the fact that it is clearly possible to improve recovery in specific situations that occur only at the limit of human ability."[32] The fact that anabolic steroids can play both therapeutic and performance-enhancing roles for elite athletes has complicated their image, and thus their social and legal status, ever since it became widely known during the 1970s and 1980s that they were effective doping drugs. The ambiguity of their status in this respect opened the door to a legitimizing of their use on therapeutic grounds. From the perspective of some physicians, another way to rationalize the physician's supervision of steroid use was to point to the athletes' inability to supervise their own drug use. "If steroids were legalized," Wilfried Kindermann said in August 1988, "then at least we physicians would have an opportunity to talk with the athletes about responsible doses."[33] What we may call the "lesser harm" argument had been endorsed often by West German sports physicians during the 1970s, and it is conceivable that this sort of medical conduct will be regarded as an acceptable practice at some point in the future.[34] But the idea of adopting medically supervised doping as official policy in August 1988 was consigned to oblivion less than two months later when Ben Johnson tested positive for the anabolic steroid stanazolol at the Seoul Olympic Games.

One consequence of this scandal, as we have seen, was the Dubin Commission report that pointed to physicians in Canada as a major source of the doping drugs that were being used by elite Canadian athletes. Another consequence of the newly stigmatized status of doping drugs was that it became riskier to function as a "frontline" sports physician to the stars. To some extent this depended on the nationality of the ambitious sports physician. The early 1990s saw the release in the newly reunited Germany of a tidal wave of information about the illicit and sometimes criminal conduct of the former East German doping doctors. This exposé of unethical behavior by sports physicians went on for years and further intensified German awareness of doping among elite athletes. In Italy, long regarded as a doping paradise for professional cyclists and other elite athletes, the role of doping doctor has usually been easier to bear, due both to less judgmental attitudes toward doping and to an inefficient legal system that works to the advantage of many defendants, including notorious doping doctors such as Francesco Conconi and Michele Ferrari, whose clients have included professional cyclists, in particular. Interestingly, the notoriety of these doctors in anti-doping circles has not deterred many world-class athletes from seeking their expert counsel on how to achieve world-class performances.[35] We are reminded once again that expecting sports physicians to oppose the doping practices of elite athletes on medical or ethical grounds has often proved to be unrealistic. Indeed, many of the pronouncements and behaviors of West German sports doctors during the 1970s and 1980s confirm this assessment.[36]

Today's practitioners of "frontline" elite sports medicine belong to the category of "entrepreneurial" physicians who supply and/or prescribe controlled hormone drugs to athletes, policemen, firefighters, bodybuilders and others who want to acquire additional muscle mass, sex drive or mental energy. Given the broad dimensions of the anti-doping campaign and the larger "war on drugs" to which it belongs, it is not surprising that these doctors often run afoul of the law.[37] The final sections of this chapter look, therefore, at the careers and medical or pseudo-medical behaviors of five of these practitioners from four countries. Their diverse nationalities are basically irrelevant, because they are all practitioners of a libertarian pharmacology that is global, often lucrative and typically based on what are traditionally recognized as nonmedical motives.

Dr. Lothar Heinrich was a sports physician at the University of Freiburg (Germany) when the anti-doping façade of this prestigious sports-medical clinic began to crumble in 2006. Heinrich served as a medical supervisor of elite cyclists for the German Cycling Association (BDR) during the period 1996–2006, attending world championships and Olympic Games in this capacity. His Freiburg colleague, Dr. Andreas Schmid, served in the same role over the same period of time, and both were also attached to the professional Team Telekom. Both eventually confessed to facilitating the doping of cyclists under their care, citing their actions as "mistakes" or "lapses" (*Verfehlungen*).[38] Heinrich lied his way through published interviews in August 2006 and February 2007. In May 2007 he made his public confession.[39]

Dr. James Shortt, a practitioner of "longevity medicine" in Greenville, South Carolina, was charged in November 2005 with forty-three counts of improperly providing anabolic steroids and human growth hormone (HGH) to a group of patients that included professional football players. In March 2006, he pleaded guilty to one count of conspiracy to distribute anabolic steroids and human growth hormone. The other forty-two counts were dropped in exchange for the guilty plea.[40] His medical license was revoked and he was ordered to pay a $10,000 fine. According to assistant US Attorney Winston Holliday, from January 2001 until June 2004 Shortt authorized at least 139 anabolic steroid prescriptions, dispensing at least 1,217 milliliters of injectable anabolic steroids; 1,110 milliliters of anabolic steroid cream; 246 anabolic steroid lozenges; and 225 anabolic steroid tablets. The grand jury that indicted Shortt stated, for example, that he had dispensed the anabolic steroid testosterone "not for a legitimate medical purpose and outside the usual course of professional practice."[41] The South Carolina Board of Medical Examiners stated that Shortt had prescribed the drugs "in doses and frequencies that were extremely unlikely to have been prescribed with any medical justification, and that were not consistent with any acknowledged indication for this drug, such as wasting syndromes, recovery after burns or trauma, or hypogonadism." What is more, Shortt's dispensing of presumed performance-enhancing drugs occurred in the larger context of flagrant and multifaceted medical malpractice. He often infused patients with intravenous hydrogen peroxide. He prescribed testosterone for a terminally ill cancer patient. He diagnosed and treated patients for Lyme disease "based only on the results of tests by an unaccredited laboratory with a 100% positive rate for Lyme disease." These behaviors prompted the Board of Medical Examiners to declare that Shortt's actions rendered him "unfit to practice medicine."[42]

Dr. Eufemiano Fuentes was one of two doctors arrested during "Operation Puerto" after Spanish police confiscated steroids, hormones and EPO from a Madrid clinic in May 2006. The police also found one hundred bags of frozen blood, blood-doping equipment and documents naming cyclists and other athletes. The cyclists included stars such as Jan Ullrich, Alejandro Valverde and Ivan Basso, all of whom were suspended by their professional teams.[43] The doping charges against Fuentes were dismissed in 2008 because his alleged doping services were not illegal before the new Spanish doping law came into effect in December 2006, and the law could not be applied retroactively.[44] The previous law penalized only doping practices considered medically harmful. For this reason, the 2006 legal charges alleged "offenses against public health."[45] In December 2010, Fuentes was interrogated and arrested once again on doping charges as a result of "Operation Greyhound" (*Operacion Galgo*), a series of raids across Spain by the Spanish police that were aimed at the doping trade. Fuentes's attempt in 2007 to dissociate himself from doping should have convinced no one.[46]

Dr. Anthony Galea is a Canadian physician and sports medicine specialist whose Toronto clinic, the ISM Health & Wellness Centre, was raided by the Royal Canadian Mounted Police (RCMP) on 15 October 2009. There they found and confiscated a controversial substance called Actovegin, an extract of calf's blood that is produced in Austria by the Swiss company Nycomed and is not on the banned substances list of the WADA. Galea's legal troubles began in September 2009 when his assistant's car was stopped and searched by US border-crossing guards, who found HGH and other drugs.[47] Galea has treated many prominent professional athletes and has earned a reputation as a "Miracle Man" among some of them. In December 2010, the RCMP charged Galea with four crimes: "criminal conspiracy to smuggle human growth hormone and Actovegin into the United States; criminal conspiracy to smuggle 'prohibited, controlled or regulated' goods into Canada; unlawfully selling Actovegin, under the Food and Drugs Act; and smuggling goods into Canada, under the Customs Act."[48] At the time, one of Galea's attorneys, Mark J. Mahoney of Buffalo, New York, issued a statement: "I can tell you categorically that this investigation is not about performance enhancement. There is absolutely no evidence—there is no basis—for anyone with knowledge of this case to say that it has anything to do with performance-enhancing drugs."[49] This statement was a politically astute attempt to place Galea firmly and publicly on the therapeutic side of the therapy–enhancement divide. The doctor's prescribing of HGH to patients over forty years of age as "antiaging therapy," however dubious it might be from a scientific standpoint, was much less problematic from a public relations standpoint than being branded as a physician who had facilitated the doping of elite athletes.

Dr. Joseph Colao "ran a thriving illegal drug enterprise that supplied anabolic steroids and human growth hormone to hundreds of law enforcement officers and firefighters throughout New Jersey" before he died in 2007 at the age of forty-five. Like many other rule-bending physicians in the US who offer patients illegal hormone therapies, Colao concocted false diagnoses of low testosterone levels or adult growth hormone deficiency to legitimate these prescriptions.[50]

None of these men trained to become doping doctors.

Lothar Heinrich trained as a sports orthopedist and osteopath and became an expert on traumatic sports injuries and high-altitude training.[51] James Shortt was a family practitioner before he lost his medical license in 2006. At the time of his arrest, he had not been sanctioned for any form of malpractice. He earned his medical degree at the American University of the Caribbean on the island of Montserrat and did a residency in family medicine in Wisconsin. It is unclear how long he had been active in his "longevity" practice prior to his involvement in doping professional football players.[52] Eufemiano Fuentes's official medical status as a gynecologist has served as a façade behind which he has practiced his own version of enhancement medicine for elite athletes.[53] Anthony Galea earned his medical degree at McMaster University Medical School in Hamilton, Ontario, and has been involved in sports medicine since he graduated in 1986. He has been registered as a physician since 1987 and "has not been involved in any disciplinary hearings resulting in a finding of misconduct or any impropriety" since that time.[54] Of the five physicians under discussion, Galea is the one among them who has built a career as a celebrity sports doctor in the style of the West German media stars of the 1980s. He appears to be a high-functioning and even charismatic extrovert who has made the most of his obsession with the preservation of youthful vigor in himself and others. Joseph Colao moved out of a declining pain-management practice several years before his death, when he traveled to Las Vegas to attend "a crash course in hormone therapy." He had studied medicine at the University of Medicine and Dentistry of New Jersey and developed an interest in physical therapy. Having undergone triple bypass surgery at thirty-eight, Colao became a self-injecting hormone user and built an impressively muscled body. Like some other doctors who role-model transformative hormone therapy for their patients, Colao became an enthusiastic advocate of this form of enhancement.[55]

The careers of these five men are separated from those of the West German celebrity sports physicians by two decades during which the anti-doping campaign developed into a juggernaut compared to the disorganized and ineffectual doping control measures of the 1980s. The establishment of WADA in 2000, following two decades of neglect and inadequate efforts on the part of the IOC, gave the anti-doping campaign an authority and a credibility it had never had before. For this reason, the global campaign to oppose the use of performance-enhancing drugs by elite athletes eventually achieved a politically correct status that rules out overt collaborations between elite athletes and physicians who want to dope while preserving their reputations and their licenses to practice medicine. That is why the careers of four of these five doctors were interrupted or terminated by legal or medical authorities. The fifth, Joseph Colao, would certainly have been indicted and stripped of his license had he not died before his prescribing practices were exposed by investigative journalists in 2010. In summary, it is much riskier today than it was in the 1980s to be a celebrated sports physician who publicly favors or is suspected of doping elite athletes.

What connects these two eras is the attitude of defiance that rejects and even disdains anti-doping regulations in the name of the patient's wellbeing. Heinz Liesen, for example, was openly contemptuous of the anti-doping rules of the 1980s. A generation later, Eufemiano Fuentes expressed the same lack of interest in anti-doping measures: "The health of a sportsman is far more important than any sporting rule. If I can't stick to the rules I close my eyes and think only about safeguarding the health of my patients."[56] Lothar Heinrich took the same line: "That is what is decisive for the physician, that my athletes are and stay healthy. I'm not an anti-doping expert, I'm responsible for their health." He added, "My job is to be a team physician, not a doping commissar."[57] Both of these compromised physicians found it expedient to suggest that not giving hormones to athletes might endanger their health, and that this possibility legitimated the practice of what sports authorities regard as illicit hormone doping. Interestingly, the "lesser harm" argument on behalf of "medically supervised" doping seems to have disappeared. Today's doping doctors do not legitimate their own roles by describing their clients as being unable to control their own steroid habits. The doctor–client relationship is now represented as a medically advantageous collaboration that should be shielded from the prying eyes of regulators.

Although such private medical relationships have become notorious in the sports world, they are flourishing in the subspecialty known as "anti-aging" medicine. Alan D. Rogol, a pediatric endocrinologist at the University of Virginia who has published on the abuse of steroids and growth hormone, points out: "Nobody's watching. Each patient sees his doctor, and his doctor has a doctor–patient relationship, and if he's diagnosed as deficient—however that's done—then a legitimate prescription is written." This absence of surveillance has encouraged expansive interpretations of conditions that have been treated by means of hormone therapy. "We're not turning a blind eye to it, but we don't tell doctors how to be doctors," a Special Agent for the Drug Enforcement Administration said in 2010. "It's not our mission to stand guard at every doctor's door to make sure they do their due diligence. That's where the Hippocratic Oath comes in."[58] The problem is that a significant number of doctors do not do their due diligence. One motivation is the easy money a doctor can make by writing large numbers of fraudulent prescriptions for hormones. Another motivation may be the intention to "enhance" the life of the patient by means of a hormone treatment that is likely to be more experimental than reliably therapeutic. Potential risks are ignored, and the Hippocratic injunction to "do no harm" fades into the background of the doctor–patient relationship.

The irony is that it was FIFA's head doctor, the custodian of a sports-medical culture in which conflicts of interest are well-known, who called upon his World Cup colleagues to reaffirm the Hippocratic Oath. One hears precious little of such scruples in the wider world that has now embraced various "enhancements" of the human organism.

NOTES

1. See, for example, John Hoberman, *Mortal Engines: The Science of Performance and the Dehumanization of Sport* (New York: Free Press, 1992), 131–145.
2. Otto Riesser, "Über Doping und Dopingmittel," *Leibesübungen und körperliche Erziehung* 17 (1933): 393–394.
3. Otto Riesser, "Ist medikamentöse Beeinflussung im Sport möglich?" *Die Leibesübungen* 18 (1930): 537.
4. World Anti-Doping Agency, *World Anti-Doping Code* (Montreal: World Anti-Doping Agency, 2009), 14. http://www.wada-ama.org/Documents/World_Anti-Doping_Program/WADP-The-Code/WADA_Anti-Doping_CODE_2009_EN.pdf (accessed 7 January 2011).
5. Ove Bøje, "Doping: A Study of the Means Employed to Raise the Level of Performance in Sport," *Bulletin of the Health Organization of the League of Nations* 8 (1939): 452.
6. For a contemporary account of what track-and-field athletes were taking during the 1930s, see Bøje, "Doping."
7. See, for example, Hoberman, *Mortal Engines*, 243; John Hoberman, "Sports Physicians and the Doping Crisis in Elite Sport," *Clinical Journal of Sport Medicine* 12, no. 4 (2002): 203–208.
8. "Proceedings of the New York Meeting: Abstract of Proceedings of the House of Delegates of the American Medical Association at the Annual Meeting in New York, June 3–7, 1957." *Journal of the American Medical Association* 164, no. 11 (1957): 1231–1251.
9. Quoted in Michael Sehling, Reinhold Pollert and Dieter Hackfort, *Doping im Sport: Medizinische, sozialwissenschaftliche und juristische Aspekte* (Munich: BLV Verlagsgesellschaft, 1989), 100.
10. Quoted in "Hemmungslos," *Süddeutsche Zeitung*, 17–18 November 1984.
11. Committee on Sports Medicine and Fitness, "Use of Performance-Enhancing Substances," *Pediatrics* 115, no. 4 (2005): 1103.
12. "Sports Medicine—Is There Lack of Control?" *Lancet* 332, no. 8611 (1988): 612.
13. Charles L. Dubin, *Commission of Inquiry into the Use of Drugs and Banned Practices Intended to Increase Athletic Performance* (Ottawa: Canadian Government Publishing Centre, 1990), 385.
14. "When Pressure to Win Collides with Doctors' Oath," *New York Times*, 31 August 2010.
15. "Sportmediziner uneins," *Süddeutsche Zeitung*, 2 February 1988.
16. Ivan Waddington, *Sport, Health and Drugs: A Critical Sociological Perspective* (New York and London: E & F Spon, 2000), 7.
17. "Die meisten Zuschauer sprechen Johnson frei," *Frankfurter Allgemeine Zeitung*, 16 January 1989.
18. Brigitte Berendonk, *Doping-Dokumente: Von der Forschung zum Betrug* (Berlin: Springer-Verlag, 1991), 43, 45.

19. See Hoberman, *Mortal Engines*, 252–265.
20. See, for example, John Hoberman, "How Drug Testing Fails: The Politics of Doping Control," in *Doping in Elite Sport: The Politics of Drugs in the Olympic Movement*, ed. Wayne Wilson and Edward Derse, 241–274 (Champaign, IL: Human Kinetics, 2000).
21. Hoberman, *Mortal Engines*, 258–259. See "Ich mache meine eigene Medizin," *Der Spiegel*, 1 April 1991, 196.
22. "Frontmann, Guru, Zielscheibe: Klümper öffnet die Tür," *Süddeutsche Zeitung*, 19 July 1988.
23. "Typen wie aus dem Panoptikum," *Der Spiegel*, 23 July 1984, 71.
24. "Sportmediziner uneins," *Süddeutsche Zeitung*, 2 February 1988.
25. "Doping mit erlaubten Mitteln," *Süddeutsche Zeitung*, 22 January 1987.
26. "Wider die Doping-Mentalität der Scharlatane," *Süddeutsche Zeitung*, 24 May 1988.
27. "Liesen: Rufmord," *Süddeutsche Zeitung*, 11 June 1999.
28. "Zuviel Theater um Anabolika," *Süddeutsche Zeitung*, 23 January 1985.
29. See, for example, John Hoberman and Charles E. Yesalis, "The History of Synthetic Testosterone," *Scientific American* 272, no. 2 (1995): 60–65.
30. John Hoberman, *Testosterone Dreams: Rejuvenation, Aphrodisia, Doping* (Berkeley: University of California Press, 2005), 35.
31. "Trinken, um Leistung zu bringen," *Süddeutsche Zeitung*, 7–8 June 1986.
32. "Der Sport ist wie ein ungepflügtes Land," *Süddeutsche Zeitung*, 4 February 1985.
33. "Kontrollen in den Trainingsphasen," *Süddeutsche Zeitung*, 11 August 1988.
34. See, for example, "Doping und deutsche Ärzte (West und Gesamtdeutsch)—ein Überblick." http://www.cycling4fans.de/index.php?id=4455 (accessed 25 January 2011). This web essay is based on many credible journalistic sources.
35. On the relationship of Francesco Conconi to the politics of doping in Italy, see John Hoberman, "Introduction: 'Doping and Public Policy,'" in *Doping and Public Policy*, ed. John Hoberman and Verner Møller (Odense: University Press of Southern Denmark, 2004), 10–11.
36. See, for example, "Doping und deutsche Ärzte (West und Gesamtdeutsch)—ein Überblick." http://www.cycling4fans.de/index.php?id=4455 (accessed 25 January 2011). This web essay is based on many credible journalistic sources.
37. On the "entrepreneurial" hormone-prescribing physician, see Hoberman, *Testosterone Dreams*, 190–191.
38. "Der Arzt, der Betrug und die Ethik," *Berliner Zeitung*, 25 May 2007.
39. "Meine Arbeit ist Teamarzt, nicht Dopingkommissar," *Süddeutsche Zeitung*, 19–20 August 2006; Andrew Hood, "The Sunday Interview: T-Mobile's Dr. Lothar Heinrich," http://velonews.competitor.com/2007/02/road/the-sunday-interview-t-mobiles-dr-lothar-heinrich_11681 (accessed 6 February 2011).
40. "Shortt Enters Guilty Plea in Steroids Case," *USATODAY.com*, 6 March 2006.
41. See http://www.casewatch.org/doj/short/indictment.shtml (accessed 10 February 2011).
42. See http://www.casewatch.org/board/med/short/suspension.shtml (accessed 10 February 2011).
43. "Operation Puerto Doctor Speaks Out against Doping at Sporting Conference," Associated Press, 4 July 2007.
44. "'Operacion Galgo' in Spanien," *FAZ.NET*, 12 February 2011 (accessed 11 February 2011). http://www.google.de/#hl=de&gs_nf=1&cp=30&gs_id=3g&x

hr=t&q=%22'operacion+Galgo'+in+Spanien%22&pf=p&sclient=psy-ab
&oq=%22'operacion+Galgo'+in+Spanien%22&aq=f&aqi=&aql=&gs_
l=&pbx=1&bav=on.2,or.r_gc.r_pw.r_qf.,cf.osb&fp=998f4d8e1aaa52c2&bi
w=1108&bih=978

45. "Inside the Blood Doping Investigation," *SPIEGEL.ONLINE*, 10 July
2006 (accessed 31 December 2010). http://www.google.de/#hl=de&gs_
nf=1&cp=38&gs_id=7p&xhr=t&q=%22inside+the+blood+doping+investig
ation%22&pf=p&sclient=psy-ab&oq=%22inside+the+blood+doping+inves
tigation%22&aq=f&aqi=&aql=&gs_l=&pbx=1&bav=on.2,or.r_gc.r_pw.r_
qf.,cf.osb&fp=998f4d8e1aaa52c2&biw=1108&bih=978
46. "Operation Puerto Doctor."
47. "Sports Medicine Pioneer Subject of Doping Inquiry," *New York Times*, 14
December 2009; "Doctor under Investigation for Doping Is Charged," *New
York Times*, 16 December 2009.
48. "Charges Link Doctor to 3 Years of Smuggling," *New York Times*, 19
December 2009.
49. "Canadian Doctor Dispensed Drugs to Athletes, Assistant Tells Investigators," *New York Times*, 18 December 2009.
50. Amy Brittain and Mark Mueller, "NJ Doctor Supplied Steroids to Hundreds of Law Enforcement Officers, Firefighters," *Star-Ledger*, 12 December
2010.
51. See http://www.gots.org/deutsch/News/GOTS_News_Archiv_Detail.php5?
det=pres_0064 (accessed 16 February 2011).
52. See http://www.healthgrades.com/directory_search/physician/profiles/dr-
md-reports/dr-james-shortt-md-cfd6ca57 (last accessed May 6, 2012).
53. See http://www.velonation.com/News/ID/6762/Could-Eufemiano-Fuentes-
lose-his-medical-licence.aspx (accessed 18 December 2010).
54. See http://www.zoominfo.com/search#search/profile/person?personId=849
38824&targetid=profile (accessed 16 February 2011).
55. Brittain and Mueller, "NJ Doctor."
56. "Doctor Puts Clients' Health before Doping Regulations," http://daily-
dosearchive.wiredin.org.uk/sport_archives2006/july1106.htm (accessed 10
July 2006).
57. "Meine Arbeit ist Teamarzt."
58. Amy Brittain and Mark Mueller, "Booming Anti-Aging Business Relies
on Risky Mix of Steroids, Growth Hormone," *Star-Ledger*, 14 December
2010.

BIBLIOGRAPHY

Berendonk, Brigitte. *Doping-Dokumente: Von der Forschung zum Betrug*. Berlin:
Springer-Verlag, 1991.
Bøje, Ove. "Doping: A Study of the Means Employed to Raise the Level of Perfor-
mance in Sport." *Bulletin of the Health Organization of the League of Nations*
8 (1939): 439–469.
Brittain, Amy and Mark Mueller, "Booming Anti-Aging Business Relies on Risky
Mix of Steroids, Growth Hormone," *Star-Ledger*, 14 December 2010.
"Canadian Doctor Dispensed Drugs to Athletes, Assistant Tells Investigators,"
New York Times, 18 December 2009.
"Charges Link Doctor to 3 Years of Smuggling," *New York Times*, 19 December
2009.
Committee on Sports Medicine and Fitness. "Use of Performance-Enhancing Sub-
stances." *Pediatrics* 115, no. 4 (2005): 1103–1106.

"Der Arzt, der Betrug und die Ethik," *Berliner Zeitung*, 25 May 2007.
"Der Sport ist wie ein ungepflügtes Land," *Süddeutsche Zeitung*, 4 February 1985.
"Die meisten Zuschauer sprechen Johnson frei," *Frankfurter Allgemeine Zeitung*, 16 January 1989.
"Doctor Puts Clients' Health before Doping Regulations," http://dailydosearchive.wiredin.org.uk/sport_archives2006/july1106.htm (accessed 10 July 2006).
"Doctor under Investigation for Doping Is Charged," *New York Times*, 16 December 2009.
"Doping mit erlaubten Mitteln," *Süddeutsche Zeitung*, 22 January 1987.
"Doping und deutsche Ärzte (West und Gesamtdeutsch)—ein Überblick." http://www.cycling4fans.de/index.php?id=4455 (accessed 25 January 2011). This web essay is based on many credible journalistic sources.
Dubin, Charles L. *Commission of Inquiry into the Use of Drugs and Banned Practices Intended to Increase Athletic Performance*. Ottawa: Canadian Government Publishing Centre, 1990.
"Frontmann, Guru, Zielscheibe: Klümper öffnet die Tür," *Süddeutsche Zeitung*, 19 July 1988.
Hoberman, John. "How Drug Testing Fails: The Politics of Doping Control." In *Doping in Elite Sport: The Politics of Drugs in the Olympic Movement*, edited by Wayne Wilson and Edward Derse, 241–274. Champaign, IL: Human Kinetics, 2000.
———. "Introduction: 'Doping and Public Policy.'" In *Doping and Public Policy*, edited by John Hoberman and Verner Møller, 10–11. Odense: University Press of Southern Denmark, 2004.
———. *Mortal Engines: The Science of Performance and the Dehumanization of Sport*. New York: Free Press, 1992.
———. "Sports Physicians and the Doping Crisis in Elite Sport." *Clinical Journal of Sport Medicine* 12, no. 4 (2002): 203–208.
———. *Testosterone Dreams: Rejuvenation, Aphrodisia, Doping*. Berkeley: University of California Press, 2005.
Hoberman, John, and Charles E. Yesalis. "The History of Synthetic Testosterone." *Scientific American* 272, no. 2 (1995): 60–65.
Hood, Andrew. "The Sunday Interview: T-Mobile's Dr. Lothar Heinrich," http://velonews.competitor.com/2007/02/road/the-sunday-interview-t-mobiles-dr-lothar-heinrich_11681 (accessed 6 February 2011).
"Ich mache meine eigene Medizin," *Der Spiegel*, 1 April 1991, 196.
"Inside the Blood Doping Investigation," *SPIEGEL.ONLINE*, 10 July 2006 (accessed 31 December 2010).
"Kontrollen in den Trainingsphasen," *Süddeutsche Zeitung*, 11 August 1988.
"Liesen: Rufmord," *Süddeutsche Zeitung*, 11 June 1999.
"Meine Arbeit ist Teamarzt, nicht Dopingkommissar," *Süddeutsche Zeitung*, 19–20 August 2006.
"'Operacion Galgo' in Spanien," *FAZ.NET*, 12 February 2011 (accessed 11 February 2011).
"Operation Puerto Doctor Speaks Out against Doping at Sporting Conference," Associated Press, 4 July 2007.
"Proceedings of the New York Meeting: Abstract of Proceedings of the House of Delegates of the American Medical Association at the Annual Meeting in New York, June 3–7, 1957." *Journal of the American Medical Association* 164, no. 11 (1957): 1231–1251.
Riesser, Otto. "Ist Medikamentöse Beeinflussung im Sport Möglich?" *Die Leibesübungen* 18 (1930): 537–539.
"Sportmediziner uneins," *Süddeutsche Zeitung*, 2 February 1988.

———. "Über Doping und Dopingmittel." *Leibesübungen und Körperliche Erziehung* 17 (1933): 393–394.

Sehling, Michael, Reinhold Pollert and Dieter Hackfort. *Doping im Sport: Medizinische, sozialwissenschaftliche und juristische Aspekte*. Munich: BLV Verlagsgesellschaft, 1989.

"Shortt Enters Guilty Plea in Steroids Case," *USATODAY.com*, 6 March 2006.

"Sportmediziner uneins," *Süddeutsche Zeitung*, 2 February 1988.

"Sports Medicine—Is There Lack of Control?" *Lancet* 332, no. 8611 (1988): 612.

"Sports Medicine Pioneer Subject of Doping Inquiry," *New York Times*, 14 December 2009.

"Trinken, um Leistung zu bringen," *Süddeutsche Zeitung*, 7–8 June 1986.

"Typen wie aus dem Panoptikum," *Der Spiegel*, 23 July 1984, 71.

Waddington, Ivan. *Sport, Health and Drugs: A Critical Sociological Perspective*. London: E & FN Spon, 2000.

"When Pressure to Win Collides with Doctors' Oath," *New York Times*, 31 August 2010.

"Wider die Doping-Mentalität der Scharlatane," *Süddeutsche Zeitung*, 24 May 1988.

World Anti-Doping Agency. *World Anti-Doping Code*. Montreal: World Anti-Doping Agency, 2009. http://www.wada-ama.org/Documents/World_Anti-Doping_Program/WADP-The-Code/WADA_Anti-Doping_CODE_2009_EN.pdf (accessed 7 January 2011).

"Zuviel Theater um Anabolika," *Süddeutsche Zeitung*, 23 January 1985.

Part IV

Sports and Medicine Contested

13 Doctors without Degrees

Michael Atkinson

MUST WE PUT INFORMATION ON A DIET?[1]

We are sat at a restaurant table, five triathletes physically and emotionally spent after a grueling day of competition in Ontario's sweltering summer heat. My body is slumped into a wooden Adirondack chair, with my remaining energy squarely focused on the volume of food I will consume in the next hour in the hopes of recovery. A waitress approaches us, trying to keep hold of five supersize menus and a plastic jug of much needed water. Without a word or hesitation I shoot my hand out in a forty-five-degree angle, clutching at the top menu. I snatch and open it midair and scan the entire appetizer and entrée columns. The time between the end of the waitress' scripted recounting of the daily specials and my exuberant order for nachos, five bean soup and a vegan shepherd's pie could have only been measured in milliseconds. My friends, however, take much more time to decide. They always do. They comb over the selections, aggressively counting calories, macronutrient contents and the physiological consequences of the food for their bodies. I feel like apologizing to our waitress, who is dressed all in black and is now clearly thinking about the other customers and orders she must process, as beads of sweat pour down her forehead. They predictably order several jugs of water and the lowest calorie options on the menu. What they do next is both impressively disciplined and decisively pathological.

Here we are stationed in one of the most beautiful environs in northern Ontario, blessed to be able to devote an entire day to the pleasure of sporting competition. The pine trees, smell of bark mulch and lilacs fill the air. I have nowhere to be other than right here, and neither does Stan, David, Rob or Ian.[2] Our race has concluded, we fared well and will race again another day. This is a space without care or worry or anxiety . . . at least in theory. But the four of them fret. Stan leans over to Ian and asks, "Should we do it now? Now? Now, Ian?" Ian glances right and left as if he is worried someone is watching. Their arms slink and slither toward the ground, and then underneath our table with timed synchronicity. Pausing only for the briefest moment, they each extract two sandwich bags from tactically stationed racing duffel bags and slide them into the pockets on their cargo shorts. Contained in the satchels are postrace recovery tonics, protein powders and a mix of branched chain amino potions. All contraband foods, they think anyway, on the restaurant patio. "Ian," whispers Rob, "you have enough for all of us, right?" Within seconds the waitress lugs four more clear pails of ice water to our table, the condensation dripping with pace from each. After quickly pouring glasses for the table, mixing well-measured amounts from each magic packet of nutritional goodness, Ian distributes the elixirs to all. I laugh and partially taunt them with, "Fucking hell, guys, not for me, I'm going to eat today." Rob seamlessly quips back, "Think about that when you look at the race stats posted over there, my brother." He knows full well I finished behind all of them.

The boys constantly tease me for *eating without calculation* before, during or after a day of racing or training. I have neither delusions nor fantasies of becoming a professional and tend to, perhaps quite irresponsibly to them, justify my penchant for eating fun foods with references to my training load and volume. David pipes in with, "Mike, you know this; if the body is not refueled properly you'll never get better, and probably worse. The shit they serve here might taste great, but it's garbage energy." I get a little cheeky. "Yeah, but you fucking guys are not lab researchers or nutritionists, okay? At best your info and recipes are based on trial and error or what some coach says to you, right? You might think you have a science of eating nailed down, but I bet you're doing a hundred things wrong. Do you even know exactly what is in all of that shit?" We've been down this conversational road a million times. We'll debate food and exercise supplements until the final check arrives in its fake leather wrapped case, which I offer to pay, as I ordered the bulk of the food. Their measly salads and paltry sundry items account for little, as always.

Maybe it's just me, but I cannot eat out of a bag or wash down white powders and scientifically engineered crystalline concoctions with tap water and refer to such a process as nourishment. I find little pleasure or satiety in what I have come to refer to as *plastic eating*. But many other triathletes I know integrate plastic eating into their weekly nutrition regimens. Some passively consume drinks, bars, powders and other sports-performance liquids, whereas others integrate them meticulously into their gastronomic schedules. The latter consume information about eating for performance as voraciously as a post-event meal. Five years of ethnographic immersion in triathlon and duathlon cultures forced me to examine, among other things, my and others' constructions of eating, the body and health. In what follows, I discuss how the emergence and diffusion of plastic eating in sports cultures like triathlon exemplifies a sort of death of subjective eating in healthist or performance-oriented cultures. Here, both the fleshy bodies and engineered foods have potentially triumphed as objects over the human subject in triathlon culture, with participants increasingly constructing and promulgating their own pseudo-medical understandings of the link between food, bodies and health. Such sports enthusiasts drive plastic eating and self-objectification to the logic of extremes as a *fatal strategy*.

THE TRIATHLETES

I clip my shoes into my pedals and glide my bike over the cracks at the end of my driveway. Briefly scanning down at the computer perched on the handlebars, I notice the time; it is precisely 5:45 p.m. I'm hungry, so hungry in fact that I think about skipping the two-hour training session and gorging at a local vegetarian restaurant. Before my brain convinces my feet to decouple from the pedals, I hear a voice, "Hey, are you ready?" It's Chris, whose belly is most likely empty too, but he's smiling from ear to ear. "Ready for the brick [workout]?" "What do you think, home boy!" I say back without thinking. "All right, let's do it, then," he says before slugging down three or four mouthfuls of orange sports drink. Within ten minutes of leaving my house, we are sat with twenty or so other members of a triathlon group that trains together four or five times a week throughout the year. Comprised of mainly age-group (a nice way of saying nonelite) athletes and racers, this cabal of triathlon enthusiasts seems equally energized for the workout. I've been working out and competing alongside them for about six months now and have come to relish our weekly sessions in both physical and social ways. John and Carl lean on a car and mull over world events. Alison and Jim talk about an upcoming half-Ironman in the US. Susan meticulously checks all of her training kit for the evening, laying it out on the grass beside her bike. At one point or another, everyone pulls out a sports drink, gel or some ergogenic to make it through the workout. A 6:00 p.m. training session, like those at 7:00 a.m. or noon, challenge the culinary scheduling ability of even the most seasoned athlete. The answer is *supplementation*. Our coach, a former police officer and now full-time triathlon enthusiast, leads us through the evening's ordeal. "Right, then, do two laps on the bike around the course (an 800-meter loop) and then run a lap at about 70 percent. We'll do that for ninety minutes and then cool down. Remember to drink a lot of E-load [an electrolyte drink] because it's hot tonight." For the next ninety minutes, lawyers, real estate agents, salespeople, design consultants and, of course, one professor whizz around the course under the late July sun. Gears click, bodies drip, pedals purr, breath billows, wheels hum and running shoes slap in a Fordist assemblage of sport.

Membership in a triathlon club is worth its ethnographic weight in gold in terms of learning the phenomenology of the activity, grasping the social aspects of the culture and observing nutritional strategies *in situ*. My degree of involvement in triathlon remains, to date, at the age-group level. My wife, Lindsey, facilitated my ethnographic foray into the world of triathlon, herself a somewhat accomplished age-group athlete in Ontario. She introduced me to one of her training clubs in 2005 and encouraged me to participate as both a recreational athlete and researcher. Age-group athletes do not compete as professionals or elites, and pay entrance fees at events and race against individuals in a common age and gender classification (typically, a range of five to ten years within each category). From 2005 to 2007, I competed in seventeen duathlons, including three half-Ironman distances (8 kilometers run, 90 kilometers bike, 21 kilometers run) and one international Powerman (10 kilometers run, 50 kilometers bike, 5 kilometers run). In 2005, I competed in Ontario Provincial Championships in duathlon and, in 2006, both the Ontario Provincial and Canadian National Duathlon Championships. From 2005 to 2008, I competed in seventeen short-distance triathlons in Ontario. Through the process of participant observation with triathletes in southern Ontario, I spent over six hundred hours training with them, hanging around at competitions (fifty-seven separate events over three years) and socializing within a variety of nonsporting contexts. Copious hours were devoted to the discussion of performance in endurance sport, with much debate about appropriate styles of eating for athletes. Notes regarding these conversations were transcribed after our interactions and logged into a database.

Sixty-two triathletes in the southern Ontario region were interviewed in addition to gathering participant observation data. By using the chain referral technique common in qualitative research, social networks in the sport were tapped.[3] I trained with two triathlon clubs in one Canadian city and used members from each, including my wife, as initial sponsors. Through friendship networks tapped in competition and socialization at races, I developed a series of additional informant chains. Although no theoretical or purposive sampling procedures were structured into the process, participants with a range of endurance sport abilities and backgrounds were purposefully targeted for interviews. All of the participants reside, train and mainly compete in the province of Ontario, Canada.

With a population exceeding four million and a burgeoning endurance sport culture, the number of triathletes and triathlon races in the southern Ontario region is increasing exponentially. Triathlon enthusiasts interviewed for this study range in age from twenty-four to sixty-five years of age (a mean age of thirty-six years) and were equally represented by gender status (thirty male, thirty-two female). A slight majority were single (58 percent), most were middle class (94 percent), had a mean household income of approximately CDN$88,000 and shared predominantly Canadian/European heritages (86 percent). Experience with, and weekly commitment to, triathlon varied in the group. Most trained four to six days per week, devoted a mean of 14.5 hours to training/competition per week and had a mean of seven years' involvement in triathlon. Active competition also varied, with the number of races entered per year ranging from one to seventeen. Finally, a handful of the triathletes had competed at both national and international levels (eleven in the study), with the rest competing locally in age-group races. Interviews were conducted in a variety of settings, such as my university office, a coffee shop, in a car on the way to a race, a local park and a restaurant. Interviews were semi-structured by a list of approximately twenty-five questions designed to elicit subjects' narratives concerning their backgrounds and experiences with triathlon over time—including, of course, questions about their dietary regimens. I used a tape recorder or video camera during some of the interviews. Interviews were (within several hours, or at maximum, one day) transcribed onto computer files and filled in considerably (in the tradition of theoretical memoing) as I conceptually analyzed the texts. Interviews ranged in length from forty-five minutes to three and a half hours. In all cases, pseudonyms are employed to protect the participants' identities.

ETHNOPHARMACOLOGY

"Hi, Oliver, what are you hunting for today?" A twentysomething store clerk clad in a black training suit asks with a sort of enthusiasm I find suspicious. "I'm looking for a new BCAA [branched chain amino acid] stack I saw advertised in a magazine last week. A friend of mine says you have it," responds one of my best training buddies. Here we go, the next thirty-five or forty minutes of my life will be spent listening to overly loud dance music piping into my ears from the store stereo system intermingled with the tedium of Oliver and this girl (who, if we can trust her name tag, is actually called "Destiny") going over the newest innovations in sports supplements. Oliver convinced me it would be a quick in and out of the shop, but I knew better. He's here at least twice a week chatting with Destiny about supplements. I think he is in love with her; she seems incredibly sexy and funny, but just maybe he's more in love with the supplements she peddles. Oliver is a very curious guy. At thirty-two years old, he is having the best triathlon season of his life—few injuries, great competition results and phenomenal body shape. His attitude is positive, and he seems to genuinely enjoy the daily grind of training and racing. He attributes all of his recent success to shifts and experimentations with his eating plan. Oliver avoids eating whole foods prior, during and after training and engages in plastic eating. "Have you tried ZMA capsules as well?" remarks Destiny. "They give you a great recovery boost." "No, because I know a few guys who've taken them and they have warned me I'll just end up with seriously dark pee. None of our experiences back up the [medical] claims about testosterone-boosting effects." This conversation will well and truly go on for a long time. I glance around, desperately searching for something interesting to read. There must be one thousand or so products in this sport and health nutrition mega-chain. I've only dabbled with a few gels, electrolyte drinks and protein powders in the past, so the cacophony of products in this Christmas store for the athlete is dizzying. Where do you even start? Do I need everything in the store to be fit, to be able to do my best? Just to be a pain in the ass I intrude with, "Does any of this really work?" Deathly silence, two brows furrow, a moment of disbelief and their conversation scarcely skips a beat. We leave thirty minutes later, Oliver is $150 lighter and yet so much happier.

"What the hell was the comment all about? What are you playing at?" I knew he would ask before our seat belts were even clipped, and so I had rehearsed my response in anticipation. "Mate, why do you spend so much money on that stuff? Do you really believe all of the shit you read in magazines?" I'm only a year into the ethnography at this point and I am still learning about what makes triathletes tick. My fractious probe is a deliberate "bad cop" technique for stimulating dialogue through confrontational gestures, questions and claims.[4] "No, I don't because I've probably done more field-testing with the products than all of the scientists combined. I bet none of them have ever used any of it in real life. I'd stack my knowledge of eating for performance against theirs any day." He's probably right, I think to myself. "What I do is read as much as I can and then take bits and pieces from here and there which make sense. I try things out, ask other people what works for them and go from there." Research bells start to ring in my ears. Where is a notepad when you need one? "What you'll learn is that people on the inside [triathlon, in this case] share a knowledge base about eating and what works. It's not really written down anywhere, but you'll get glimpses of it in triathlon magazines from time to time." Oliver has just nicely described the sports version of ethnopharmacology, a cultural science of eating based on local rather than medically authoritative knowledge bases.

For many triathletes, carefully followed eating regimens crystallize beyond the boundaries of clinical observation, testing, discourses and practices. Sociologists of sport and physical culture are paying moderate attention to the social dynamics of ethnopharmacology. The sociological literature detailing ethnopharmacology in sport is still very much in its infancy, but several key pieces are worth mentioning. Most of the core articles and chapters in the extant field tend to focus on illicit drug use rather than the full panorama of over-the-counter performance-enhancing foods and supplements or simply, *ergogenics*. For example, Lee Monaghan is arguably the godfather of ethnopharmacological research within recreational athlete and bodybuilder cultures. Across his corpus of research, Monaghan characterizes bodies in sport as "chemistry experiments."[5] Monaghan's call for awareness regarding athlete sensibilities about self-doping and performance enhancement encourages researchers to view subcultural penchants for doping as an ethic of self-care rather than strict violations of health norms in sport. Sociologists of sport, including Dunning and Waddington; Beamish and Ritchie; Waddington, Malcolm, Roderick and Naik; Atkinson and Young; Beamish; and Waddington and Smith all illustrate the complex sociocultural dimensions of drug (and food) consumption in sport;[6] each documenting how knowledge of how, when and why to use particular ergogenics springs from athlete cultures now as much as from so-called detached medical circles.[7]

Through an ethnographic study of recreational athlete and gym members' use of over-the-counter ergogenics, I previously illustrated the rather blasé attitude many recreational athletes possess toward supplementation. The men I studied almost unanimously value athletes' own organic knowledge of sports-performance aides over clinicians or other medical authority figures.[8] My findings ring with Tscholl, Junge and Dvorak's exposure of the prevalence, and general lack of concern over, the widespread use of medications, supplements and nutritional/performance aides among football elites at the respective 2002 and 2006 football World Cups.[9] Huang, Johnson and Pipe noted a similar trend of ambivalence and ethnopharmacology in Canadian athletes participating in recent Olympic Games.[10] Schwenk and Costley note how trends of increasing self-directed supplementation might be systematic indicators of sports cultures that no longer promote cautious or holistic eating per se, but a wider range of plastic eating and drug supplementation practices in both legal and illegal forms.[11]

Cultures engrained with intense logics and practices of "slimming for sport" are replete with ethnopharmacological ideologies and discourses. The rapidly developing literature on anorexia in sport or *athletica anorexia* provides glimpses and insights on how regimes of self-starvation become entrenched as a cultural norm in gymnastics, figure skating, distance running and other sports worlds. Unfortunately, the lion's share of existing research tends to focus on the highly individualized characteristics, mood states, self-perceptions and body orientations of at-risk or clinically diagnosed athletes rather on the cultures that systematically and generationally breed eating attitudes.[12] Rarely do analyses of anorexia in sport focus on the cultural logics of eating in specific sports clusters, or the ethnopharmacological norms underpinning athletes' physical regimens. For example, a meta-review of the literature indicates that a general biographical or psychological composite of the athlete with an emaciation eating disorder, or at risk of developing such a disorder, has been cobbled. The emaciator in sport is (stereo)typically female (9:1 or 10:1 ratio to males),[13] participates in sports overemphasizing performance-related thinness ideologies or aesthetics[14] and is pathologically preoccupied with physical appearance.[15] The emaciator's psychological profile is easy to deconstruct, as an individual with low-self esteem,[16] an obsessive compulsion toward self-monitoring, high anxiety,[17] a drive toward perfectionism,[18] moodiness and negative affect state,[19] exhibiting exercise dependence or *athletica anorexia*[20] and has body dysmorphia.[21] Athletes with emaciation-related eating disorders are not as likely to have experienced past histories of physical and sexual abuse as their nonathlete counterparts,[22] but links between domineering or hyper-authoritarian family structures are common.[23] Although much of this biographical or pathway information is fascinating and telling, it reveals little regarding the physical cultural norms and ideologies of dangerous eating within sports cultures, or the manners by which emaciators in sport tend to believe their experientially derived knowledge of eating and sports bodies is vastly superior to dieticians', nutritionists' and other medical experts'.

Notwithstanding the preceding, ample evidence exists to suggest that so-called cultures of expert medical knowledge are heavily scrutinized, negotiated or subverted in some sports settings.[24] Kim quite clearly argues that physicians' knowledge of eating and the body is under attack by elite athletes in particular.[25] Here, the athletes might take direction from sports physicians and their diagnoses/suggestions, but do whatever they wish (in a pastiche manner) with such advice. Pike's research on women rowers illustrates how, when particular athletes become disgruntled with normal pain treatment protocols in sport, they will perform their own homework, seek and then practice alternative treatment methods (see also Pike's contribution to this collection).[26] Porucznik, Reeser and Willick's research on the use of pain medication by athletes attests to the frequency at which sports participants' may even ignore doctors' orders and pursue their own supplementation strategies.[27] Safai's acknowledgment that the field of sports medicine is at ideological odds with athletes is especially important in the study of ethnopharmacology.[28] For although sport clinicians (including nutritionists or dieticians) often promote caution with regard to eating, athletes have developed risky ethnopharmacology practices in the pursuit of high performance and sporting distinction. On these grounds and others, traditional boundaries of medical/scientific authority over the performing athletic body are being negotiated, redrawn and in some cases erased in sport cultures.

My friend Oliver describes learning how to eat and supplement properly as a "bit by bit" process. Discovering "the [scientific] bits" is far more self-directed than in previous eras, and the ubiquity of sports nutrition information is but one factor fueling the overall entrenchment of ethnopharmacology in recreational and elite-level sports like triathlon. Ironically, and perhaps quite unintentionally, the mass marketing and distribution of scientifically designed sports supplements provides an opportunity for considerable innovation and knowledge formation on the part of athletes. For the remainder of this chapter, we delve deeper into the movement toward athletic self-stylization through supplementation and inspect the contestation of medical/traditional authority posed by athlete ethnopharmacological beliefs and practices as a fatal strategy deeply symbolic of broader trends in late modern social life.

FATALLY STRATEGIC SUPPLEMENTATION

The absolute object is one that is worthless, whose quality is a matter of indifference, but which escapes objective alienation in that it has made itself more of an object than the object—this gives it a fatal quality.[29]

The ongoing implosion of medical or scientific subjectivity and out-right control regarding nutrition in sports cultures and elsewhere is no mere accident or coincidence. Do not be fooled by the ubiquity of plastic, laboratory-designed food everywhere and athletes' increasing reliance on plastic eating; such is not the seductive triumph of the biomedical over the everyday! Neither does the commercialization of sports supplements sug-gest a victory of the market economic over a hapless athlete mob. Bound-ary erosion processes so characteristic of late modernity produce *doctors without degrees* in sports places. The more *scientifically generated* nutri-tional information that is distributed, mediated, promoted and packaged to consumers, the more eating becomes locally ecstatic; that is, people are able to become doctors without degrees because of the sheer "obesity," or what Baudrillard might refer to as the *obscenity*, of eating information in the media.[30] These doctors without degrees deploy plastic foods—the sports gel, the energy bar, the magic recovery shake, the body-rebuilding tablet—over real foods as everyday ritual. The plastic, more perfect than natural food, triumphs over the imperfect "whole" food. James (age thirty-four) says to me one afternoon on a car ride home from a race, "Thank God I had my wonder food in the silver wrapper [his sports energy bar]. I can't even stomach real food while racing, eh." Where one once supplemented with sports products at the advice of a trainer, nutritionist or sports doc-tor (to prevent illness, guard against vitamin deficiency or enhance short bursts of embodied performance), triathletes and others now often design massive portions of their eating programs around specially designed sports products on their own accord. Jim (age twenty-seven) says: "I don't need a doctor, and I don't need a dietician. With the right mix of training and experimentation, you learn how to eat. I schedule and organize my own diet, and, yes, supplements are a major part."

Baudrillard paints a recurring picture of a do-it-yourself society spiral-ing in the ecstasy of communication; a world of oversaturated meanings, de-centered subjects and so much information that any single piece of infor-mation is rendered irrelevant.[31] In the mosaic of popular circulated food information, every athlete extracts his or her own secret from the litany of "medical recommendations" and more perfect-than-perfect recipe for supplementation. Jennifer (age twenty-four) tells me one day in the middle of a five-hour bike ride: "A lot of people ask me what I eat and I sort of half tell them the truth. 'I eat this.' 'What's that?' You know, and it works, but I'm not ready to share it with everyone." Most of these dietary plans are based on little knowledge of the biomechanisms of performance, the relationship between chemicals and movement or their long-term effects. Being able to self-customize and self-medicate as one sees fit, using one's own cobbled knowledge and reflexive experience, has far more meaning to the triathletes than scientifically legitimated evidence about nutrition and sports performance. Becoming a doctor without a degree and self-stylizing one's nutritional regimen, thus producing the aura of control and mastery of both the body and the self, is a consequence of information overload—of the saturation and obesity of food knowledge everywhere:

> When I first started into triathlon, our coach gave us some advice [about eating and supplementing], I spoke with a nutritionist and a local sports dietician. What a waste of fucking money, going to the experts. What they do is take some basic information about how much you train and the sorts of foods you eat on a weekly basis and spit back to you a preprogrammed eating plan. So, I read more magazine articles, some books on eating for long-distance running and triathlon, spoke to a couple more coaches, and like hundreds of other athletes. Everyone will tell you something interesting and useful, I guess, in a certain way. All of the knowledge at once is sort of confusing. Who do you trust and what do you trust? One person will tell you not to eat this or that, while the next suggests that should be a staple of your diet . . . I finally realized that no one has the best knowledge about eating, you have to learn for yourself and find the right foods that work for you. All of the books are fine and good for basic information, but they don't replace intimate knowledge about what really works for you, personally, in sport. (Justine, 29)

When I reflect on Justine's comments, "the art of [late modern] life" that Bauman describes ring true:

> In our individualized society we are all artists of life—whether we know it or not, will it or not and like it or not, by decree of society if not by our own choice. In this society we are all expected, rightly or wrongly, to give our lives purpose and form by using our own skills and resources, even if we lack the tools and materials with which artists' studios need to be equipped for the artist's work to be conceived and executed. And we are praised or censured for the results—for what we have managed or failed to accomplish and for what we have achieved and lost.[32]

Whereas Foucault advocates care of the self as the practice of emancipation, freedom and the fulfillment of desire,[33] Baudrillard, like Bauman, might point to the primacy of the object rather than subject-orientation in contemporary modalities of self-care. Self-crafting as an art of existence has become object and simulation oriented. Athletes' diets simulate and hyperbolize doctors' proscribed diets; ergogenics mimic and supplant whole foods in the practice of self-care. Doctors and their knowledge become merely commodities in the self-stylization process. Their subjectivities are de-centered in the process and transform into signs for production and signification in the process of doing athlete identity. John, a forty-three-year-old veteran triathlete tells me: "Triathletes are funny because many of us are far more clinical and regimented about eating than the most militant doctor. But we don't eat in a way that a doctor might tell you to eat! They [doctors] provide the basic information, and that's it really." *Doctors without degrees* are flesh artists in this sense, seduced by the ruse of biological liberation (that is, the controlled and predictable performance of the object body) offered by plastic foods. More information about eating leads not to an art (of eating) for all in an emancipatory manner. Baudrillard argues we live in an "excremental world" categorized by increasing amount of information but less meaning.[34] Here, modernity collapses under the weight of information with catastrophic implications for meaning where we think that information produces meaning, but the opposite occurs. Clint (age forty-five) says to me one day in the middle of an interview: "In some strange way, I think I've lost any sense of what is real about food, and who knows what to eat. About half the time I'm eating something, I look down at it and say, 'What the hell is this really, anyway?' The contents mean something to me, but the process of eating just doesn't. I don't seriously desire to eat; I just want to eat properly." The meaning, truth and the real regarding food are reversed by doctors without degrees, and partially become restricted to local, partial and seductive objects like nutritional supplements. This world of real food and real eating—which we inhabit like living phantoms in the desert—is a place where we may not have a politics of the desiring subject, but we do have *fatal strategies*.

At first glance, a common desire to perform well among triathletes leads to an ethnopharmacological science of eating, to be better, to perform and to be predictable—quintessential modernist thinking and performance strategy. But as triathletes progress through Baudrillard's third-order simulacrum (into the realm of eating for the image or thought of performance), chemically designed superfoods seduce beyond performance terms alone.[35] Perfectly engineered (at least in theory) foods call people to eat through a unique logic, the logic of calculation and mastery. Real knowledge of their embodied effects is no longer sought out as the promise or simulation of perfection is enough and ethnopharmacology flourishes.

> As a triathlete, supplements and sports products are so everywhere that they become regarded as logical. The more you consume them, the more normal it becomes. I had to laugh a year ago at this . . . I went out to a restaurant with a few friends for lunch, about a week away from Nationals. They ordered whatever—typical choices like burgers and nachos and sandwiches, and I ordered small garden salad and a Perrier. I was starving, but nothing on the menu looked appetizing. I didn't want to be rude to the waiter so I ordered the salad. We were sitting on a patio, and I noticed a GNC (nutrition) store across the street and down a hundred yards or so. I grabbed my cell phone right after we ordered, said I had to make a call, and then ran down [to GNC]

and bought a protein bar. I scoffed it down running back to the restaurant. . . . You might laugh, but when it's how you eat all the time,
and how you need to eat to stay fit, it's hard to compromise because it's
necessary, you know. (Gwen, 36)

Objects of plastic eating in the hands of triathletes do not simply liberate
them to self-style and craft their own regimens of eating, but rather pave
the way for the triumph of the hyperreal diet—plastic diets that are viewed
as more real versions of food than raw, unprocessed, organic food. Baudrillard writes: "The fetish performs this miracle of erasing the accidentiality
of the world and substituting for it an absolute necessity."[36]

Yet Baudrillard might not, and somewhat surprisingly to some, decry the
triumph of the object in sports nutrition. In *Fatal Strategies*, Baudrillard
writes that within obscenely obese information cultures individuals should
thus surrender to the world of objects, learning their ruses and strategies,
and should give up the project of sovereignty and control. He appears to
base this strategy on the idea that the subject has shown it cannot dominate
the object. Modern progress is associated with the domination of nature
and directs the natural and social world in a progressive direction, but
surely this has all imploded and become impossible in the current era where
subject cannot be distinguished from object—where reality and image cannot be separated, and society takes on a new dynamic. Baudrillard, like
Kroker,[37] associates this new society with the victory of the object and proposes that we ourselves become more like things, like objects, and eschew
the illusion and hubris of the control of subjectivity. Likewise, he proposes
that it is useless to change or control the world and that we should give
up such subjective strategies and adopt the *fatal strategies* of objects. He
argues for taking things to their extreme and, by so doing, surpassing the
limits and subverting the tendencies because, "only the subject desires; only
the object seduces."[38] We must, therefore, become more like objects in our
increasingly pataphysical society.

Serious recreational triathletes often engage plastic eating to the extreme,
to its extensive object-orientation. Just as the body is objectified through
rigorous training and competition, that which enters the body through
the act of digestion is objectified; as such the ritual of eating as a form of
group/cultural life is similarly objectified with incredible precision. Finn
(age twenty-seven) recounts: "Not only can I tell you what I'll eat today,
but for like the next month. Almost by the hour, really." The more fake
fooding encompasses one's daily corporeal regime, the more their ethics of
self-care become objectified in an almost transhumanist (i.e., quasi-cyborg)
manner. Fake food and tastes of the synthetic become better than the real,
especially in a world in which people fear or suspect raw, unprocessed and
natural foods for their deficiencies or excesses. Ferne (age thirty) states, "I
tried a bit of pure chocolate at a coffee shop the other day, and I dunno, it
just doesn't taste as good as the chocolate they put into [energy] bars." As I
write the past few lines, I am reminded of an excerpt from my field notes:

The basement of Greg's house is bursting with of blue, orange and grey boxes. I mean he usually has stacks and stacks of them, but even more than usual tonight. Probably four hundred or so neatly lined up around the walls, hiding the fake wood paneling of the basement. We're down here playing a game of a pool at a party he's hosting for us [a triathlon team] . . . People are talking to me, asking what races are coming up, I stop to take a shot every minute or so, and I just cannot take my eyes of the boxes. They are protein bars and energy gels Greg buys in bulk to pass on to the group. They are astonishing, so neatly packed up and uniform and perfect in athletic content. It's like the first time I saw a naked woman in a *Playboy* magazine. My gaze is fixed and I'm not quite sure how to process the visual as a neophyte. All of the bars will be, eventually, eaten by friends of mine over the course of the summer. Someone is asking me, I think Stuart, about my new racing rims, but I lean over to Greg and say, "Mate, I just have to ask about these bars. What the hell? Does it ever bother you to have all of them in the basement?" "They'll only be here for a couple of weeks. Most people ordered five or six boxes a long time ago. Wait and see, half of them will be gone after the party tonight!" As the last two words come from his mouth, my eyes shoot across the room. Sure enough, three or four people are already sizing up the lot, placing bits of tape with their names imprinted on them to mark their ergogenic territory. There is party food all around—which I notice is not being eaten—but thoughts are on the bars, as always.

REFLECTIONS [REFRACTIONS]

The degree to which triathletes incorporate fake foods into their diets is by no means at the extreme end in high-performance sports cultures. Groups like professional bodybuilders, for example, take sports supplementation to a level not yet reached in triathlon circles. But the degree to which even recreational athletes replace whole or unprocessed foods with ergogenics is noteworthy nevertheless. Additionally, the manners by which athletes are replacing real with fake foods mirrors and dovetails with the processes by which sports doctors, nutritionists and others are being replaced as hegemonic "experts" in sports contexts. The increasing disappearance of "regular" food and medical monitoring of nutrition practices in triathlon is perhaps a harbinger of transhumanist eating tendencies and a bioethic of radical libertarianism in sport and elsewhere. The do-it-yourself nature of triathlon diets and the manners by which the athletes tend to eschew eating advice "from the outside" is sociologically fascinating. Curiously enough, at a time when kinesiological borders within the university are expanding, and when sports nutritionists (among others therein) are in high demand, it seems that those with officially sanctioned medical knowledge have never been more subculturally challenged.

Indeed, the homeopathic logics underpinning ethnopharmacological practices in triathlon cultures and elsewhere are outcroppings of life in a late modern society. Conditions of difference, bio-liberation and knowledge/information ubiquity hail individual and collective triathletes to fashion their own systems of dietary production as an ethic of self-care. Here, *doctor's orders* regarding food and diet are only shards of advice to be used in manners the athletes see fit. Objectified, routinized and blankly rationalized forms of plastic-eating-for-performance comprise one but many of the bioethical standards upheld within many modern triathlete formations, and, in some ways, typify the sorts of fatal strategies of complete triumph of the object Baudrillard outlines. The *oeuvre* toward self-customization and styling (through diet or any other personal practice) and the systematic challenges it poses to the authority of any one group's biopower (such as licensed doctors or dieticians) may be, as Baudrillard comments, somewhat post-political.[39] The growing distrust of doctors' and dieticians' prescriptions for proper food intake among triathletes is not an overt political contestation focusing on identities or signifying practices at odds within a hierarchy of social control. Ethnopharmacology is, rather, a gesture of outright indifference or ambivalence toward more modern knowledge bases and recommendations. Sports nutritionists, dieticians and others, of course, from time to time, recommend a handful of sports supplements to the athletes, but triathletes themselves transform and hyperbolize the recommendations in their own ways. Such is an interesting trend in shifting power relations between people in the triathlon figuration: such that important challenges to the outright biopower of medical experts have been initiated. In becoming *doctors without degrees* and relishing their group's own preferences for and knowledge bases regarding plastic eating, triathletes illustrate how locally produced, existential knowledge has considerable cultural capital in late modern physical cultures.

I burned out today in what will probably be my last long-distance triathlon of the year. A mix of physical and mental fatigue have finally conquered my resolve to run or bike or swim for now. I'm sitting here, slumped down in the back of Donna's minivan on the ride home and the combination of dried sweat and sunburn on my skin reminds me how much my body has taken a beating over the past eight months. Helen is passing around a bunch of homemade recovery bars and the smell is almost sickeningly sweet. "Eat, you need to eat, Michael," she says to me like a priest forcing Communion. I grab three squares from the plastic container and gobble them down. About 60 percent of my diet is now "performance food." A year ago I laughed at Stan, Dave and Rob for basing their diet on sports foods. But here I am, dying for nourishment and my first thought of an ideal food is a sports bar comprised mainly of protein power. I've changed a lot, my body has changed a lot and I have a totally different relationship with food now.

I remember thinking this just before the race today. Glancing across the race zone [at the starting line], all I could see were booths containing ergogenics. No bananas, natural juice drinks or anything resembling grown food. I wonder what my body is becoming. Eating food out of tins and plastic wrappers and things you need to mix isn't so crazy to me anymore, but it still doesn't seem real. But I'm hungry now and eat protein bars because it makes sense, and just feels like the right thing to do sitting here in Donna's car.

NOTES

1. Baudrillard, *Fatal Strategies*, 29.
2. In all cases, pseudonyms are employed to protect participants' identities.
3. Atkinson, "Triathalon."
4. Hathaway and Atkinson, "Active Interview Tactics."
5. See Bloor, Monaghan and Dobash, "Body as a Chemistry Experiment"; Monaghan, "Challenging Medicine?"; "Looking Good Feeling Good"; "Vocabularies of Motive."
6. Dunning and Waddington, "Sport as a Drug"; Beamish and Ritchie, "Performance and Performance-Enhancement"; Waddington et al., "Drug Use"; Atkinson and Young, *Deviance and Social Control*; Beamish, "Social Construction"; Waddington and Smith, *Addicted to Winning*.
7. Mottram, *Drugs in Sport*.
8. Atkinson, "Playing with Fire."
9. Tscholl, Junge and Dvorak, "Use of Medication."
10. Huang, Johnson and Pipe, "Use of Dietary Supplements."
11. Schwenk and Costley, "When Food Becomes a Drug."
12. Sherman and Thompson, "Athletes and Disordered Eating"; Smolak, Murnen and Ruble, "Female Athletes."
13. Sundot-Borgen, "Prevalence of Eating Disorders"; Tiggemann and Kuring, "Role of Body Objectification."
14. Pritchard and Tiggemann, "Objectification in Fitness Centers."
15. Thøgersen-Ntoumani and Ntoumanis, "Self-Determination Theory Approach."
16. Bas, Karabudak and Kiziltan, "Vegetarianism and Eating Disorders."
17. Vardar, Vardar and Kurt, "Anxiety."
18. Arguete, Gold and Schwartz, "Eating Attitudes."
19. Tiggemann and Kuring, "Role of Body Objectification."
20. Reinking and Alexander, "Prevalence."
21. Mountford, Haase and Waller, "Body Checking."
22. Calam and Slade, "Sexual Experience."
23. Atkinson, "Playing with Fire."
24. Theberge, "We Have All the Bases Covered"; Malcolm, "Unprofessional Practice?"
25. Kim, "Conventional Medicine."
26. Pike, "Doctors Just Say." See also Pike in this collection.
27. Porucznik, Reeser and Willick, "Use of Pain Medication."
28. Safai, "Healing the Body."
29. Baudrillard, *Simulations*, 146.
30. Baudrillard, *Fatal Strategies*.

31. Baudrillard, *Simulations*; *Ecstasy of Communication*; *Fatal Strategies*; *Transparency of Evil.*
32. Bauman, *Art of Life*, 9.
33. Foucault, "Ethics of the Concern."
34. Baudrillard, *Ecstasy of Communication*; *Fatal Strategies.*
35. Baudrillard, *Fatal Strategies*, 140.
36. Baudrillard, *Simulations.*
36. Baudrillard, *Fatal Strategies*, 145.
37. Kroker, *Will to Technology.*
38. Baudrillard, *Fatal Strategies*, 141.

BIBLIOGRAPHY

Arguete, M., E. Gold and H. Schwartz. "Eating Attitudes, Body Satisfaction, and Perfectionism in Female College Athletes." *North American Journal of Psychology* 7 (2005): 345–352.

Atkinson, Michael. "Playing with Fire: Masculinity, Health and Sports Supplements." *Sociology of Sport Journal* 24 (2007): 165–186.

———. "Triathlon, Suffering and Exciting Significance." *Leisure Studies* 27 (2008): 165–180.

Atkinson, M., and K. Young. *Deviance and Social Control in Sport.* Champaign, IL: Human Kinetics, 2008.

Bas, M., E. Karabudak and G. Kiziltan. "Vegetarianism and Eating Disorders: Association between Eating Attitudes and Other Psychological Factors among Turkish Adolescents." *Appetite* 44 (2005): 309–315.

Baudrillard, Jean. *The Ecstasy of Communication.* New York: Semiotext(e), 1988.

———. *Fatal Strategies.* New York: Semiotext(e), 1990.

———. *Simulations.* New York: Semiotext(e), 1983.

———. *The Transparency of Evil.* London: Verso, 1993.

Bauman, Zygmunt. *The Art of Life.* Cambridge: Polity, 2008.

Beamish, Rob. "The Social Construction of Steroid Subcultures." In *Tribal Play: Sport Subcultures and Countercultures*, edited by Michael Atkinson and Kevin Young, 273–294. London: Elsevier Press, 2008.

Beamish, R., and I. Ritchie. "Performance and Performance-Enhancement in Sport: The Paradigm Shift in the Science of 'Training' and Performance-Enhancing Substances." *Sport in History* 25 (2005): 434–451.

Bloor, M., L. Monaghan and R. Dobash. "The Body as a Chemistry Experiment: Steroid Use among South Wales Bodybuilders." In *The Body in Everyday Life*, edited by S. Nettleton and J. Watson, 27–44. London: Routledge, 1999.

Calam, R., and P. Slade. "Sexual Experience and Eating Problems in Female Undergraduates." *International Journal of Eating Disorders* 8 (1989): 391–397.

Dunning, E., and I. Waddington. "Sport as a Drug and Drugs in Sport." *International Review for the Sociology of Sport* 38 (2003): 351–336.

Foucault, Michel. "The Ethics of the Concern for Self as a Practice of Freedom." In *Foucault Live (Interviews, 1961–1984)*, edited by Sylvère Lotringer, 432–449. New York: Semiotext(e), 1996.

Hathaway, A., and M. Atkinson. "Active Interview Tactics in Research on Public Deviance: Exploring the Two Cop Personas." *Field Methods* 15 (2004): 161–185.

Huang, S., K. Johnson and A. Pipe. "The Use of Dietary Supplements and Medications by Canadian Athletes at the Atlanta and Sydney Olympic Games." *Clinical Journal of Sports Medicine* 16 (2006): 27–33.

Kim, H. "Do Not Put Too Much Value on Conventional Medicine." *Journal of Ethnopharmacology* 100 (2005): 37–39.

Kroker, A. *The Will to Technology and the Culture of Nihilism: Heidegger, Nietzsche & Marx*. Toronto: University of Toronto Press, 2004.

Malcolm, Dominic. "Unprofessional Practice? The Status and Power of Sports Physicians." *Sociology of Sport Journal* 23 (2004): 376–395.

Monaghan, Lee. "Challenging Medicine? Bodybuilding, Drugs and Risk." *Sociology of Health & Illness* 21 (1999): 707–734.

———. "Looking Good, Feeling Good: The Embodied Pleasures of Vibrant Physicality." *Sociology of Health & Illness* 23 (2001): 330–356.

———. "Vocabularies of Motive for Illicit Steroid Use among Bodybuilders." *Social Science & Medicine* 55 (2002): 695–708.

Mottram, David. *Drugs in Sport*. London: Routledge, 2005.

Mountford, V., A. Haase and G. Waller. "Body Checking in the Eating Disorders: Associations between Cognitions and Behaviours." *International Journal of Eating Disorders* 39 (2006): 708–715.

Pike, Elizabeth. "Doctors Just Say 'Rest and Take Ibuprofen.'" *International Review for the Sociology of Sport* 40 (2005): 201–219.

Porucznik, C., J. Reeser and S. Willick. "Use of Pain Medication among Collegiate Club Volleyball Players." *Medicine and Science in Sports Exercise* 39 (2007): S394–S395.

Pritchard, I., and M. Tiggemann. "Objectification in Fitness Centers: Self Objectification, Body Dissatisfaction, and Disordered Eating in Aerobic Instructors and Aerobic Participants." *Sex Roles* 53 (2005): 19–28.

Reinking, M., and L. Alexander. "Prevalence of Disordered Eating Behaviors in Undergraduate Female Collegiate Athletes and Non-Athletes." *Journal of Athletic Training* 40 (2005): 47–51.

Safai, Parissa. "Healing the Body in the 'Culture of Risk': Examining the Negotiation of Treatment between Sports Medicine Clinicians and Injured Athletes in Canadian Intercollegiate Sport." *Sociology of Sport Journal* 20 (2003): 127–146.

Schwenk, T., and C. Costley. "When Food Becomes a Drug: Nonanabolic Nutritional Supplement Use in Athletes." *American Journal of Sports Medicine* 30 (2002): 907–916.

Sherman, R., and R. Thompson. "Athletes and Disordered Eating: Four Major Issues for the Professional Psychologist." *Professional Psychology: Research and Practice* 32 (2001): 27–33.

Smolak, L., S. Murnen and A. Ruble. "Female Athletes and Eating Problems: A Meta-Analysis." *International Journal of Eating Disorders* 27 (2000): 371–380.

Sundot-Borgen, J. "The Prevalence of Eating Disorders in Elite Female Athletes." *International Journal of Sports Nutrition* 3 (1993): 29–40.

Theberge, Nancy. "'We Have All the Bases Covered.' Constructions of Professional Boundaries in Sport Medicine." *International Review for the Sociology of Sport* 44 (2009): 265–282.

Thøgersen-Ntoumani, C., and N. Ntoumanis. "A Self-Determination Theory Approach to the Study of Body Image Concerns, Self-Presentation and Self-Perceptions in a Sample of Aerobic Instructors." *Journal of Health Psychology* 12 (2007): 301–315.

Tiggemann, M., and J. Kuring. "The Role of Body Objectification in Disordered Eating and Depressed Mood." *British Journal of Clinical Psychology* 43 (2004): 299–311.

Tscholl, P., A. Junge and J. Dvorak. "The Use of Medication and Nutritional Supplements during FIFA World Cups 2002 and 2006." *British Journal of Sports Medicine* 42 (2008): 725–730.

Vardar, E., S. Vardar and C. Kurt. "Anxiety of Young Female Athletes with Disordered Eating Behaviors." *Eating Behaviors* 8 (2004): 143–147.

Waddington, I., D. Malcolm, M. Roderick and R. Naik. "Drug Use in English Professional Football." *British Journal of Sports Medicine* 39 (2005): 18–23.

Waddington, I., and A. Smith. *Addicted to Winning: An Introduction to Drugs in Sport*. London: Routledge, 2009.

14 Pre-Participation Screenings in Sports

A Review of Current Genetic/Nongenetic Test Strategies[1]

Arno Müller

Sport, or at least regular physical activity, is by evidence-based criteria seen as primary and secondary prevention for illnesses such as cardiovascular diseases. Analysis suggests that benefits of regular physical activity outweigh potential health costs.[2] So-called pre-participation examinations may reduce the potential health risks for athletes. Because current pre-participation examinations—either mandatory or voluntary—do not consider genomics to contribute to the reduction of those risks, sports medicine can be seen as both an emerging field of application and an area of marked uncertainty. The expectation of scientists worldwide is that in the next decades the world of sport will be confronted with a variety of *promises*, varying from preventive screening to the genetic selection of talent and the enhancement of athletic performance with *gene doping*.

The chapter reports some of the findings from a project conducted by researchers at Maastricht University investigating how physicians, athletes and organizations in sport and medicine frame ethical and societal issues raised by preventive and selective applications of genomics in sports and sport medicine. The chapter starts by looking at how mass electrocardiogram (ECG) screening of athletes is organized in different national and continental contexts. It explores the controversial role of the Italian model of *mandatory* mass screening as a standard bearer. The chapter then discusses some of the broader debates about whether genetic testing might be introduced alongside or instead of existing screening, before addressing the concerns voiced by various stakeholders about the implementation of such technological developments. The chapter draws on literature in sports medicine and cardiology journals and data from interviews with over twenty high-performance athletes, coaches, sport cardiologists, etc., as well as three workshops/focus group discussions with various stakeholders.[3] The chapter concludes by arguing that there is no agreement on nongenetic screening strategies and therefore genetic screenings should (if at all) be performed only as a test on demand. Future decisions should be guided by the respect for the athlete's autonomous decision.

PRE-PARTICIPATION SCREENING IN SPORT

In many European countries athletes have to undergo a health examination, the so-called *pre-participation examination* or *pre-participation
screening* (PPS).[4] Physical activity and sport especially cause stress to the
cardiovascular system so medical clearance is sometimes required for athletes to participate in organized competitive sports. Screenings primarily
consist of examinations of cardiological features, physical aspects and personal and family (medical) history. Although the current standard of PPS
is *nongenetic*, the analysis of family history can be seen as a reverse form
of genetic screening. However, as we shall see, the rigor of the screening
procedure varies across Europe.

The current PPS *standard* is that there is *no standard*. However, in most
European countries a distinction is made between amateurs and high-performance or elite athletes. In some countries nonelite athletes do not receive
regular PPS (e.g., Denmark) or only a basic medical checkup such as a review
of medical history and an ECG at rest (e.g., Germany). In the case of high-
performance-level athletes (e.g., Olympic squad members), sports federations
may *demand* certain examinations to allow athletes to participate.[5] National
and continental sport medical associations, such as the European Society
for Cardiology (ESC), the American College of Cardiology (ACC) and the
American Heart Association (AHA)[6] also *recommend* specific examinations.
A third form of the institutionalization of PPS is to oblige athletes to undergo
those examinations by a *national law*. For example, in France national regulations about PPS only apply to high-performance athletes, whereas in Italy
national law obliges high-performance athletes *and* amateurs to undergo
PPS. The Italian case is, however, exceptional within Europe.

Evidence suggests that most cases of sudden death due to hypertrophic
cardiomyopathy (HCM) occur between the ages of twelve and thirty-five
years. Thus, for example, the Study Group of Sport Cardiology of the ESC
stated in their 2005 Consensus Statement that "screening should start at
the beginning of competitive athletic activity, which for the majority of
sports disciplines corresponds to an age of 12–14 years."[7] Other bodies
have issued similar recommendations. For example, the so-called "Lausanne Recommendations," which were formulated under the umbrella of
the International Olympic Committee (IOC) Medical Commission, recommend pre-participation cardiovascular screening for all participants at the
beginning of competitive activities until the age of thirty-five years.[8] An
AHA task force recommends that PPS should start for athletes aged fifteen
years old.[9] Östman-Smith et al. argue in favor of introducing screening
even earlier.[10] The UK-based initiative Cardiac Risk in the Young (CRY)
also argues for screening to start at an early age, but states that "for the
screening programme to be fully effective, all young people (aged 35 and
under) involved in sporting activities should undergo an ECG."[11]

The Italian PPS model, where PPSs are *mandatory* and abnormal findings lead to *exclusion* from competitive sports, is held by some to be the most rigorous model of examination. It was established in Italian law in 1982,[12] and Italy remains the only country in the world where all citizens (i.e., professionals *and* amateurs) aged twelve to thirty-five years, participating in organized and competitive sports, are required to undergo preventive general medical and cardiovascular evaluation. This routinely includes 12-lead ECG, in addition to a review of personal and family history, and a physical examination (with measurement of blood pressure). Italian physicians who carry out PPS are licensed specialists in sports medicine who have undergone a full-time postgraduate residency program for four years.[13] PPS evaluations are usually performed in sports clinics and private offices, which are present in virtually all communities with populations above ten thousand. An estimated three million sportspeople are evaluated annually throughout Italy.

Athletes judged to be free of cardiovascular disease[14] (or other limiting conditions) obtain a certificate of eligibility for competitive sports. Others are referred to major clinical centers for the purpose of diagnosis and assessment of eligibility for competitive sports. Athletes cleared in national PPS may become members of the Italian national teams. Of these elite athletes, about five hundred per year are selected and referred to the Institute of Sports Medicine and Science in Rome for a medical and physiological evaluation before their participation in national or international events. This protocol routinely includes echocardiography.[15]

Abnormal PPS findings lead to a subject being declared unfit and mean that the athlete is no longer allowed to participate in sport at the club or federation levels. The athlete can file a complaint against a positive test result, but it is strictly forbidden for a club to allow such an athlete to participate in organized activities because a health-damaging pathology could be existent. Even if the club has the written consent of the athlete or his/her parents, it cannot disclaim liability. Athletes can only participate with PPS validation.[16]

The ESC recommendations mark the first attempt to standardize screening programs across Europe. These recommendations were dominated by the Italian screening strategy. Although Pelliccia et al. labeled their recommendation a *consensus document*, there was disagreement on the screening strategy, especially within Scandinavian countries (e.g., Denmark,[17] Norway). Firstly, the Danish Task Force on Sudden Death argued that the Italian data were limited because it was only based on the Veneto region. Second, the cost-effectiveness was questioned because of the rare occurrence of sudden death in athletes under thirty-five years (i.e., one to two per one hundred thousand per year). Others questioned the efficacy of ECG examinations that form the core element of the Italian PPS model and the ESC recommendations. Lawless and Best note:

Although some authorities advocate the use of ECG screening of young athletes, further studies are required to define what constitutes a normal ECG in athletes, and to determine whether ECG-based screening protocols truly are superior, not only in finding disease, but also saving lives. For those who either choose ECG-based screening or interpret ECG in athletes, we propose a simple interpretation scheme and decision tree.[18]

Besides *technical controversies*, some *conceptual weaknesses* within the European recommendations can also be identified. Even though Pelliccia et al. have continued to show "evidence" for their screening program,[19] de Wert and Vos[20] and also Wren criticize the 2005 recommendations for being unclear on key terms like "pre-participation," "young" and "competitive." The foundation of the screening program can be regarded as weak if conceptual uncertainties guide the recommendations.

Some of the Scandinavian opposition might be related to the use of *mass* screenings. Hernelahti et al. cite costs, logistics, inefficiency and the risk of false-positive findings (i.e., a test result that incorrectly suggests the presence of a disease) as arguments against the general cardiovascular screening of athletes.[21] In Sweden, the Board of Health and Welfare recommends examination of certain risk groups only; for example for first-degree relatives to patients with familial cardiac diseases associated with a risk of Sudden Cardiac Death (SCD), and young people with exercise-related symptoms, as well as top athletes. [22]

Whereas the ESC recommendations aim for *European-wide* implementation, in 2007 Corrado et al. suggested a *worldwide* approach.[23] Others, such as Douglas, repeated this call:

> Although both US and European guidelines recommend screening athletes for suspected heart disease before participation in competitive sport, they disagree on which findings are associated with increased risk as well as those athletes whose activities should be restricted. Recent Italian data suggest that screening programs can save lives, but few countries have fully adopted such practices. It is time to develop an international consensus on who should receive pre-participation screening, who should perform the screening, what tests the screening should consist of, and what criteria should be used to restrict participation.[24]

Such was the momentum of this movement that, in 2008, the Bethesda Conference #36 made a further appeal for a global approach.[25]

PROPOSALS FOR GENETIC TESTING/SCREENING

Genetic testing includes a wide range of tests: for example, testing for treatable and nontreatable conditions, for conditions that are present at different stages of life and for so-called "carrier testing" of healthy individuals to determine their reproductive risks. In order to avoid forms of *genetic overgeneralization* (i.e., the lack of differentiation between different genetic tests, different test results and different forms of genetic information), it is necessary to be clear about key terms and the way they are meant to be understood within this chapter.

It is important to distinguish between *genetic tests* and *genetic (population) screenings*. Although a range of definitions exist, in the context of this chapter *genetic testing* is to be understood as the testing of individuals who request such a test because they already have a medical problem or are worried that they may be at risk. In the literature we can find the following definition: tests that are "offered to individuals known to be at increased risk of a condition in order to answer the question, 'Does this person have this disease?'"[26] *Genetic screening* is to be understood as a systematic offer of tests to a larger group of people (for example, the population of competitive athletes) that are free of symptoms and have not voiced concerns about their genetic makeup/propensity to illness. The literature defines *screenings* as examinations that "are offered to a population of apparently healthy persons in order to find those few at increased risk."[27]

Genomics (the study of genomes) can be seen as an additional tool to improve health checkup standards. In order to illustrate the potential impact of genomics and predictive medicine upon the future of public health, interviewees were asked about two sport-related examples for application: (a) genetic screening for *cardiovascular risks*, and (b) genetic screening for *neurological risks*. Although the identification of so-called *athletic genes* was not the primary focus of this study—the project had a clear stress on the *preventive* aspect of genomics in the field of sports—performance-related genetic testing is an expanding market, not only economically, but also with regard to (sport) science (see also Kondo and McNamee's contribution to this collection).[28] Thus it cannot be completely neglected here also because the distinction between preventive genetic tests and performance-related genetic tests is unclear. For instance, the angiotensin-converting enzyme (ACE) is related to general physical performance but is also associated, for example, with coronary heart disease and hypertension.[29]

HCM is one of the leading causes of SCD in sports settings. The position of the UK-based Cardiomyopathy Association (CMA) serves as a general introduction into the medical assumptions underlying screening strategies. The CMA assumes that gene testing will help future treatment. Although carrying a gene is not the same as suffering the disease, the earlier a condition is diagnosed the more effectively a disease can be managed, with side effects minimized and patient quality of life improved. Family screening, which allows early diagnosis and prevention of SCD, becomes of increasing importance. However, the interpretation of the subtle findings can be difficult in the general population, and the risk of false positive results is high. It is therefore important to understand the familial pattern of the cardiomyopathies and intensify efforts to recognize and manage the people who *are* at risk of having or later developing these

conditions. Increased awareness among families and medical professionals is a cornerstone for that.[30]

The CMA remains cautious about the predictive power of genetic tests:
"to date a positive result in gene testing in cardiomyopathy cannot predict if
the individual is going to develop the disease when it is going to develop or
what the prognosis is going to be."[31] But what role could preventive genetic
testing play in the context of sports? The case of the Italian gold medal–
winning swimmer Domenico Fioravanti, who in 2004 was banned from
competitive sport because of his health status, is illustrative. Fioravanti
was diagnosed HCM in nongenetic PPS, but because exercise may lead to
similar changes to the heart muscle the diagnosis could not be definitive.
Because genetic testing is assumed to have the potential to more accurately
diagnose HCM than existing procedures Fioravanti was reported as hoping
that their introduction "may one day weed out those who have a high risk
of suffering sudden death from those with a low risk, and so allow people
like him to compete."[32] Italian cardiologists, however, expressed their reservations about the introduction of genetic screenings to identify HCM.

> HCM is characterized by large genetic heterogeneity; 19 genes and 2
> loci have been associated with the disease, and hundreds of different
> mutations have been identified. As a consequence, searching for muta-
> tions in so many genes is unlikely to become the preferred approach for
> the introduction of genetic screening for HCM in clinical practice.[33]

Yet genetic testing remains a hot topic within (sport) medicine and among
policy makers in a variety of countries. In Germany a law has recently
been implemented that addresses the aspects of "genetic diagnosis," the so-
called "Gendiagnostikgesetz—GenDG."[34] German policy makers are usually relatively reluctant to address genetic issues (compared, e.g., to those in
the Netherlands), and guidelines for PPS in sports (*Leitlinie Vorsorgeuntersuchung im Sport*) published by the German Society for Sports Medicine
and Prevention (DGSP) should be seen within that tradition.[35] The DGSP
has sought to avoid *genetic issues* so far; only *Familienanamnese* (family
history) is explicitly mentioned. For Wildor Hollmann, a German sports
medicine expert and honorary president of the Fédération Internationale de
Médecine du Sport (FIMS), "further genetic screenings do not seem to be
sensible at the moment."[36]

The UK government's position on the relationship between genetic testing and HCM is stated in the Department of Health's framework document. It notes a potential value of genetic testing:

> Clinical evaluation of first degree relatives is recommended annu-
> ally through adolescence and every 5 years thereafter. The ongoing
> need for clinical evaluation underscores one of the potential values of
> gene testing to establish disease risk status. Probands should undergo

mutation analysis and when a probable disease causing mutation is identified, cascade screening of the family will identify those individuals who require ongoing clinical evaluation and permit reassurance of the remainder.[37]

The French position on genetic testing is that it "is not needed for every case; only if there are indications, e.g., family history."[38] There is, however, some interest in exploratory research on genetic testing of larger groups of athletes. In many other European countries genetic testing plays no role in the current PPS context. During interviews with Danish experts, for example, a strong opposition was expressed to genetic and nongenetic mass screening approaches.[39]

In the US, Barry Maron, a sports medicine expert and director of the Minneapolis Heart Institute Foundation, has been reported as having "serious doubts about the usefulness of this genetic test for diagnosis." In his view, "It misses not only 25% of the genes already linked to the condition . . . but also the many other genetic mutations that are probably involved but have not yet been discovered." The costs of comprehensive testing, even if it were available, would prohibit its use for young athletes.[40] Conversely, American cardiologists Ng and Maginot hold that some cases should be referred to appropriate specialists such as a geneticist or a genetic counselor because absence of a positive family history does not rule out cardiac abnormality.[41]

Australia's National Health and Medical Research Council (NHMRC) explicitly addresses sports medicine concerns on its website.[42] Asking, "Can genetic screening be used to determine predisposition to illness or injury?" the NHMRC position reads as follows:

> The use of genetic testing to determine whether an individual has a predisposition to sports-related illnesses or injuries is still experimental. It is known that some genetic disorders (e.g. Marfan syndrome—associated with tallness, and an abnormality of the aorta that can lead to rupturing and death) can represent a serious health risk in someone undertaking strenuous activity. In, for example, the professional basketball associations, physical appearances of Marfan syndrome or features of this disorder detectable by a test such as echocardiography might be looked for in professional athletes.

A second important question addresses the *legal* concerns about genetic testing in the sporting area.

> The use of genetic testing and genetic information to exclude people from participation in sport, directly or indirectly, will become a bigger issue in future, especially where there is a genetic predisposition to a condition, rather than evidence of an existing disease. The Australian

Law Reform Commission and the NHMRC through the 2003 *Essentially Yours* report recommended that, as a general rule, predictive genetic information should not be used to make decisions affecting employment (this would extend to sport).[43]

Thus, on the one hand, they deem the applicability of genetic tests as "experimental"; on the other hand, the NHMRC speculates that issues linked to genetic testing will increase in the future.

Some experts are more positive about genetic testing, noting that current (nongenetic) screening strategies seem insufficient for detecting cardiovascular diseases in athletes. For example, Dutch sports cardiologists Panhuyzen-Goedkoop and Verheugt affirm that "sudden cardiac death in young athletes (12–35 years) is usually caused by inherited or congenital cardiac disorders." They note that HCM is a genetic disease with a mutant gene variation, which "develops during adolescence where there is rapid hypertrophy during fast growth and development of the human body."[44] As a result they see "recommendations on future screening by gene analysis in an athlete suspected of HCM, other electrical cardiac diseases, or even in athletes coming for pre-participation cardiovascular screening will be a great step forward."[45] Additionally, findings of associations between certain genes and heart diseases as well as special gene pools nourish speculation about the feasibility of genetic screening strategies to protect athletes from SCD:

> Physicians should be aware of the emerging role of genetic testing for cardiovascular diseases in athletes with a family history of heart disease or sudden death. Advances in the diagnosis and understanding of cardiovascular disease may provide better tools for preventing sudden death of young athletes in the future.[46]

But again there are other voices, such as Michels et al., that urge against overestimating the usefulness of genotyping.[47] Another report argues, "With a few exceptions . . . prognosis based solely on genotype is premature and inappropriate, since exceptions for several initially identified genotype-phenotype associations were found."[48]

And some are clearly ambivalent about whether genetic tests will provide a solution to the uncertainties and costs of traditional (nongenetic) mass screening strategies. For example, Neish expresses doubts about the feasibility of "mass screening of asymptomatic athletes with no clues on physical examination," and argues that there are many risks involved in finding the right diagnosis. At the same time, however, he identifies the potential benefits of genetic screening of athletes: "Eventually, DNA testing may be a cost-effective way to screen for many cardiac diseases, including cardiomyopathies and many life-threatening arrhythmias."[49]

The ESC clearly expresses such dilemmas:

> Genetic analysis has the potential to provide a definitive diagnosis should any one of the most common mutant Genes be identified; however, important limitations remain, i.e. the substantial genetic heterogeneity of the disease with the potential of false-negative results, and the complex, time consuming and expensive techniques needed which, so far, limit routine implementation of genetic testing in clinical practice.[50]

Furthermore the ESC supports genetic testing of asymptomatic at-risk family members but again foresees problematic consequences. "As family genetic screening for HCM will largely be implemented in clinical practice, physicians will face the dilemma of making recommendations regarding sports participation for subjects who have only preclinical evidence of HCM (i.e. genotype positive—phenotype negative)."[51]

The comparison by Pelliccia et al. of US and European criteria for eligibility and disqualification of competitive athletes with cardiovascular abnormalities represents a *state-of-the-art* survey of PPS with a focus on genetic aspects. The authors did not aim for an exhaustive and comprehensive comparison of the European and American consensus documents, but focused their attention:

> on those areas that present the most relevant differences between the 2 documents with respect to risk evaluation and recommendations for competitive sports participation, as viewed through the prism of different medical, legal, and social backgrounds in the US and Europe. These considerations largely relate to those genetic cardiovascular diseases that are most relevant to sudden death in young athletes.[52]

Pelliccia et al. conclude that although "genetic testing" [*sic*] could be a helpful tool to diagnose congenital heart diseases, it is not routinely performed in either the US or in Europe.

> Current diagnosis of inherited arrhythmogenic cardiomyopathies might be greatly improved by the genetic testing of asymptomatic athletes. However, molecular analysis is currently not routine testing, either in the European or US screening programs, but is performed selectively (e.g., when LQTS or Marfan syndrome is suspected). Moreover, protocol [*sic*] for protecting the personal genetic information of highly visible athletes is not specifically discussed in either the European or US recommendations.[53]

Thus, within the scientific community a wide range of views exist on the value and feasibility of genetic testing as a countermeasure to HCM.

STAKEHOLDERS' VIEWS: ISSUES IN PREVENTIVE GENETIC TESTING/SCREENING

In the following section, the issues and problems raised by stakeholders (e.g., athletes, coaches, sport physicians, sport cardiologists) are addressed. These can be put into four categories: technological issues, issues related to prioritization of resources and testing, regulatory issues and concerns with genetic testing in general.

Technological Issues

Concerns about the accuracy of genetic tests were expressed by all stakeholder groups. The multidimensional character of defining "accuracy" is expressed in the following quote:

> Analytical validity of a genetic laboratory test is a measure of how well the test detects what it is designed to detect. It encompasses analytical sensitivity (the probability that the test will detect a gene variant it is designed to detect when present in a sample) and analytical specificity (the probability that the test will be negative when a specific variant tested for is not present in a sample). Clinical validity measures the extent to which an analytically valid test result can diagnose a disease or predict future disease. For predictive genetic tests, it includes positive predictive value (the ability to predict that an individual will develop a disease) and negative predictive value (the ability to predict that an individual will not develop a disease).[54]

In the eyes of some stakeholders genetic testing is seen as "science fiction." It is not only regarded as being a possibility for the future, but also as something that is not sophisticated enough for application today. It was said, for instance, that there is not enough supporting evidence and that current testing is unable to deal with "the complexity of certain cardiological diseases." Stakeholders further think of the test as something that creates rather than resolves *uncertainty* and is thus "of limited value" because of the inability to predict every abnormality. According to one sport cardiologist, "Cardiac deaths are not preventable, you can't find all of them by screening." Stakeholders that completely oppose genetic testing hold strong doubts about the validity and the predictive quality of the tests. There was a concern that the prospect of both *false-negative* (i.e., a result which incorrectly suggests that the disease is not there) and *false-positive* test results "might ruin the athletes' lives."

Prioritizing Resources

In setting priorities, a range of considerations were expressed. Some stakeholders questioned whether, if performance sport is an unhealthy activity, money should be allocated to it from the broader health care budget. Others argued that it is not only top athletes who are at risk, but people in all walks of life. If there are risks in life in general (e.g., from traffic), what is the rationale for genetic testing of athletes? The underlying assumptions here are that: (a) athletes are a rather small (sub)population of society; and (b) the number of incidents that could be detected by genetic testing is relatively low.

Stakeholders also identified a lack of adequate education and training of medical experts as influencing priorities. For instance, if not all cardiologists can fully read and interpret the ECG of performance athletes,[55] should resources be devoted to educating the medical experts? Closely connected to the supposed lack of training in interpreting the results of traditional tests, it was stated that the "real problem" is the gap of knowledge between the nonsport doctors with their "perfect knowledge in biochemistry and genetics" on the one side, and sport physicians who are not very well trained on this and might be vulnerable to lobby groups (like lobbyists from the pharmaceutical industry) on the other.

In advocating priorities the question of traditional (nongenetic) screening versus genetic testing was also raised. As we have seen, there is no standard PPS throughout Europe, and no general acceptance on what *should* be the standard. Sport cardiologists see this as a "question of information," of "how to convince people that this is a good thing to do." It is, thus, something that is felt likely to be implemented in future, with genetic testing coming after that. Thus, as a sport cardiologist put it, "We have to go step by step: first is to standardize the current screening program and implement it as widely as possible and then we can use genetic testing as an additional tool to identify genetically transmitted diseases." Yet debates about existing screening standards create *societal pressures* on politicians and policy makers, for none of them would want to be criticized for not taking the right measures to prevent sudden death in (young) athletes. With reference to the Italian model, one UK politician raised his concerns about falling behind some of the UK's European partners.

Although similar pressures regarding genetic testing will potentially emerge, their creation relates to whether or not genetic testing is regarded as being *essentially different* to nongenetic testing.56 What is seen to be different is the applicability of genetic testing for the two possible cases: (a) the neurological case (e.g., genetic testing of boxers to assess their risk of developing Parkinson's or Alzheimer's disease); and (b) the cardiological case (e.g., genetic testing for HCM). Here the view of some stakeholders was that it might be suitable to do genetic tests for cardiological problems, because they are "emergency," or life-and-death issues. For neurological problems—which might (or might not) come to expression in twenty or thirty years from now—such a test is regarded as less feasible.

Stakeholders also repeatedly mentioned economic pressures and the *cost-effectiveness* of genetic screenings. The majority of nonmedical stakeholders expressed the view that genetic screening is not cost-effective. Some sport physicians also doubt whether the small number of sudden deaths that do occur justify the high costs of mass testing or screening. Yet one neurologist involved in genetic testing in his daily practice stressed that genetic testing "is very easy and very cheap . . . it is not a financial question." A sports cardiologists similarly argued that compared, e.g. to the high cost of HIV prevention, "I think, when it is these young people . . . who die, and it's preventable. I think the price is not really a problem."

However, recognition of competing health care costs meant that several stakeholders see the implementation of genetic tests for athletes as unlikely and the lack of resources for traditional screening for athletes in some European countries is cited as supporting evidence. Although it is not entirely true that there are "no resources," the decision is highly political. One sport cardiologist confirmed this view by using the term *political reason* to describe (or even blame) the politicians and federations for not making traditional (nongenetic) PPS their first priority. Besides the pressures on the national economy in general and on the health care budget in particular there are financial pressures within the sport system itself. Neurologists involved in boxing mentioned that "of course we have to protect the players and boxers, but we have to be honest," because commercial pressures mean that efforts to protect the athlete's health might be ignored if the athletes stand to lose out financially. Yet although the (financial) impact on the health care system of a sudden death may be no greater than that of a patient who is in a persistent vegetative state,[57] the impact on the sport community, as one cardio-geneticist remarked, might be huge. Sudden death of an athlete live on TV would radically alter the parameters of this debate.

Regulation of Genetic Testing

How did stakeholders think testing in sport should be regulated? Those interviewees who were aware of the distinction between testing and screening suggested that the former should only be performed if other indicatory factors existed (e.g., family history). Testing of asymptomatic athletes was rejected because "genetics should be kept for disease."

Sport administrators argued that a genetic screening program for state-supported athletes (i.e., mainly top-level athletes) could more easily be justified for high-performance athletes than amateurs. More generally, a neurologist suggested that mandatory genetic testing can be justified if it is clearly linked to a profession. This would, e.g., include a profession like boxing in which the genetic risk of brain disease is increased by the activity. One coach felt that a genetic screening program of all athletes would be too paternalistic. In relation to testing minors, a sports scientist with legal expertise noted that, as in many other areas, decision-making responsibility lay with the parent/guardian. Nevertheless, there have been documented cases in which minors have been allowed to make their own decision.[58]

A majority of stakeholders argued that genetic testing should only be introduced on a voluntary basis. One reason for doing so is apparently the respect for the freedom and autonomy of the individual athlete. One athlete compared this issue to smoking, which, although not recommended, is a matter of personal liberty. In that context another athlete was concerned about team physicians that are prepared to do things to athletes that they wouldn't do to themselves.

It was also felt that mandatory screening might do more harm than good because it might deter people from taking part in what is, after all, "a very healthy activity and pursuit." Following this rationale genetic testing should be done only with the permission of the athletes. Whereas some athletes argued against any mandatory genetic tests, most elite athletes were highly pragmatic. Olympic athletes who were interviewed stated that as long as it did not hurt and as long as such genetic tests would not be too time-consuming, they would not object. Similarly an Olympic boxing coach said that genetic testing would be fine "as long as it helps to improve the image of our sport."

Others were concerned that genetic testing in the field of sports might effectively become a so-called *coercive offer*. That is to say, athletes might be given what appears to be a free choice, but the consequences of declining would effectively force the athlete to take the test; e.g., athletes who do not do the test will not get the license to compete. Moreover, the possibility of getting the athlete's *informed consent* [59] on such complex issues like genetic testing was questioned, as was the "inappropriate" medicalization of athletes through genetic testing. One position advocated was simply that "it's not a sports question, it's always a general recommendation." Other interviewees pointed out that the result of a genetic test should only be used to give advice to athletes.

Some stakeholders (including athletes) saw justification for a mandatory genetic screening for athletes. They argued that in high-performance sport human rights cannot be fully applied, for currently associations can "force" athletes to undertake other forms of regulatory testing (e.g., for drugs). The underlying argument is that athletes volunteer to be members of sports clubs or federations and have the freedom to go elsewhere to practice their sport. One athlete (a former Olympic champion from Eastern Europe) stated: "If you don't like to compete—don't compete! So if you do not want to do a genetic test don't engage, for example, in high-performance sports." One medical doctor suggested that genetic testing should be mandatory for all athletes (amateur and professionals), but exclusion should only be mandatory for professionals.

And what about the right *not* to know?[60] One medical doctor claimed this for himself: "I simply think that I really don't want to know." Is it possible to deny this right to the athlete? However, another doctor asserted that although the right not to know generally exists, "the athletes cannot claim to have this right because it seems inapplicable here."

A further area of regulation addressed the consequences for athletes with a positive genetics test. Although leading cardiological associations agree on the exclusion of athletes with HCM from competitive sports, a number of interviewees were in favor of leaving the decision to withdraw from competition to the individual athlete. Others wanted physicians to have the ultimate decision, whereas another group suggested that athletes *and* physicians should decide as a "team." Some interviewees stressed that as tests only address risk factors, uncertainties inevitably remain, and thus the legitimacy of a mandatory ban is questionable.

General Concerns about Genetics and Genetic Testing

A great number of genetic testing concerns expressed by stakeholders were not particularly linked to genetic testing in the field of sports but related to genetics in general. Interviewees noted that genetic tests generated "hugely sensitive data," which required considerable protection. Such direct interference with the privacy of athletes demanded that athletes' consent should be gained. There was also concern that this information could be misused for illegal enhancement, i.e., doping purposes, thus the primary aim of the tests had to be clear. From a coach's perspective, genetic tests could identify performance-relevant features. As one noted, "the more information I have to do my job—the better!" But it was also stated that a coach should not judge an athlete solely on the basis of a genetic test because, it was argued, application can compensate for genetic inheritance.

A further precondition for the implementation of routine genetic testing was that the infrastructural capacity should be equally available in all participating countries. As one official commented, "We cannot implement things that can be done in Finland but not in Ethiopia." Yet genetic screening of a large population was also seen to be impossible to implement because of religious, ethical and legal reasons. It was questioned whether people would be able to deal with genetic knowledge and if sufficient genetic counseling would be available. Others recommended extensive education programs because of the "extremely complicated ethical problems" involved. It was argued that the public should be better informed about the consequences of participating in elite sport; that if athletes were pushed to the limit, turned into gladiators, society would have to accept that from time to time such things like sudden death on the pitch might occur. As one sport cardiologist put it, we have to ask ourselves, "Does society really need this high-level sport?"

CONCLUSION

The data presented in this chapter serve as foundational work for a deeper ethical analysis in the future. For this reason the chapter has mainly focused on the technical and conceptual debates rather than the normative controversies. However, we can conclude that mandatory *nongenetic* cardiological screenings (as they are implemented in Italy for high-performance athletes as well as for leisure-time athletes) are not accepted through all European countries; hence, European-wide *genetic* screening does not seem implementable. Generally some stakeholders argued that if genetics comes into PPS in the future, it should rather be introduced as a *test* for individuals who ask for it and not as a mass *screening*. An important argument against screenings is the respect for the athlete's autonomous choice. Nonetheless, some athletes indicated that screenings might be justifiable if a high-performance athlete's health was at stake. Although the predictive power of genetic tests are regarded as limited, it can further be concluded that they should only constitute advice to athletes who are at risk, and that no one should be banned because of his/her health status (cf. respect athletes' autonomy, especially for the right of self-harm). We can finally conclude that the decision to implement such screenings (genetically or nongenetically) is a highly political one and not solely guided by empirically informed medical evaluations. This is particularly the case where there is no agreement on what medical data mean, as seems to be the case with existing PPS models.

NOTES

1. This chapter is the result of a research project (2007–2009) of the Centre for Society and Genomics in the Netherlands, funded by the Netherlands Genomics Initiative. Thanks to Guido de Wert and Agnes Meershoek for helpful comments.
2. See Deutsche Gesellschaft für Sportmedizin und Prävention, "S1—Leitlinie Vorsorgeuntersuchung im Sport," http://www.dgsp.de/_downloads/allgemein/S1_Leitlinie.pdf (accessed 12 October 2009).
3. Qualitative data were recorded and transcribed and processed with the qualitative data analysis tool NVivo 7.
4. The terms *pre-participation examination* or *pre-participation screening* are used synonymously in the literature.
5. See, e.g., World Boxing Council, "Rules and Regulations," http://wbcboxing.com/downloads/WBCRULES.pdf (accessed 01 March 2009).
6. Pelliccia et al., "Recommendations"; Pelliccia, Zipes and Maron, "Bethesda Conference #36."
7. Corrado et al., "Cardiovascular Pre-Participation Screening", 521.
8. IOC Medical Commission, "Sudden Cardiovascular Death in Sport. Lausanne Recommendations," http://www.olympic.org/Documents/Reports/EN/en_report_886.pdf (accessed 01 February 2009).
9. Maron et al., "Cardiovascular Preparticipation Screening."
10. Östman-Smith et al., "Age- and Gender-Specific Mortality Rates."
11. Cardiac Risk in the Young, http://www.c-r-y.org.uk/simplicity.htm (accessed 01 September 2009). .
12. Italian Ministry of Health, "Norme Per La Tutela Sanitaria Dell'attività Sportiva Agonistica"

13. This is different in Germany as well as in the Netherlands where sport physician/sport cardiologist is not a "full" specialization. Just a few additional courses are required after the standard medical education meaning that after the completion of 240 hours additional education (120 hours Sports Medicine and 120 hours Physical Education) and a year's works experience, one can apply to receive the additional title "Sportmedizin."
14. Apart from the evaluation of the family history, no further genetic risk factors are taken into consideration. No further genetic testing is carried out unless an abnormal finding occurs.
15. Pelliccia et al., "Evidence for Efficacy."
16. Verband der Sportvereine Südtirols (VSS), "Die Sportmedizinischen Untersuchungen." http://www.vss.bz.it/fileadmin/user_upload/rundschreiben/Sportmed_Unters.pdf. Athletes who test positive have thirty days to appeal.
17. Prescott, "Cardiovascular Pre-Participation Screening."
18. Lawless and Best, "Electrocardiograms in Athletes", 787. See also Dubrawsky, "Sudden Cardiac Death"; Sen-Chowdhry and McKenna, "Is There a Role?"; Shephard, "Mass ECG Screening."
19. Pelliccia et al., "Evidence for Efficacy."
20. de Wert and Vos, "Sport Als Gezondheidsrisico?"; Wren, "Cardiovascular Pre-Participation Screening."
21. Hernelahti et al., "Sudden Cardiac Death."
22. Ibid.
23. Corrado et al., "How to Screen Athletes."
24. Douglas, "Saving Athletes' Lives", 1997.
25. Pelliccia, Zipes and Maron, "Bethesda Conference #36."
26. Post, *Encyclopedia of Bioethics*, 998.
27. Ibid.
28. See also Müller, "Gendiagnostik Zur Talentsuche?"
29. Jones, Montgomery and Woods, "Human Performance"; Rankinen et al., "Human Gene Map"; Zintzaras et al., "Angiotensin-Converting Enzyme"; Tanabe et al., "Angiotensin-Converting Enzyme Gene."
30. CMA, "Knowledge of Inheritance Patterns Grows," http://www.cardiomyopathy.org/Knowledge-of-inheritance-patterns-grows.html (accessed 01 March 2009).
31. Ibid. See also de Wert, "Cascade Screening."
32. Spinney, "Heart-Stopping Action", 606.
33. Priori and Napolitano, "Role of Genetic Analyses", 1132. A further interesting aspect about the research dynamics is addressed by Priori and Napolitano: "The discovery of new disease-related genes is usually applauded with great enthusiasm by the scientific community and is chased by the most prestigious journals. On the contrary, identification of additional mutations in the same gene is regarded as a 'less innovative' research, so expanding the knowledge of the number of genetic variations and their link to the clinical phenotype has not been adequately promoted. Unfortunately, too much of this type of research has been discouraged and perceived as having a lower priority for both publication in leading journals and funding. As a consequence, fewer investigators have been involved in these areas of research, and it has become progressively more difficult to find financial support for collecting this 'orphan knowledge'", 1134.
34. Deutscher Bundestages, "Gesetz Über Genetische Untersuchungen Bei Menschen (Gendiagnostikgesetz—Gendg)," http://www.zhma.de/fileadmin/content/downloads/gesetze/GenDG_Gesetzesbeschluss.pdf (accessed 01 March 2010).

35. Deutsche Gesellschaft für Sportmedizin und Prävention, "S—Leitlinie Vorsorgeuntersuchung Im Sport."

36. Personal communication, 30 July 2007 and 6 September 2007.

37. Department of Health (UK), "Hypertrophic Cardiomyopathy," http://www.dh.gov.uk/en/Healthcare/NationalServiceFrameworks/Coronaryheartdisease/DH_4117048?IdcService=GET_FILE&dID=13497&Rendition=Web (accessed 12 October 2009). See also de Wert, "Cascade Screening."

38. Interview Sport Cardiologist (8), 3 September 2007.

39. Personal communication, 10 September 2007.

40. Spinney, "Heart-Stopping Action," 607.

41. Ng and Maginot, "Sudden Cardiac Death."

42. The NHMRC is "Australia's peak body for supporting health and medical research; for developing health advice for the Australian community, health professionals and governments; and for providing advice on ethical behaviour in health care and in the conduct of health and medical research" (see http://www.nhmrc.gov.au/about/index.htm) (accessed 05 October 2009).

43. NHMRC, "Genetics and Sport," http://www.nhmrc.gov.au/node/327 (accessed 05 October 2011).

44. Panhuyzen-Goedkoop and Verheugt, "Sudden Cardiac Death", 2152.

45. Ibid., 2153. The Dutch optimism seems to be based upon *founder family effects* in the Netherlands that reduce HCM to the level of an (almost) mono-genetic disease. That means that the number of HCM candidate genes to be detected through a screening program is reduced in the Dutch gene pool to almost two genes only.

46. Seto, "Preparticipation Cardiovascular Screening", 23.

47. Michels et al., "Familial Screening."

48. van Spaendonck-Zwarts, van den Berg and van Tintelen, "DNA Analysis", S48.

49. Neish, "Sudden Death" 52.

50. Pelliccia et al., "Recommendations", 878.

51. Ibid. , p. 878.

52. Pelliccia, Zipes and Maron, "Bethesda Conference #36", 1991.

53. Ibid., 1993.

54. Department of Health (New York State), "Genetic Testing and Screening in the Age of Genomic Medicine," http://www.health.state.ny.us/nysdoh/task-fce/screening.htm (accessed 1 December 2008).

55. It is important to note that some countries offer education in sports medicine as full specialty whereas others offer it as a subspecialty only. The recommended time for the education ranges from two up to four years. See Ergen et al., "Sports Medicine."

56. This issue (is genetic data different from other medical data) is described in the scientific literature as the *exceptionalism debate*.

57. A persistent vegetative state is a condition where the patient, due to severe brain damage, is in a coma that has progressed to a state of wakefulness without detectable awareness.

58. See, for example, the case *Gillick v. West Norfolk and Wisbech Area Health Authority*, http://www.hrcr.org/safrica/childrens_rights/Gillick_WestNorfolk.htm (accessed 1 November 2008).

59. Informed consent can be defined as a decisionally capable patient's legally binding treatment decision reached voluntarily and based on information about risks, benefits and alternative treatments gained from discussion with a health care practitioner.

60. Chadwick, "Right Not to Know."

BIBLIOGRAPHY

Chadwick, Ruth. "The Right Not to Know: A Challenge for Accurate Self-Assessment." *Philosophy, Psychiatry & Psychology* 11, no. 4 (2004): 299–301.

Cardiomyopathy Association. "Knowledge of Inheritance Patterns Grows," http://www.cardiomyopathy.org/Knowledge-of-inheritance-patterns-grows.html (accessed 01 March 2009).

Corrado, Domenico, Pierantonio Michieli, Cristina Basso, Maurizio Schiavon and Gaetano Thiene. "How to Screen Athletes for Cardiovascular Diseases." *Cardiology Clinics* 25, no. 3 (2007): 391–397.

Corrado, Domenico, Antonio Pelliccia, Hans Halvor Bjornstad, Luc Vanhees, Alessandro Biffi, Mats Borjesson, Nicole Panhuyzen-Goedkoop, Asterios Deligiannis, Erik Solberg, Dorian Dugmore, Klaus Peter Mellwig, Deodato Assanelli, Pietro Delise, Frank van-Buuren, Aris Anastasakis, Hein Heidbuchel, Ellen Hoffmann, Robert Fagard, Silvia G. Priori, Cristina Basso, Eloisa Arbustini, Carina Blomstrom-Lundqvist, William J. McKenna and Gaetano Thiene. "Cardiovascular Pre-Participation Screening of Young Competitive Athletes for Prevention of Sudden Death: Proposal for a Common European Protocol. Consensus Statement of the Study Group of Sport Cardiology of the Working Group of Cardiac Rehabilitation and Exercise Physiology and the Working Group of Myocardial and Pericardial Diseases of the European Society of Cardiology." *European Heart Journal* 26, no. 5 (2005): 516–524.

Corrado, Domenico, and Gaetano Thiene. "Protagonist: Routine Screening of All Athletes Prior to Participation in Competitive Sports Should Be Mandatory to Prevent Sudden Cardiac Death." *Heart Rhythm: The Official Journal of the Heart Rhythm Society* 4, no. 4 (2007): 520–524.

Department of Health (New York State), "Genetic Testing and Screening in the Age of Genomic Medicine," http://www.health.state.ny.us/nysdoh/taskfce/screening.htm (accessed 1 December 2008).

Department of Health (UK), "Hypertrophic Cardiomyopathy," http://www.dh.gov.uk/en/Healthcare/NationalServiceFrameworks/Coronaryheartdisease/DH_4117048?IdcService=GET_FILE&dID=13497&Rendition=Web (accessed 12 October 2009).

Deutsche Gesellschaft für Sportmedizin und Prävention. "S1—Leitlinie Vorsorgeuntersuchung im Sport." http://www.dgsp.de/_downloads/allgemein/S1_Leitlinie.pdf (accessed 12 October 2009).

Deutscher Bundestages, "Gesetz Über Genetische Untersuchungen Bei Menschen (Gendiagnostikgesetz—Gendg)," http://www.zhma.de/fileadmin/content/downloads/gesetze/GenDG_Gesetzesbeschluss.pdf (accessed 01 March 2010).

de Wert, Guido. "Cascade Screening: Whose Information Is It Anyway?" *European Journal of Human Genetics* 13, no. 4 (2005): 397–398.

de Wert, Guido, and Rein Vos. "Sport Als Gezondheidsrisico? Een Ethische Verkenning Van Voorspellend Genetisch Onderzoek Bij Sporters." In *Beter Dan Goed: Over Genetica En De Toekomst Van Topsport*, edited by Ivo van Hilvoorde and Bernike Pasveer, 44–62. Diemen: Veen Magazines, 2005.

Douglas, Pamela S. "Saving Athletes' Lives a Reason to Find Common Ground?" *Journal of the American College of Cardiology* 52, no. 24 (2008): 1997–1999.

Dubrawsky, Chagai. "Sudden Cardiac Death in the Young." *Cardiology* 109, no. 2 (2008): 143–143.

Ergen, Emin, Fabio Pigozzi, Norbert Bachl and Hans Herrmann Dickhuth. "Sports Medicine: A European Perspective. Historical Roots, Definitions and Scope." *Journal of Sports Medicine and Physical Fitness* 46, no. 2 (2006): 167–175.

Hernelahti, Miika, Olavi Jussi Heinonen, Jouko Karjalainen, Eva Nylander and Mats Borjesson. "Sudden Cardiac Death in Young Athletes: Time for a Nordic

Approach in Screening?" *Scandinavian Journal of Medicine & Science in Sports* 18, no. 2 (2008): 132–139.

IOC Medical Commission. "Sudden Cardiovascular Death in Sport. Lausanne Recommendations." http://www.olympic.org/Documents/Reports/EN/en_report_886.pdf (accessed 01 February 2009).

Italian Ministry of Health. "Norme Per La Tutela Sanitaria Dell'attività Sportiva Agonistica (=Rules Concerning the Medical Protection of Athletic Activity. Decree of the Italian Ministry of Health), February 18, 1982." *Gazzetta Ufficiale della Repubblica Italiana* March 5 (1982): 63.

Jones, Alun, Hugh E. Montgomery and David R. Woods. "Human Performance: A Role for the Ace Genotype?" *Exercise and Sport Science Review* 30, no. 4 (2002): 184–190.

Lawless, Christine E., and Thomas M. Best. "Electrocardiograms in Athletes: Interpretation and Diagnostic Accuracy." *Medicine and Science in Sports and Exercise* 40, no. 5 (2008): 787–798.

Maron, Barry J., Paul D. Thompson, James C. Puffer, Christopher A. McGrew, William B. Strong, Pamela S. Douglas, Luther T. Clark, Matthew J. Mitten, Michael H. Crawford, Dianne L. Atkins, David J. Driscoll and Andrew E. Epstein. "Cardiovascular Preparticipation Screening of Competitive Athletes: A Statement for Health Professionals from the Sudden Death Committee (Clinical Cardiology) and Congenital Cardiac Defects Committee (Cardiovascular Disease in the Young), American Heart Association." *Circulation* 94, no. 4 (1996): 850–856.

Michels, Michelle, Yvonne M. Hoedemaekers, Marcel J. Kofflard, Ingrid Frohn-Mulder, Dennis Dooijes, Danielle Majoor-Krakauer and Folkert J. Ten Cate. "Familial Screening and Genetic Counselling in Hypertrophic Cardiomyopathy: The Rotterdam Experience." *Netherlands Heart Journal* 15, no. 5 (2007): 184–190.

Müller, Arno. "Gendiagnostik Zur Talentsuche? Ethische Anmerkungen." In *Talentdiagnose Und Talentprognose Im Nachwuchsleistungssport: 2. Bisp-Symposium: Theorie Trifft Praxis*, edited by Gabriele Neumann and Bundesinstitut für Sportwissenschaft, 443. Cologne: Sportverl Strauß, 2009.

Neish, Steven. R. "Sudden Death in Competitive Athletes." *Medscape General Medicine* 9, no. 4 (2007): 52.

Ng, Benton, and Kathleen R. Maginot. "Sudden Cardiac Death in Young Athletes: Trying to Find the Needle in the Haystack." *World Medical Journal* 106, no. 6 (2007): 335–342.

NHMRC, "Genetics and Sport," http://www.nhmrc.gov.au/node/327 (accessed 05 October 2011).

Östman-Smith, Ingegerd, Goran Wettrell, Barry Keeton, Daniel Holmgren, Ulf Ergander, Steven Gould, Colene Bowker and Mario Verdicchio. "Age- and Gender-Specific Mortality Rates in Childhood Hypertrophic Cardiomyopathy." *European Heart Journal* 29, no. 9 (2008): 1160–1167.

Panhuyzen-Goedkoop, Nicole M., and Freek W.A. Verheugt. "Sudden Cardiac Death Due to Hypertrophic Cardiomyopathy Can Be Reduced by Pre-Participation Cardiovascular Screening in Young Athletes." *European Heart Journal* 27, no. 18 (2006): 2152–2153.

Pelliccia, Antonio, Domenico Corrado, Hans Halbor Bjørnstad, Nicole Panhuyzen-Goedkoop, Axel Urhausen, Fracois Carré, Aris Anastasakis, Luc Vanhees, Eloisa Arbustini and Silvia Priori. "Recommendations for Participation in Competitive Sport and Leisure-Time Physical Activity in Individuals with Cardiomyopathies, Myocarditis and Pericarditis." *European Journal of Cardiovascular Prevention and Rehabilitation* 13, (2006): 876–885.

Pelliccia, Antonio, Fernando M. Di Paolo, Domenico Corrado, Cosimo Buccolieri, Filippo M. Quattrini, Cataldo Pisicchio, Antonio Spataro, Alessandro Biffi,

Maristella Granata and Barry J. Maron. "Evidence for Efficacy of the Italian National Pre-Participation Screening Programme for Identification of Hypertrophic Cardiomyopathy in Competitive Athletes." *European Heart Journal* 27, no. 18 (2006): 2196–2200.

Pelliccia, Antonio, Douglas P. Zipes and Barry J. Maron. "Bethesda Conference #36 and the European Society of Cardiology Consensus Recommendations Revisited a Comparison of US and European Criteria for Eligibility and Disqualification of Competitive Athletes with Cardiovascular Abnormalities." *Journal of the American College of Cardiology* 52, no. 24 (2008): 1990–1996.

Post, Stephen G. *Encyclopedia of Bioethics*. 3rd ed. New York: Macmillan Reference USA, 2003.

Prescott, Eva. "Cardiovascular Pre-Participation Screening of Young Competitive Athletes for Prevention of Sudden Death: Proposal for a Common European Protocol." *European Heart Journal* 27, no. 23 (2006): 2904–2905.

Priori, Silvia G., and Carlo Napolitano. "Role of Genetic Analyses in Cardiology: Part I: Mendelian Diseases: Cardiac Channelopathies." *Circulation* 113, no. 8 (2006): 1130–1135.

Rankinen, Tuomo, Molly S. Bray, James M. Hagberg, Louis Perusse, Stephen M. Roth, Bernd Wolfarth and Claude Bouchard. "The Human Gene Map for Performance and Health-Related Fitness Phenotypes: The 2005 Update." *Medicine and Science in Sports and Exercise* 38, no. 11 (2006): 1863–1888.

Sen-Chowdhry, Srijita, and William J. McKenna. "Is There a Role for the 12–Lead ECG in Pre-Participation Screening of Athletes?" *Cardiology* 109, no. 2 (2008): 144–144.

Seto, Craig K. "Preparticipation Cardiovascular Screening." *Clinical Sports Medicine* 22, no. 1 (2003): 23–35.

Shephard, Roy J. "Mass ECG Screening of Young Athletes." *British Journal of Sports Medicine* 42, no. 9 (2008): 707–708.

Spinney, Laura. "Heart-Stopping Action." *Nature* 430 (2004): 606–607.

Tanabe, Yuji, Ryo Kawasaki, Jie Jin Wang, Tien Y. Wong, Paul Mitchell, Makoto Daimon, Toshihide Oizumi, Takeo Kato, Sumio Kawata, Takamasa Kayama and Hidetoshi Yamashita. "Angiotensin-Converting Enzyme Gene and Retinal Arteriolar Narrowing: The Funagata Study." *Journal of Human Hypertension* 16 (2009): 16.

van Spaendonck-Zwarts, Karin Y., Maarten P. van den Berg and J. Peter van Tintelen. "DNA Analysis in Inherited Cardiomyopathies: Current Status and Clinical Relevance." *Pacing Clinical Electrophysiology* 31, no. 1 (2008): S46–S49.

Wren, Christopher. "Cardiovascular Pre-Participation Screening of Young Competitive Athletes for Prevention of Sudden Death: Proposal for a Common European Protocol." *European Heart Journal* 26, no. 17 (2005): 1804.

World Boxing Council. "Rules and Regulations of the World Boxing Council." http://wbcboxing.com/downloads/WBCRULES.pdf (accessed 01 March 2011).

Zintzaras, Elias, Gowri Raman, Georgios Kitsios and Joseph Lau. "Angiotensin-Converting Enzyme Insertion/Deletion Gene Polymorphic Variant as a Marker of Coronary Artery Disease: A Meta-Analysis." *Archives of Internal Medicine* 168, no. 10 (2008): 1077–1089.

15 Sports Medicine beyond Therapy
Genetic Doping and Enhancement

Yoshitaka Kondo and Mike McNamee

In postmodernity, it is said, there is an increasing tolerance of the widely divergent lifestyles of individuals. Within the processes that comprise this trend is an increasing skepticism toward, and at times the total rejection of, the possibility of universal value standards, whether religious or secular. These processes are evidenced both in body-practices as well, of course, as intellectual ones.[1] As proof of the bodily instantiations of this trend, we can look to nonclinically indicated body modification through plastic surgery. Traditionally, cosmetic surgery had helped victims of car crashes or facial disfigurement by dog attacks or the amelioration of genetic defects. The use of biotechnologies has not, until recently, extended beyond therapy except in science fiction. Now these technologies are being used for the purposes of autonomously chosen body modifications/enhancements. This trend must be seen alongside other aspects of physical and cognitive enhancement, chosen for either aesthetic reasons or functional gains.[2]

Sports science and sports scholarship more generally has witnessed much "gene talk,"[3] which suggests either that genetic enhancement is around the corner,[4] or already being practiced surreptitiously. Of course, whether this gene talk is idle and speculative chatter, current practice or even genuine possibility is a matter of much debate.[5]

It is necessary, however, to conceptualize the expansion of genetic technologies in the broader context of the long-standing, pharmacologically driven doping problem. How this is to be evaluated, whether as (at least potentially) therapy and/or enhancement is the object of this chapter. Yet discussions relating to genetic technologies are not restricted to academic milieu. Governments across the globe have commissioned reports not merely on the pros and cons of genetic technologies in sports, but also explicitly as to the range of normative issues they raise for humanity as a whole.[6] Perhaps the most prominent of these reports emanates from the US where the then president, George W. Bush, commissioned a group of highly regarded, conservatively inclined scholars and scientists to report on the use of biotechnology beyond therapeutic aims; titled *Beyond Therapy*.[7] Its third chapter, "Superior Performance," considered the problem of doping as it relates to enhancement through biotechnology, and thus is pertinent to the present chapter. At least in this respect, sports-related discussion has come to the forefront of scientific (featured in a *Nature* editorial in 2008)[8] and political discourses. In the latter case, the discussion has typically been framed as a contest between what are sometimes referred to as "bio-liberals" or "bio-conservatives."[9]

The aim of this chapter is critically to discuss the stance of the president's commission and to explore its ramifications for sporting practices and institutions.[10] First, we articulate the conceptual boundaries of the problem and focus particularly on the blurred distinction between *therapy* and *enhancement*. Second, we review the shift between pharmacological and genetic doping. Following a recent trend in moral philosophy, we draw upon a literary work to frame the discourses of enhancement, especially a prophetic novel from 1955 written by the Danish writer Knud Lundberg, and compare this to empirical research that illustrates the genetic technological revisioning of athletic excellence. Third, we explore the key ethical issues arising from that section of *Beyond Therapy* that deals directly with enhanced performance. We conclude that the sources for critically evaluating the nature and purposes of sports medicine, including its moral boundaries, are multidisciplinary in nature, extending (at least) to historical, literary and philosophical scholarship.

MEDICAL ETHICS, SPORTS MEDICINE AND BIOMEDICAL ENHANCEMENT

Bioethics is said to be the field of systematic research that comprises a range of ethical methodologies and theories in various interdisciplinary contexts (including moral perspectives, decision making, conduct and policies regarding ethical problems) involved in biosciences, biotechnology and health care. Traditionally it has dealt with concrete ethical issues such as those that relate to end-of-life care, euthanasia, the (competing) definitions of death, the ethics of organ donation and selling, the just allocation of therapeutic resources, caregiver–patient relationships and the nature and scope of informed consent. More recently the rise of biotechnology has extended the scope of bioethics. Increasingly academic articles and policy makers are engaged in discussions on the use of embryonic stem cells, the mis/use of prenatal and preimplantation genetic diagnoses and, most dramatically, the future of human nature. It is against this trend that doping has most recently become a focus of shared interest between medical philosophers/ethicists and sports philosophers/ethicists.[11]

Among the international community of sports philosophers the stance toward doping and anti-doping is mixed. Although there is no doubt that doping is an effective technology for improving competitive performance, its illegitimacy is argued by leading scholars.[12] At least as many scholars, however, argue that it represents an arbitrary imposition on the available means of performance enhancement. Their arguments tend to be skeptical, in the philosophical sense.[13] They rarely, if ever, announce the value of doping-permitted sports,[14] but rather point to analogies where what is thought to be objectionable about doping (e.g., potential harm) is permissible in other circumstances (e.g., boxing, American football, rugby).[15] Typically their moral perspective is a utilitarian one where what counts is the maximum amount of good consequences distributed impartially among all those affected. They characteristically dismiss talk of duties or of the virtues of sportsmen and sportswomen unless they are productive of good consequences. And along with this moral theoretical perspective is a deep-rooted commitment to liberalism, where individuals' autonomous choices are to be respected—even those that harm the individual who chooses them, though not where harms extend involuntarily to others. Where their argument has been positive, philosophers and scientists have attempted to shift the focus from ethical terrain (the so-called "spirit of sport" criterion) to one based solely on harm minimization.[16] A clear example is the use of establishing safe hematocrit levels to safeguard against excessive blood viscosity and its potential for causing heart attacks in professional cycling, or the use of brain scans for boxers.[17]

Writers from medical perspectives are more uniform in their public declaration that doping is unacceptable at both an individual and institutional level (e.g., International Federation of Sports Medicine [FIMS], World Medical Association [WMA]). Although there are exceptions,[18] it is clear that medical technologies in sports have extended beyond therapy and that this may call into question their status as medicine.[19] Under a traditional therapeutic conception, (sports) medicine is restricted to treating disease, injury or infection; preventing injury or illness; and to recovering health.[20] Clearly, doping is contrary to these goals and is at odds with the decision-making standards for the validity of medical treatment.[21] Countering this position within the shared fields of medical and sports ethics, Juengst has disputed whether the therapy/enhancement distinction can mark the moral boundary between the permissible and the impermissible that conservatives attribute to it.[22]

Within global anti-doping sports policy, the World Anti-Doping Agency (WADA) has successfully sought international support from governments (via UNESCO), sports medicine organizations (such as FIMS) and international sports federations (e.g., IAAF). Despite achieving widespread intergovernmental support (128 countries have national anti-doping organizations as signatories), some sports remain either outside the agreement (e.g., baseball) or have publicly queried the powers of WADA's Code (e.g., soccer). Nevertheless, concessions for the use of what might be used as doping products are allowed exceptionally in recognition of the fact that athletes' rights to health care take precedence over sporting rules that govern fair contests.[23] Thus Section 4.4. of the World Anti-Doping Code (2003) stipulates:

> Each International Federation shall ensure, for any Athlete who is entered in an International Event, that a process is in place whereby Athletes with documented medical conditions requiring the Use of a Prohibited Substance or a Prohibited Method may request a therapeutic use exemption.[24]

This has established the "International Standard for Therapeutic Use Exemptions" of the World Anti-Doping Code.

Compliance with this regulation, however, potentially facilitates the use of substances both as a means for medical therapy *and* for enhancement.[25] In other words, the physician makes the decision regarding the use of products for treatment aware that there may be performance-enhancement consequences. Therefore, the ethics of physicians themselves regarding the use of medical means must be subject to governance policy.[26]

In one form or another medical ethics has existed in the West since the fifth century BC when Hippocrates laid down the oath that has taken his name. It attempted to lay out a proto-code of conduct to govern physicians' commitment to their art and their dealings with patients. It is, however, far from clear which norms, rules or principles ought to apply in twenty-first-century sports medicine,[27] when for more than a century it has been at the service of elite sports among other pursuits.[28] The source of potential confusion arises partly because of the heterogonous contexts of sports (e.g., amateur versus professional) and the roles and services provided to the athlete patient (by, e.g., orthopedic surgeons, sports physiotherapists, masseuses, team doctors, event physicians). Although there will be strong resemblance to other spheres of medicine (especially military medicine and occupational medicine), there are also likely to be certain unusual role-related norms (see Waddington in this collection).

The most widely utilized medical ethical model in the West is that of Beauchamp and Childress. Their *Principles of Biomedical Ethics* is included in medical education throughout the Western world.[29] Their account of medical ethics comprises four principles: respect for patient autonomy, acting toward the patient's good, not harming the patient and acting justly. It is widely thought that where there is tension or conflict among the principles, primary importance ought to be placed on respect for patient autonomy.[30] Medical interventions that are in compliance with these principles are *ipso facto* considered to be legitimate medical conduct.

Some critics challenge the traditional therapeutic conception of medicine. They argue that there exist practices widely recognized as belonging to medicine that involve enhancement. Take, for example, the practice of immunization. This boosts the human body's normal capabilities to withstand viruses or bacteria. Within sports, critics sometimes mention hip replacement surgery (e.g., the American cyclist Floyd Landis), which though therapeutic may also enhance performance. In both cases, it may be said that the goal of the intervention is more properly seen as preventative and the enhancement effects are mere by-products.

The use of medical technology to bring about enhancement beyond normal function has been one of the most discussed issues in medical ethics in recent years.[31] Enhancement, however, is not a straightforward concept. Nor is it absolutely clear that it can always be distinguished from its conceptual antonym therapy. We discuss these problems in the following section.

WHAT IS ENHANCEMENT?

There has been mounting ethical interest in the use of medical science for enhancement due to the rapid development of genetic science and progress in neuroscience in recent years. Yet precisely how we are to understand enhancement is not always sufficiently clear. First, let us accept a broad conception of enhancement that includes any development that improves a function(s) of a human body without (net) deleterious side effects. Some enhancements are sought, or are useful, for specific purposes and some for much more general purposes. Nevertheless, articulating more precisely the concept of improvement invites two further problems, for typically there are two intersecting accounts of improvement that are at play in discussions about enhancement: one that makes a distinction between objective (or intersubjective) and subjective improvements and a second that makes a distinction between improvement in relation to a norm and improvement purely in relation to the *status quo ante*. It is helpful to keep these apart at least for analytical purposes.

The first distinction is concerned with who is to judge whether a certain change is an improvement. Thus we can ask of any purported enhancement whether it is determined objectively (or intersubjectively at least) or whether it is exclusively a matter for personal judgment. The second distinction is concerned with establishing the baseline for judging or measuring improvement. Is it, for instance, a species-based norm or is it the function of one specific individual?

These two intersecting distinctions give rise to four different ways of (mis)understanding improvement and *a fortiori* enhancement. The most restrictive of these is the objective, norm-based account that usually underlies arguments making a distinction between therapy in the sense of bringing a person (or restoring them) to a normal level of functioning, and enhancement in the sense of improving function above the normal.[32] The most expansive account is the subjective, *status quo* account, which essentially entails that any physical change a person deems to be an improvement of his function is an improvement.[33] Although this conception is widely employed in medical ethics, it is clear that the kinds of enhancements that are troublesome in elite sports are more likely to be captured in supra-subjective terms—either as an improvement on the whole class of human beings or the specific reference class of elite athletes, or indeed of previous athletic potential of an individual.[34]

In the recent bioethics literature, doping is frequently cited as a typical example of enhancement (without specifying the kind of enhancement alluded to in the preceding) and there is thought to be a possibility that gene doping, in particular, as a form of genetic engineering enhancement, will come to be used before long because gene sequencing has already identified over one hundred genes associated with athletic performance (for an assessment of the current state of genetic knowledge, see also Müller's contribution in this collection). It is thought, in principle, that via genetic engineering clinicians may either upregulate "desirable" genetic expression or, as is the case with myostatin (which prevents excessive muscular growth), downregulate or inhibit "undesirable" genetic expression. The extent to which the latter is merely a self-serving fabrication, pejoratively labeled "gene talk," is a moot point.[35] Even conservative estimates about the possibility of gene doping do not rule out its possibility, though they do question how realistic estimations are as to the possibilities of the technique. Yet speculation of gene doping is not by any means, as we shall see, a new phenomenon.

FORGING AHEAD: FROM PHARMACOLOGICAL TO GENETIC DOPING

We can see reports in the media nearly every week regarding suspected doping and violators. Most likely the report will be accompanied by a sense of inevitability or resignation that the doping problem is here to stay and will never be eradicated or resolved. Support for this pessimistic (realistic?) view is evidenced by the fact that WADA so frequently adds different products and methods to their banned list as novel doping strategies are uncovered or anticipated. This has been repeated over and over again since 1968, when the first anti-doping code came into effect at the Grenoble Winter Olympic Games.[36]

In 2003, WADA policy was amended to outlaw "methods applying genetic treatment" to its already lengthy list of banned substances and techniques. As far as anti-doping policy makers were concerned, the age of "gene doping" had finally emerged. Although this phenomenon raises many and varied questions, in this chapter, we focus on the relationship between bioscience/biotechnology and sports that has given birth to the possible emergence of genetic doping. To do this we must look backward as well as forward. We therefore consider the period of transition from the age in which substances were used to improve muscular strength to the age when natural capacities themselves can be transformed.

Following Martha Nussbaum's groundbreaking work *The Fragility of Goodness*, recent philosophical discussions in ethics have drawn on fiction

for ethical insight. Nussbaum drew upon the genre of ancient Greek trag-
edies to draw attention to the limitations of human reason to dictate and control the search for, and living of, the good life. Since modernity, human kind
has invested its faith in human reason (at its zenith, experimental science) to
describe, predict and control human living. Equally, modernist morality, following the ancient Greek philosopher Protagoras more than two thousand
years earlier, held man to be the master of all things so that in being rational
we were at the same time morally responsible for our actions.

More than fifty years ago, the Danish novelist Knud Lundberg anticipated the rise of biotechnology and its potentially transformative effects on
the ethics of elite sports. His account of an Olympic Men's 800m Race—
Det Olympiske Håb (English translation: *The Olympic Hope*; Japanese
translation: *Tragedy of the Olympic Spirit*) can be interpreted as both
prophesy of elite sport's futuristic development and the present-day perils
of drugs and other doping. The latter interpretation was taken in a Japanese newspaper article, which described the novel as follows:

> The stage is the Olympic Games. The 800m finals are about to start.
> There are six runners at the starting line. A giant who has continued
> to take growth hormones since youth, a young man who has injected a
> drug that enables rocket-like spurts and a man who was born through
> artificial fertilization of the sperm and egg of famous runners . . . The
> starting pistol sounds and the race begins.[37]

Karaki, who cited this novel, expressed surprise that this science fiction
appeared in a magazine issued prior to the 1964 Tokyo Olympics and published by the Japan Amateur Sports Association. Yet the novel had already
been published for nearly a decade by then and had received critical support in the English-speaking world at least.[38] Moreover, the book's fame and
insight cannot be disconnected from Lundberg's own familiarity with elite
sports. Not only did he represent Denmark in basketball and handball (a
sport of enormous popularity across Scandinavia), but he captained the Danish Olympic team and was captain of the Olympic football (soccer) team in
a time when the gap between national amateur and professional teams was
nowhere near as marked as it is today. He was still playing international football in 1956, a year after the book was published in Denmark.[39]

The context of the Cold War between the superpowers looms large over
the text (reflected in the choice of national characters), but is not of present
concern. More significantly, the close interaction of athletes and scientists
depicted in the novel foresees the current sports world almost to the extent
that it now scarcely reads like fiction. The six finalists who appear in the novel
include two black Americans, a giant named Jackson and small-statured
Stoker; two Russian athletes, Konev, a gladiator type with a body consisting only of bones, sinew, muscle and skin, and Vlasov, a human locomotive;
followed by Hasenjäger (literally, hare hunter), a supreme masterpiece who is

the offspring of German folk ideology; and finally the Danish athlete Erling, castigated by the media as a dilettante. Lundberg cleverly sets out five of his characters, with the exception of Erling, as prototypes of excess that will undermine the integrity of sports as wholesome competition.

Jackson, an American, is a black athlete who was created by chemist Dr. Lamond taking advantage of hormone manipulation in a project in the past in which giants were forced to marry. His externally administered hormone regime has, however, had the effect of preventing his intellectual and sexual development beyond that of a twelve-year-old. Though his father was a tall world-class basketball player, the American athlete Stoker is thought to be the illegitimate offspring of his mother's adulterous relationship. He receives injections of drugs just prior to races. Konev of Russia is the winner of the All-Soviet Union Baby Championships and his parents were given medals and lifelong pensions. In a truly interesting scenario, he is supreme in real athletic power but he falls, problematically, in love with a swimmer (Sonja). He thinks that if their love is to flourish his only recourse is to intentionally lose and be eliminated as a national team member in order to break out of the surveillance and management regime to pursue his amorous goal. He decides to do just that. The sports physicians/scientists are totally mystified about why he is not able to win given his perfect physical condition. It would seem that the force of state-sponsored science is incapable of intervening in matters of love. Vlasov, also a Russian athlete, was placed second in the All-Soviet Union Baby Championships behind Konev. Apparently destined always to be placed second behind Konev, he has reconciled himself to his fate (though it now appears that he may be able to beat the smitten Konev). Hasenjäger of Germany was born as the result of a eugenics experiment. He has 399 siblings by other mothers and was born through artificial fertilization between a father who was an Olympic runner and a mother who was among Germany's top one thousand middle-distance runners. He was injected with a chemical substance just prior to the race. Unlike the other five, Erling of Denmark, though it may seem a piece of excessive patriotism or romanticism, emerges into the novel alongside his grandfather. Whereas in the novel there are athletes who strongly back the spirit of amateurism and do not receive any support at all from a specialized scientific entourage, the Danish character is prominently different from the other finalists.

It is also possible to catch a glimpse of the values that were held in the 1950s. In the novel, presaging real life, doping is banned. There was rumor and innuendo even in the 1950s as to widespread use of enhancement products such as amphetamine or Benzedrine.[40] Nevertheless, though there are rules to prohibit it, there is no hesitation whatsoever in breaching them by athletes and their nationalistic scientific and sports medicine entourages.

The sports world of the future depicted in the 1955 science fiction novel is, then, in some ways prescient. Clearly Lundberg did not foresee the fall of the Berlin Wall and the lessening of tensions between capitalist and communist superpowers. Yet more recent advances in science and technology have progressed sufficiently far to make some of the earlier speculation imminently feasible. But we ought not to get carried away. It cannot be insignificant that in one of the world's leading medical journals, the *New England Journal of Medicine*, a relatively recent review article neglected even to mention professional athletics and sports medicine in its discussion of ethical, legal and social implications of genetic medicine.[41] It is necessary to be somewhat more circumspect than others have been in proclaiming that—on the evidence of the identification of certain genetic precursors to muscular contraction and growth—we are only a step away from gene doping. It is not yet clear precisely how genetics will alter our understanding of athletic potential and performance.[42] Some of the claims made by sports ethicists and scientists regarding the potential for human enhancement seem to blur the lines between fact and science fiction.[43] But among other things this novel shows that gene talk in sports is not new. Neither is it uniform. Whereas some embrace the prospect of genetic technologies, others are more wary of its potentially Promethean character.[44]

In 1991, Laura spoke of the potential for using genetic engineering such as that given in the following within the context of the discussion of the doping problem in sports. First of all, Laura points out that, even if the pharmacological problem could be resolved, it would be no more than a superficial solution appearing in a different form. In other words:

> If a competitive advantage that is harmless and undetectable is created through technological innovation in genetic engineering that is currently usable or possibly usable in the future or if marksmanship athletes use "eyes" that are designed through biotechnology or genetic engineering, it is difficult to see, for instance, how a competitive advantage such as a bionic or genetically engineered eye used by an athlete in the shooting competition could legitimately be prohibited.[45]

Laura's predictions give further evidence of the need for skepticism. He draws upon the history of advances in genetic engineering in detail and in envisaging the completion of gene mapping, leaping to the conclusion that it will become possible in the near future to artificially regulate virtually all human characteristics induced by major genes. As examples, he cites skin color, eyes, hair color, head hair, stature, skeletal structure and muscles. Contrast this optimism with a more recent analysis of commercial genetic profiling for health risks and interventions that suggests:

> Although genomic profiling may have potential to enhance the effectiveness and efficiency of preventive interventions, to date the scientific evidence for most associations between genetic variants and disease risk is insufficient to support useful applications.[46]

From the vantage point of 1991 one could be forgiven for thinking that a brave new world of genetically modified athletes and sports was just around the corner. In addition, in the section on gene therapy, Laura states that "It is possible in principle, that is to say, to splice into the relevant cells of an adult human being a gene for muscle-cell augmentation" and contends that muscle augmentation would be possible without using drugs.[47] In the section on cloning, he states that it would be possible to use embryo-freezing technology to choose clones of Olympic athletes to produce one's own children. He concludes by saying that super-cloned athletes would no longer be a dream but could actually be created.

The vision of Laura's brave new sports world, paradoxically exaggerated beyond Lundberg's sports science fiction, is not hopelessly naïve. He argues that, insofar as genes are considered the foundation for the formation of humans, once Pandora's box of gene manipulation is opened, there will be no way of knowing how far such manipulation will proceed. As a case example, he cites research to genetically modify sensory function in the form of a modified sense of smell and research for embedding the uterus in the body of a male and inducing pregnancy by inserting embryos created through artificial fertilization.

In Lundberg's novel, sports science and medicine go hand in hand, whereas Laura's remarks prefigure the recent debates about whether medicine ought to aim exclusively at therapy or if it should embrace enhancement goals. Like Lundberg he is skeptical of genetically determined athletic champions, but he nevertheless recognizes that "a transformation from an intention to eliminate genetic defects to an intention to incorporate genetic improvements in body building athletes is like the two sides of a coin" and that "the technological capacity to eliminate 'bad genes' cannot be rigidly distinguished in practice from the object of genetic improvement or 'positive eugenics'."[48] He predicts that people will probably lean in the direction of positive eugenics. Laura points out that, as an extension of this, techniques for improving competitive capabilities will ultimately be taken over by positive eugenics engineering, and thus declares the end of the current problem of drug-based doping. Of course Laura's contentions naturally give rise to objections regarding his excessive expectation of continued genetic control over life (often referred to as genetic determinism), which must be tempered by actual advances in genetic science. It is not credible, however, to deny the possibility that the science and technology of genetic engineering will be introduced into sports medicine and sports science. Nevertheless, principled discussion of the pros and cons of such introduction cannot avoid a clear discussion of the goals of sports medicine set out earlier that extend beyond traditional therapeutic ones.[49]

SUPERIOR PERFORMANCE, BEYOND THERAPY

Despite the existence of both fictional and scientific futuristic predictions, the first genuinely substantial philosophical discussion of the enhancement goals of medicine is a report of the President's Council on bioethics entitled

Beyond Therapy. It scrutinizes the enhancement debate from the perspective of bioethics amid the emergence of enhancement in American society. A purview of its contents reveals how considerations of sports ethics are central to the debate. It comprises discussions of "Better Children," "Superior Performance" and "Ageless Bodies, Happy Souls," the contents of which represent potential axes for enhancement medicine at all stages of the human life cycle. For present purposes we focus on "Superior Performance," which examines the effects that the desire to realize superior performance and outperform others has on individuals and society when linked to medical science and technology centered in biotechnology.

The mantra of commercialized and commodified elite sports has been said to mirror capitalist ideology: enough is never enough; perpetual progress is both possible and desirable.[50] Just as capitalism denies limits to economic growth so, it is often said, elite athletes should recognize no boundaries in their search for excellence in performance. Even Lundberg, despite his naturalism, has been trained from an early age in scientifically supported athletic preparation and training techniques. *Beyond Therapy*, however, draws our attention to the meaning of sports for humanity in a sustained way that is superior to the prospective imagination of the novelist Lundberg and the scientist Laura. It explores special differences in meaning found within intentional human activities in the pursuit of performance in sports. When pursuing superior performance through better training, the functioning of the body and the understanding and experience of the functioning body become mutually more closely knit. Meanwhile, the report contends that "with interventions that bypass human experience to work their biological 'magic' directly—from better nutrition to steroids to genetic muscle enhancements—our silent bodily workings and our conscious agency are more alienated from one another."[51] The authors draw attention to qualitative differences between performances gained through better training and those gained through the use of drugs or other illicit means.

Thus the core question that emerges in the ethical analysis is: what is the essence of humanity in that pursuit of excellence? In other words:

> Which biomedical interventions for the sake of superior performance are consistent with (even favorable to) our full flourishing as human beings, including our flourishing as active, self-aware, self-directed agents? And, conversely, when is the alienation of biological process from active experience dehumanizing, compromising the lived humanity of our efforts and thus making our superior performance in some way false—not simply our own, not fully human?[52]

Among the ethical concepts and questions involving the doping problem, whether as pharmacological or genetic enhancement, are the problems of fairness and equality among athletes using them, the problem of social pressures that coerce athletes into, or in the direction of, using them and the physical aftereffects. Nevertheless, according to *Beyond Therapy*, these ethical concepts and questions cannot be considered to be the definitive problem. Rather, the report considers whether illicitly enhanced performance "can actually be looked upon as humanly superior performance." If it is humanly superior performance, then that assumes "understanding the true dignity of excellent human activity, and how some new ways of improving performance may distort or undermine it."[53] The use of various means for improving activity capabilities—from stimulants to blood doping to genetic engineering of muscle—calls into question the dignity of the performance of those who use them.[54] What is called into question here is the meaning of human identity, that is, humanly excelling in activities as "I: myself." It is in the experience of cultivating excellent acts and activities through capabilities that are humanly nurtured, in particular, that gives meaning to competition in sports. They write:

> Even in the most competitive activities, the deepest meaning may not be honorable victory, or beating one's best human opponents in a worthy way, but rather the human agent at-work in the world—especially the lived experience, for both the spectator and doer, of a humanly cultivated gift, excellently-at-work.[55]

In short, the report's authors invoke an older concept that liberal and utilitarian bioethicists typically reject: dignity. Modern liberal and utilitarian bioethicists reject the idea of the dignity of human beings.[56] Their more common focus is on autonomous decision making and perhaps the target is often the sanctity of human life as it renders problematic choices at the beginning and end of life. Human well-being, chosen subjectively, created autonomously, is what matters most. In sharp contrast to this liberal worldview, the authors of *Beyond Therapy* argue:

> The dignity of human sport (or any other human activity) is determined not simply or predominantly by the measured and separate result, but also by who achieves it and how. Seen not as a detachable deed but as an activity of an agent, athletic performance depends on both the doing of a deed and the identity of the doer.[57]

It is a truism to say that sports activity is human conduct. It is also, of course, a platitude. But what does it mean to remind ourselves of sport's humanity? And can that meaning have significance? We paraphrase in the following the account from *Beyond Therapy*. The runners choose to run the race; they accept the goal of the activity and set their own achievement goals; they prepare themselves for it; they survey their rivals and plot strategies; acknowledging their constraints (their personal best, their present conditioning, their injury status and so on), they cultivate and discipline their body and its natural gifts in pursuit of the goal. Under this conception, sports as human endeavor, the goal, the means and the manner of striving are all matters of conscious awareness and deliberate choice, from beginning to end. In a word, what makes the racers running a human act humanly done is that it is engaged in more or less freely, and knowingly, and through conscious choice. And one can see in Lundberg's cleverly constructed prototypes the lack of such agency in all but one of the athletes.

Considered in the light of the preceding, excellent performance acquired through the practical application of biotechnology that goes "beyond therapy" is clearly ironic in the following senses:

1. In moving beyond therapy the athlete also reaches beyond their self-identity:
   By turning to biological agents to transform ourselves in the image we choose and will, we in fact compromise our choosing and willing identity itself, since we are choosing to become less than normally the source or the shapers of our own identity.[58]
2. In moving beyond therapy in genetic manipulation we undermine our dignity as humans that have their own individuality and body. Employing biotechnologies for self-transformation, we undermine the very excellence of our own individual embodiment that our enhanced performance was intended to achieve The thing we so highly prized becomes easier through biotechnological transformation and in so being becomes less valued, less excellent.
3. In deforming the character of our own desires by destroying the unique mutual relationship between the body and soul that is expressed in human desire, that is, by aiming to realize human desire.

Beyond Therapy further warns that there is in principle no limit to the desire to transcend the limits to which we are bound; that we readily lose sight of the fact that there is no way to stop that desire for superhuman capabilities; and that, ultimately, we are even deprived of the freedom to pursue human excellence and become enslaved.

In their conclusion, the report's authors draw upon an older moral language. They argue that biotechnological policies ought to follow suit of the environmentalist lobby that urges a precautionary principle.[59] Biotechnologies such as gene transfer represent "unnatural means" and thus they undermine the dignity of human activities that form a proper background for the recognition of excellence in activities such as athletics. Whether the concept of naturalness can carry the normative weight that its authors load it with is an important issue that requires detailed examination that is beyond the scope of the present chapter. Nevertheless, *Beyond Therapy* indicates that our present time is an era in which the myopic pursuit of superior performance has distorted our conception of sports as human endeavors. The worry, they argue, is that the traditional processes of enhancement—of which education is a paradigm—has developed over centuries where its guardians have kept close scrutiny on the relations between means and ends. Technicist conceptions of education where the keywords are minimizing effort in the name of efficiency are relative newcomers to pedagogical debates about the development and even perfection of our rational nature. They recognize that biotechnologies may enhance parts of our agency in terms of functionings but not the whole. They contend that difficulties would arise if the workings of medical science seek to transcend therapy. The report expresses the following concern:

> Where the goal is restoring health, the doctor's discretion is guided by an agreed-upon and recognizable target. But a physician prescribing for goals beyond therapy is in uncharted waters. Although fully armed with the means, he has no special expertise regarding the end—neither what it is nor whether it is desirable. To the extent that the patient is transformed from a sick person needing healing into a consumer of technical services, medicine will be transformed from a profession into a trade and the doctor-patient relationship into a species of contract, ungoverned by any deep ethical norms.[60]

This observation in *Beyond Therapy* is an extremely important one and has profound ramifications for sports medicine. There are concerns that the transformation of the deep ethical imperatives in the physician–patient relationship in therapy to a contractual (economic) relationship of producer-consumer in enhancement is likely to accelerate the path toward unimpeded enhancement where the individual alone can be judge and jury not only on what counts as an enhancement, but what risks may be taken irrespective of their social consequences. And the degree to which financial incentives have driven pharmacological doping behaviors is only too apparent. The extent to which more profound biotechnologies such as gene transfer will undermine our conceptions of humanly excellent activity is a serious question.

The report's authors view the movement beyond therapy as the extension of the medicalization processes highlighted by Illich and others in the 1970s.[61] They point out the risk that society may come to depend on medical practices, products and terminology to explain and "solve" what have hitherto been understood more simply and nontechnologically as problems of living. Under such a transformation, aging comes to be viewed not so much as a part of the human life cycle but rather as a disease to be ameliorated or even eradicated. They write:

> The therapeutic intention at the heart of medicine—the goal of making whole that which is broken or disabled—runs the risk of looking increasingly upon the entire human condition in this way and, as a result, of regarding biotechnological measures as the royal road to improving our lot in life.[62]

Besides considering biotechnological means as an all-purpose solution, medicalization attempts to resolve all problems that occur in everyone's life within the context of therapy. Various problems emerge when foreseeing an obsession with enhancement by viewing all situations through the lens of disease and disability (medically conceived). It would seem that the significance of transcending therapy and the importance of coming face-to-face with existential issues or what have been understood since antiquity as "problems of life" are being called into question here by imperializing medical practices and institutions.

CONCLUSION: MEDICAL TRANSFORMATION OF SPORTS AND SPORTSPERSONS

Present-day biotechnological research has enabled members of the medical professions, who are its principal gatekeepers, to fundamentally change the conventional concepts of human birth, life and death. From practices such as prenatal genetic diagnoses and in vitro fertilization, to debates about surrogate motherhood, death with dignity and voluntary euthanasia, we are constantly confronted with the increasing scope and power of medical technology. We have no great reason for thinking sports will be isolated from such trends. To the contrary, there are grounds for thinking that the Olympic logic of faster, higher, stronger invites this shift in medical self-understanding rather more readily than other branches of medicine where much greater precaution prevails. Once genetic maps are completed and disease genes are identified through human genome research, medical therapies will proceed apace. One can unproblematically see the day in the none too distant future when medical scientists target genes that, for example, predispose human obesity. It is no great conceptual leap to imagine thereafter that genetic therapy will be devised for children who have lower athletic potentials. At the time when clinical research for practical applications of genetic therapy are better recognized, one may anticipate that a veritable flood of research, clinical applications and patents will be accompanied by limited debate. The substance of many of these points, and their impact, is not based on guestimations: there are many sources that inform our insight into the future, from scientists' best guesses to science fiction.

What nourishes the critical debate surrounding the desirability, legitimacy or even propriety of these "advances" in sports medicine? There are various sources to fire the moral imagination. We have tried to show that fiction no less than scientists' future-gazing can enrich our understanding of possible future scenarios and help us to think through the conceptual and ethical aspects they entail. In some cases the debate about the future of gene doping has elided these sources. Perhaps it is best to say that we need a clear appreciation when we move from one source to the other.

The shifting nature and purposes of sports medicine cannot be seen in isolation from these broader trends. It is clear that governments, intergovernmental associations and research ethics committees continue to have an important regulatory function to play in the development of mainstream medicine. In contrast, we must suppose that the nature of at least some sports medical enterprises beyond therapy will be pioneered in elite sports in strict secrecy. Which national or professional sports medicine team would want to advertise their latest innovation or to have transparent ethical oversight if it allows competitors to nullify their nontransparent advantage? Precisely how sports medicine researchers secure ethical oversight of their activities is a moot point.

It may well be the case that the use of pharmacological drugs as a means for doping will disappear from the professional sports world once it becomes the target of ever more sophisticated biotechnology. Even so, if doping through the practical application of genetic transfer technologies becomes a means for nurturing top athletes there is no doubt that we will be confronting new challenges, including the genuine possibility of undetectability. For those of us committed to both the traditional values of medicine, vigilance of the debates about the nature and purposes of sports medicine beyond therapy is extremely important.

NOTES

1. Shilling, *Body in Culture.*
2. Sahakian and Morein-Zamir, "Professor's Little Helper"; Greely, Sahakian and Harris, "Towards Responsible Use."
3. Sheridan, Passveer and Hilvoorde, "Gene-Talk and Sport-Talk."
4. Miah, *Genetically Modified Athletes.*
5. Munthe, "Ethical Aspects"; McNamee et al., "Genetic Testing."
6. See, for example, Gerlinger, Petermann and Sauter, *Gene Doping.*
7. Kass, *President's Council.*
8. "Level Playing Field."
9. Fuller, *New Sociological Imagination.*
10. McNamee, "Sporting Practices."
11. Savulescu and Foddy, "Ethics of Performance Enhancement"; Kious, "Philosophy on Steroids"; McNamee et al., "Genetic Testing"; Murray, Maschke and Wasuna, *Performance Enhancing Technologies*; Savulescu, "Compulsory Genetic Testing"; Tamburrini and Tannsjo, *Genetic Technology and Sport.*
12. Fraleigh, *Right Actions in Sport*; Loland, *Fair Play*; Murray, Maschke and Wasuna, *Performance Enhancing Technologies*; McNamee, *Sports, Virtues and Vices*; Simon, *Fair Play.*
13. McNamee, "Anti Anti-Doping."
14. For an excellent discussion of the meaningless this can, though need not, descend to, see Todd and Todd, "Reflections."
15. Savulescu and Foddy, "Ethics of Performance Enhancement"; Harris, *Enhancing Evolution*; Kayser and Smith, "Globalisation of Anti-Doping"; Kious, "Philosophy on Steroids"; MacGregor and McNamee, "Philosophy

on Steroids"; Møller, *Ethics of Doping*; Savulescu, "Compulsory Genetic Testing"; Tamburrini, "What's Wrong?"
16. Kayser and Smith, "Globalisation of Anti-Doping"; Savulescu, "Compulsory Genetic Testing."
17. Savulescu, "Compulsory Genetic Testing." See also Müller's contribution in this collection. Of course, even this criterion entails normative judgments. What constitutes a safe enough level? When is it sufficiently safe for the athlete (cyclist) to return to training or competition? These judgments are inescapably both empirical and conceptually/ethically informed.
18. Savulescu and Foddy, "Ethics of Performance Enhancement"; Harris, *Enhancing Evolution*; Kayser and Smith, "Globalisation of Anti-Doping"; Kious, "Philosophy on Steroids."
19. Edwards and McNamee, "Why Sports Medicine Is Not Medicine."
20. Lundquist, "International Anti-Doping Policy."
21. McNamee, "Beyond Consent." We cannot address this issue in detail here but note that McNamee argues that the notion of consent is problematic when there is little reliable evidence for the harmful consequences of many (if not all) pharmacological doping practices. This is not merely that there are no systematic reviews, but the products and processes themselves have not been sufficiently reliably and transparently investigated in order to fulfill the conditions of informedness in informed consent. Although McNamee discusses the issues of pediatric doping in particular, many of the issues extend to adult populations.
22. Juengst, "Annotating the Moral Map."
23. Schneider, "Context of Performance Enhancement."
24. World Anti-Doping Agency, *World Anti-Doping Code*, 17–18.
25. There exist problematic gray areas. For example, salbutomol (which aids oxygen transport) has recently been downgraded from a doping substance to one whose use must merely be registered. Another recent medical technology to be similarly downgraded is the insertion of platelet rich plasma (Sanchez et al., "Nonunions"), which also assists the increased speed of injury recovery but might also have contributed to doping.
26. Laure and Binsinger, "Doping Prevalence."
27. Edwards and McNamee, "Why Sports Medicine Is Not Medicine;" Green, "Practice Makes Perfect"; McNamee, "Whose Prometheus?"; Stovitz and Satin, "Ethics and the Athlete"; Satin and Stovitz, "Professionalism."
28. Hoberman, *Mortal Engines*.
29. Beauchamp and Childress, *Principles of Biomedical Ethics*.
30. Gillon, "Ethics Needs Principles."
31. Savulescu and Bostrom, *Human Enhancement*; Ter Meulen, Savulescu and Kahane, *Enhancing Human Capacities*; Parens, "Goodness of Fragility"; Juengst, "Can Enhancement Be Distinguished?"
32. Daniels, "Can Anyone?"
33. Harris, *Enhancing Evolution*.
34. For a fuller account of the conceptual problems attending to the meaning of enhancement and its evaluation, see Holm and McNamee, "Physical Enhancement."
35. Sheridan, Passveer and Hilvoorde, "Gene-Talk and Sport-Talk."
36. Note, however, that the Japan Sports Association had already established a subcommittee for studying doping before doping was banned in 1968.
37. Karaki, "Age of New Heroes," 5.
38. Bale, "Deviance, Doping and Denmark."
39. Ibid.
40. Hoberman, *Mortal Engines*.

41. Clayton, "Ethical, Legal, and Social Implications."
42. See, for example, Rankinen and Bouchard, "Physical Activity."
43. See, for example, Miah, *Genetically Modified Athletes*; Williams et al., "Genetic Research."
44. McNamee, "Whose Prometheus?"; Sandel, *Case against Perfection.*
45. Laura, "Doping Problem in Sport," 92.
46. Jansens et al., "Critical Appraisal," 598.
47. Laura, "Doping Problem in Sport," 98.
48. Ibid., 107.
49. Edwards and McNamee, "Why Sports Medicine Is Not Medicine."
50. Loland, *Fair Play.*
51. Kass, *President's Council*, 148.
52. Ibid., 149.
53. Ibid., 160.
54. Ibid.
55. Ibid., 162–163.
56. Macklin, "Dignity."
57. Kass, *President's Council*, 163.
58. Ibid., 171.
59. In the context of medical ethics readers are referred to the challenging debate about the utility of the precautionary principle, its proper objects and limits (see Harris and Holm, "Extending Human Lifespan"; Sandin, "Paradox out of Context").
60. Kass, *President's Council*, 346.
61. Illich, *Medical Nemesis.*
62. Kass, *President's Council*, 346–347.

BIBLIOGRAPHY

Bale, John. "Deviance, Doping and Denmark in Knud Lundberg's *The Olympic Hope.*" *Sport in History* 29, no. 2 (2009): 190–211.
Beauchamp, Tom L., and James F. Childress. *Principles of Biomedical Ethics.* 6th ed. Oxford: Oxford University Press, 2009.
Clayton, E.W. "Ethical, Legal, and Social implications of Genomic Medicine." *New England Journal of Medicine* 349, no. 6 (2003): 562–569.
Daniels, Norman. "Can Anyone Really Be Talking about Ethically Modifying Human Nature?" In *Human Enhancement*, edited by Julian Savulescu and Nick Bostrom, 25–42. Oxford: Oxford University Press, 2009.
Edwards, Steven D., and Mike J. McNamee. "Why Sports Medicine Is Not Medicine." *Healthcare Analysis* 15, no. 4 (2006): 103–109.
Fraleigh, Warren P. *Right Actions in Sport.* Champaign, IL: Human Kinetics, 1984.
Fuller, Steve. *The New Sociological Imagination.* London: Sage, 2009.
Gerlinger, K., T. Petermann and A. Sauter. *Gene Doping Scientific Basis—Gateways—Monitoring.* Deutsche Technology Assessment, Technology Assessment Studies Number 3, 2009. http://www.bundestag.de/htdocs_e/bundestag/committees/a18/translations/gene_doping.pdf (accessed 2 March 2010).
Gillon, Raanon. "Ethics Needs Principles—Four Can Encompass the Rest and Respect for Autonomy Should Be 'First Among Equals.'" *Journal of Medical Ethics* 29 (2003): 307–312.
Greely, Hank, Barbara Sahakian and John Harris. "Towards Responsible Use of Cognitive Enhancing Drugs." *Nature* 456 (2008): 702–705.

Green, Shane K. "Practice Makes Perfect: Ideal Standards and Practice Norms in Sports Medicine." *Virtual Mentor: American Medical Association Journal of Medical Ethics* (2004). http://virtualmentor.ama-assn.org/2004/07/jdsc1–0407. html (accessed 17 December 2010).

Harris, John. *Enhancing Evolution: The Ethical Case for Making Better People.* Princeton, NJ: Princeton University Press, 2007.

Harris, John, and Søren Holm. "Extending Human Lifespan and the Precautionary Paradox." *Journal of Medicine and Philosophy* 27, no. 3 (2007): 355–368.

Hoberman, John. *Mortal Engines.* New York: Free Press, 1992.

Holm, Søren, and McNamee, Mike. "Physical Enhancement: What Baseline, Whose Judgement?" In *Enhancing Human Capacities*, edited by Julian Savulescu, Ruud Ter Meulen and Guy Kahane. Oxford: Oxford University Press, forthcoming.

Illich, Ivan. *Medical Nemesis.* London: Calder and Boyars, 1975.

Jansens, A., J.W. Cecile, Marta Gwinn, Linda Bradley, Ben Oostra, Cornelia van Duijn and Muin Khoury. "Critical Appraisal of the Scientific Basis of Commercial Genomic Profiles Used to Assess Health Risks and Personalize Health Interventions." *American Journal of Human Genetics* 82, no. 3 (2008): 593–599.

Juengst, Erich "Annotating the Moral Map of Enhancement: Gene Doping the Limits of Medicine and the Spirit of Sport." In *Performance Enhancing Technologies in Sports*, edited by Tom Murray, Karen Maschke and Angela Wasuna, 175–204. Baltimore, MD: Johns Hopkins University Press, 2009.

———. "Can Enhancement Be Distinguished from Prevention in Genetic Medicine?" *Journal of Medicine and Philosophy* 22, no. 2 (1997): 125–142.

Karaki. "Age of New Heroes 1: Doping." *Asahi Shimbun*, 8 July 1996, 5.

———. "4 Stories of Doping." *Asahi Shimbun*, 31 January 2003, 15.

Kass, Leon. *President's Council of Bioethics Beyond Therapy: Biotechnology and the Pursuit of Happiness.* New York: Dana Press, 2005.

Kayser, Bengt, and Aaron C.T. Smith. "Globalisation of Anti-Doping: The Reverse Side of the Medal." *British Medical Journal* 337 (2008): 584.

Kious, Brent. "Philosophy on Steroids." *Theoretical Medicine and Bioethics* 29, no. 4 (2008): 213–214.

Laura, Rob. "The Doping Problem in Sport: From Drugs to Genetic Engineering." In *Drug Controversy in Sport*, edited by R.S. Laura and S.W. White, 90–109. Sydney: Allen and Unwin, 1991.

Laure, Patrick, and Claudia Binsinger. "Doping Prevalence among Preadolescent Athletes: A 4–Year Follow-Up." *British Journal of Sports Medicine* 41 (2007): 660–663.

"A Level Playing Field," *Nature*, 2008, 454, 667.

Loland, Sigmund. *Fair Play.* London: Routledge, 2001.

Lundberg, Knud. *Det Olympiske håb.* Copenhagen, 1955. (*Olympic Hopeful.* London: Stanley Paul, 1958.

Lundquist, Arne. "The International Anti-Doping Policy and Its Implications." In *Genetic Technology and Sport*, edited by Claudio Tamburrini and Torbjorn Tannsjo, 13–18. London: Routledge, 2007.

MacGregor, Oskar, and M.J. McNamee. "Philosophy on Steroids: A Reply." *Theoretical Medicine and Bioethics* 29 (2010): 213–34.

Macklin, Ruth. "Dignity Is a Useless Concept." *British Medical Journal* 327 (2003): 419–420.

McNamee, Mike. "Anti Anti-Doping: Why Skepticism Doesn't Cut the Mustard." *British Medical Journal* 337 (2008): 584.

———. "Beyond Consent: The Ethics of Pediatric Doping." *Journal of the Philosophy of Sport* 36, no. 2 (2009): 111–126.

———. "Sporting Practices, Institutions and Virtues: A Critique and a Restatement." *Journal of Philosophy of Sport* 22 (1995): 61–83.

————. *Sports, Virtues and Vices*. London: Routledge, 2008.

————. "Whose Prometheus?: Transhumanism, Biotechnology and the Moral Topography of Sports Medicine." *Sport, Ethics and Philosophy* 1, no. 2 (2007): 181–194.

McNamee, Mike, Arno Müller, Ivo van Hilvoorde and Soren Holm. "Genetic Testing and Sports Medicine Ethics." *Sports Medicine* 39, no. 5 (2009): 1–6.

Miah, Andy. *Genetically Modified Athletes*. London: Routledge, 2004.

Møller, Verner. *The Ethics of Doping and Anti-Doping*. London: Routledge, 2009.

Munthe, Christian. "Ethical Aspects of Controlling Genetic Doping." In *Genetic Technology and Sport*, edited by C. Tamburrini and T. Tannsjo, 107–125. London: Routledge, 2007.

Murray, Tom, K. Maschke and N. Wasuna, eds. *Performance Enhancing Technologies in Sports*. Baltimore, MD: Johns Hopkins University Press, 2009.

Nussbaum, Martha. *The Fragility of Goodness*. Cambridge: Cambridge University Press, 1986.

Parens, Erik. "The Goodness of Fragility: On the Prospect of Genetic Technologies Aimed at the Enhancement of Human Capacities." *Kennedy Institute of Ethics Journal* 5, no. 2 (1995): 141–153.

Rankinen, Tuomo, and Claude Bouchard. "Physical Activity, Mortality and Genetics." *American Journal of Epidemiology* 166, no. 3 (2007): 260–262.

Sahakian, Barbara, and Sharon Morein-Zamir. "Professor's Little Helper." *Nature* 450 (2007): 1157–1159.

Sanchez, Mikel, Eduardo Anitua, Ramon Cugat, Juan Azofra, Jorge Guadilla, Roberto Seijas and Isabel Andia. "Nonunions Treated with Autologous Preparation Rich in Growth Factors." *Journal of Orthopaedic Trauma* 23, no. 1 (2009): 58–59.

Sandel, Michael. *The Case against Perfection*. Princeton, NJ: Princeton University Press, 2007.

Sandin, Per. "A Paradox out of Context: Harris and Holm on the Precautionary Principle." *Cambridge Quarterly of Healthcare Ethics* 15, no. 2 (2006): 175–183.

Satin, David J., and Steven D. Stovitz. "Professionalism and the Ethics of the Sideline Physician." *Current Sports Medicine Reports* 5 (2006): 120–124.

Savulescu, Julian. "Compulsory Genetic Testing for APOE Epsilon 4." In *Genetic Technology and Sport*, edited by C. Tamburrini and T. Tannsjo, 136–146. London: Routledge, 2007.

Savulescu, Julian, and Nick Bostrom, eds. *Human Enhancement*. Oxford: Oxford University Press, 2009.

Savulescu, Julian, and Brent Foddy. "Ethics of Performance Enhancement in Sport: Drugs and Gene Doping." In *Principles of Health Care Ethics: Second Edition*, edited by Richard E. Ashcroft, A. Dawson, H. Draper and J.R. McMillan, 511–520. London: John Wiley and Sons, 2007.

Schneider, Angela. "The Context of Performance Enhancement: An Athlete's Perspective." In *Performance Enhancing Technologies in Sports*, edited by Tom Murray, Karen Maschke and Angela Wasuna, 28–43. Baltimore, MD: Johns Hopkins University Press, 2009.

Sheridan, Heather, B. Passveer and Ivo van Hilvoorde. "Gene-Talk and Sport-Talk: A View from the Radical Middle Ground." *European Journal of Sport Science* 6, no. 4 (2006): 223–230.

Shilling, Chris. *The Body in Culture, Technology and Society*. London: Sage, 2005.

Simon, Robert L. *Fair Play*. Boulder, CO: Westview Press, 1991.

Stovitz, Steven D., and David J. Satin. "Ethics and the Athlete: Why Sports Are More Than a Game but Less Than a War." *Clinics in Sports Medicine* 23 (2004): 215–225.

Tamburrini, Claudio. "What's Wrong with Genetic Inequality? The Impact of Genetic Technology on Elite Sports and Society." *Sport, Ethics and Philosophy* 1, no. 2 (2007): 229–238.

Tamburrini, Claudio, and Torbjorn Tannsjo, eds. *Genetic Technology and Sport.* London: Routledge, 2007.

Ter Meulen, Ruud, Julian Savulescu and Guy Kahane, eds. *Enhancing Human Capacities.* Oxford: Wiley Blackwell, 2010.

Todd, Jan, and Terry Todd. "Reflections on the 'Parallel Federations Solution' to the Problem of Drug Use in Sports: The Cautionary Tale of Powerlifting." In *Performance Enhancing Technologies in Sports*, edited by Tom Murray, Karen Maschke and Angela Wasuna, 44–80. Baltimore, MD: Johns Hopkins University Press, 2009.

Williams, Alan G., H. Wackerhage, Andy Miah, Roger C. Harris and Hugh Montgomery. "Genetic Research and Testing in Sport and Exercise Science." BASES Position Stand. http://www.bases.org.uk/write/documents/BASES%20position%20stand%20–%20as%20published.pdf (accessed 10 November 2010).

World Anti-Doping Agency. *World Anti-Doping Code*, Montreal: WADA, 2003.

Contributors

Michael Atkinson is Associate Professor in the Faculty of Kinesiology and Physical Education at the University of Toronto. Michael's central areas of teaching and research interest pertain to nonmainstream physical cultures, human rights and bio-pedagogical practices in physical cultures and bioethics within global and local sport cultures. Michael is author/coauthor of seven books, including *Battleground: Sports* (2008); *Deviance and Social Control in Sport* (with Kevin Young, 2008); *Boys' Bodies: Speaking the Unspoken* (with Michael Kehler, 2010); *Key Concepts in Sport and Exercise Research Methods* (2011); and *Deconstructing Men and Masculinities* (2010). He is editor of the *Sociology of Sport Journal* and director of the Sport Legacies Research Collaborative.

Jack W. Berryman, PhD, FACSM, is Professor of the History of Medicine in the Department of Bioethics and Humanities and Adjunct Professor in the Department of Orthopaedics and Sports Medicine in the School of Medicine at the University of Washington in Seattle, Washington. He is the official historian for the American College of Sports Medicine and chair of ACSM's Office of Museum, History, and Archives. Dr. Berryman was president of the North American Society for Sport History 1989–1991 and edited the *Journal of Sport History* from 1977 to 1984. His current research involves video interviews of past and present distinguished leaders in sports medicine and exercise science.

Neil Carter is a Senior Research Fellow in the International Centre for Sports History and Culture at De Montfort University, Leicester. He is the author of *The Football Manager* (2006) and his new book, *Medicine Sport and the Body*, is due to be published by Bloomsbury-Academic in 2012. Between 2004 and 2007 he was a Wellcome Trust Research Fellow for a project on the history of sports medicine. He has recently coauthored an article on the television coverage of the Special Olympics GB National Summer Games in 2009, which will be published in *Media, Culture and Society* in 2012.

John Hoberman has been active in sports studies and sports journalism for the past thirty-five years. His books include *Mortal Engines: The Science of Performance and the Dehumanization of Sport* (1992) and *Testosterone Dreams: Rejuvenation, Aphrodisia, Doping* (2005). His articles include "The History of Synthetic Testosterone" (*Scientific American*, February 1995) and "Listening to Steroids" (*Wilson Quarterly*, Spring 1995). He has taught sports studies at Harvard University, the University of Chicago and the University of Texas at Austin where he is Professor of Germanic Studies. His current research concerns anabolic steroid use by police officers and military personnel.

Yoshitaka Kondo is a Professor for the School of Health and Sport Sciences at Chukyo University, Japan. He is current secretary-general of the Japan Society of Physical Education, Health, and Sport Science and vice president of the Japanese Society of Sport Education. He is a member of International Association for the Philosophy of Sport and also an editorial member of the *Journal of the Philosophy of Sport*. He has taught the philosophy and ethics of sport and physical education for undergraduate and graduate school students at Chukyo University, Japan. Recent publications include "The Japanese Debate Surrounding the Doping Ban," in *Sport in Society*.

Joseph A. Kotarba, PhD, is Professor of Sociology and director of the Center for Social Inquiry at Texas State University-San Marcos. His theoretical orientation is symbolic interaction and his primary methodology is ethnography. Dr. Kotarba teaches and conducts research in two areas: the sociology of culture and the sociology of health. He is currently combining these interests in a study of injury prevention and management among professional artists, musicians and athletes. Dr. Kotarba has also studied health and illness phenomena such as the chronic pain experience, the wellness movement, health care needs of homeless adolescents and translational medical/scientific research.

Dominic Malcolm is Senior Lecturer in the Sociology of Sport at Loughborough University. Trained as a sociologist, the twin empirical foci of his research are the sociohistorical development of cricket and the practice of sports medicine. His recently published books include *Sport and Sociology* (2012) and *Globalizing Cricket* (2012). Recent studies of sports medicine include the analysis of the management of concussion in rugby union and the role of an Eliasian sociology of knowledge in aiding understanding of clinician–patient encounters in sport.

Fred Mason is an Associate Professor in the Faculty of Kinesiology, University of New Brunswick, where he teaches and researches broadly in the areas of sport history and sport sociology. Disability sport, in its current and historical contexts, and historical perceptions and discourses about people with disabilities are among his major research interests. His work has been published in a range of venues, including the *Canadian Bulletin of Medical History/Bulletin canadien d'histoire de la médecine*, the *International Review for the Sociology of Sport*, the *Electronic Green Journal*, and he has edited collections on science fiction.

Mike McNamee is Professor of Applied Ethics at Swansea University. He is the Founding Chair of the British Philosophy of Sport Association and former president of the International Association for the Philosophy of Sport. His books include *Research Ethics in Exercise, Health and Sports Sciences* (with S. Olivier and P. Wainwright, 2006); *Sports, Virtues and Vices* (2008); *Reader in Sports Ethics* (2010); and *Doping and Anti Doping Policy in Sport* (edited with V. Møller, 2011). He is editor of the journal *Sport, Ethics and Philosophy* and he runs (slowly) and plays football and tennis (when not injured!).

Arno Müller is Junior Professor in the Department of Philosophy of Sport and Sport History at the University of Leipzig. He previously worked at the Universities of Bielefeld and Maastricht, where he worked at the Centre for Society and Genomics in the Netherlands, on a research project on genetics and sport funded by the Netherlands Genomics Initiative. He is an executive member of the European Association for the Philosophy of Sport.

Vicky Paraschak is an Associate Professor in the Department of Kinesiology, University of Windsor, where she teaches in Sport Sociology and Outdoor Recreation. Her research has focused for many years on aboriginal peoples in sport and recreation within the context of unequal power relations and broader government policies. More recently she has incorporated a Strengths Perspective into her analysis and helped to facilitate leadership development for underserved youth in local high schools using the Teaching Personal and Social Responsibility model. She has remained active as a consultant in strategic planning for recreation and sport in the Northwest Territories of Canada.

Elizabeth C. J. Pike is head of the Department of Sport Development and Management, and chair of the Anita White Foundation (www.chi.ac.uk/awf) at the University of Chichester, UK. She has researched, published and delivered numerous national and international presentations on risk, injury, aging and gender issues in sports. Elizabeth serves on the editorial board of the journals *Revista de ALESDE, Leisure Studies* and the *International Review for the Sociology of Sport*. She is on the executive board of the International Sociology of Sport Association, serving as the president of the association from 2012 to 2015 (www.issa.otago.ac.nz).

Parissa Safai is an Associate Professor in the School of Kinesiology and Health Science in the Faculty of Health at York University. Her research interests focus on the critical study of sport at the intersection of risk, health and health care. This includes research on sports' "culture of risk" and the development and social organization of sport and exercise medicine, as well as the social determinants of athletes' health. Her work has been published in such journals as the *Sociology of Sport Journal*, the *International Review for the Sociology of Sport*, *Sport History Review* and the *Canadian Bulletin of Medical History/Bulletin canadien d'histoire de la médecine*.

Andrea Scott is Senior Lecturer in the Sport Development and Management Department at the University of Chichester, where she is responsible for teaching within the Sociology of Sport discipline. Her research interests include the occupational practices of sports medicine clinicians, including doctors, physiotherapists and sports therapists, and the consequences of sport medicine's professionalization both for the organization of medicine in sport and the quality of care provided to athletes.

Nancy Theberge is Professor at the University of Waterloo, where she is appointed to the Departments of Kinesiology and Sociology. She holds a PhD in sociology from the University of Massachusetts at Amherst. She has published widely on topics related to gender, sport and physical activity and the social organization of sport medicine. She served as the editor of the *Sociology of Sport Journal* from 2002 to 2004 and in 2005 received the Distinguished Service Award from the North American Society for the Sociology of Sport. Her current research activity includes investigations of constructions of gender in biomedical research on injuries and the professional practices of ergonomists, an occupational group whose work bears similarities to that of sport medicine practitioners.

Lone Friis Thing is an Associate Professor at the Department of Exercise and Sport Sciences, University of Copenhagen. She has an MSc in Humanities and Social Sciences of Sport and Biology and a PhD in Sociology, both from the University of Copenhagen. Lone's research focuses on the use of physical activity and sport for health promotion and illness prevention. Among others, she has worked with the elderly in relation to heart disease and lifestyle and Danish schoolchildren on innovative culture strategies for organizational change. She is a board member of the Danish Institute for Sports Studies.

Ivan Waddington is Visiting Professor at the Norwegian School of Sport Sciences, Oslo, and the University of Chester, UK. He is the author of *Sport, Health and Drugs* (2000) and a coauthor of the British Medical Association report, *Drugs in Sport: The Pressure to Perform* (2002). He has also coedited *Pain and Injury in Sport: Social and Ethical Analysis* (2006) and *Matters of Sport: Essays Presented in Honour of Eric Dunning* (2007). His most recent book (with Andy Smith) is *An Introduction to Drugs in Sport: Addicted to Winning?* (2009).

Index

A

Aboriginal peoples 126, 146
Abrahams, A. 58, 59–60, 72
Achilles Club 59
acupuncture (see complementary and
    alternative medicine)
altitude 6, 10
amateurism 65
American Association for Health,
    Physical Education and Recre-
    ation (AAHPER) 26, 37, 41
American College of Cardiology (ACC)
    33, 37, 40–41, 286
American College of Sports Medicine
    (ACSM) 2, 9, 13, 16, 25–53, 58,
    67, 78
American Congress of Physical
    Therapy 39
American Heart Association (AHA)
    25, 37, 39–40, 286
American Medical Association (AMA)
    3, 4, 6, 249
American Orthopedic Society 79
American Therapeutic Society 39
anabolic steroids 209, 248–249
Andrews, D. 2
anterior cruciate ligament (ACL) reha-
    bilitation/reconstruction 113,
    188–189, 192, 194, 196
aromatherapy (see complementary and
    alternative medicine)
Association of Chartered Physio-
    therapists in Sports Medicine
    (ACPSM) 64, 66, 70, 244
Association Internationale Medico
    Sportive (see FIMS)
athletic therapy 4
athletic training/trainers 4, 10, 25, 77,
    89, 115–116

athletica anorexia 273
Atkinson, M. 15
Ayurvedic medicine (see herbal
    medicine)

B

Bailey, S. 77, 83
Bairner, A. 17
Batt, M. 3
Baudrillard, J. 275–278
Bauman, Z. 276
Beamish, R. 10, 164
Beck, U. 193
Berryman, J. 6, 9, 13, 61, 78
Beyond Therapy 305, 315–318
Bioethics (see ethics)
biomechanics 4, 11, 25, 73, 85, 156
biotechnology 188, 305–320
Bishop, L. 39–40
Bloodgate 213
British Association of Sport and
    Exercise Medicine (BASEM) 3,
    4, 13; activities 62–63; mem-
    bership 60–62, 64–65, 69–70;
    multidisciplinarity of 62, 64,
    70; origins of 58–60; politics
    of 63–68; regional associations
    of 64
British Association of Sport and Medi-
    cine (see BASEM)
British Association of Sports Sciences
    (BASS) 67, 70, 73
British Association of Trauma in Sport
    (BATS) 65–66, 70
British Journal of Sports Medicine 62,
    63, 66
British Medical Association (BMA) 3,
    6, 205
British Medical Journal 3

For Product Safety Concerns and Information please contact our
EU representative GPSR@taylorandfrancis.com Taylor & Francis
Verlag GmbH, Kaufingerstraße 24, 80331 München, Germany